CRACK THE FINAL FRCR PART A Exam

MODULES 1, 2, 3

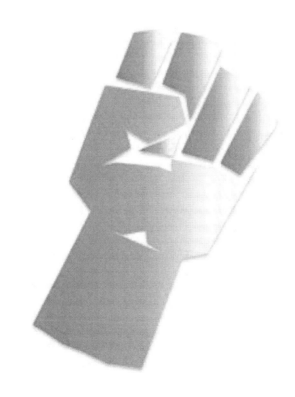

-PROMETHEUS LIONHART, M.D.

Disclaimer:

Readers are advised - this book is **NOT to be used for clinical decision making**. Human error does occur, and it is your responsibility to double check all facts provided. To the fullest extent of the law, the Author assumes no responsibility for any injury and/or damage to persons or property arising out or related to any use of the material contained in this book.

Published by: Prometheus Lionhart

Title ID: 5682544

ISBN-13: 978-1516936090

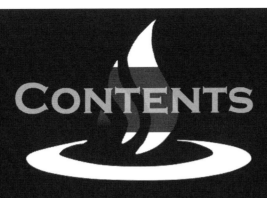

CONTENTS

All chapters were written by Prometheus Lionhart, M.D.

Introduction

The Final FRCR (Part A) is a single best answer exam ("multiple choice test" - we call it in the states). The candidates are grilled on all aspects of clinical radiology plus some physics and anatomy. The "Specialty Training Curriculum for Clinical Radiology" is referenced by the RCR as the source - but it is nothing more than a vague laundry list of radiology diagnoses and skills. The exam is held over three consecutive days. Success is measured by the ability to pass all 6 modules.

What makes this book unique?

Dr. Prometheus Lionhart is the premier Radiology board review expert in the United States. He is the sole author, illustrator, and publisher of the #1 selling and most used board review book series for the American Board of Radiology's CORE Exam (*Crack the CORE Exam Vol 1 & 2*). The "CORE Exam" is essentially the American equivalent to the FRCR Part A.

Dr. Lionhart has turned his attention to the FRCR Exam, remastering his famous American texts for direct use on the FRCR Exam.

The Impetus for this book was to not write a reference text or standard review book, but instead, strategy manual for solving multiple choice questions for Radiology. The author wishes to convey that the multiple choice test is different than an oral exam in that you can't ask the same kinds of open ended essay type questions. *"What's your differential?"*

Questioning the contents of one's differential is the only real question on oral examinations, or real life view-box work. That simple question becomes nearly impossible to format into a multiple choice test. Instead, the focus for training for such a test should be on things that can be asked. For example, anatomy facts - what is it? ... OR... trivia facts - what is the most common location, or age, or association, or syndrome? ... OR... What's the next step in management? In this book, the author tried to cover all the material that could be asked (reasonably), and then approximate how questions might be asked about the various topics. Throughout the book, the author will intimate, "this could be asked like this" , and "this fact lends itself well to a question." Included as the last chapter in each volume is a strategy chapter focusing on high yield "buzzwords" that lend well to certain questions.

This is NOT a reference book.
This book is NOT designed for patient care.
This book is designed for studying specifically for multiple choice tests

Legal Stuff

Readers are advised - **this book is NOT to be used for clinical decision making**. Human error does occur, and it is your responsibility to double check all facts provided. To the fullest extent of the law, the Author assumes no responsibility for any injury and/or damage to persons or property arising out or related to any use of the material contained in this book.

I FIGHT FOR THE USERS

-TRON 1982

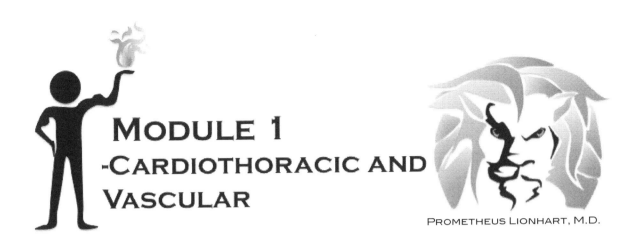

MODULE 1
-CARDIOTHORACIC AND VASCULAR

PROMETHEUS LIONHART, M.D.

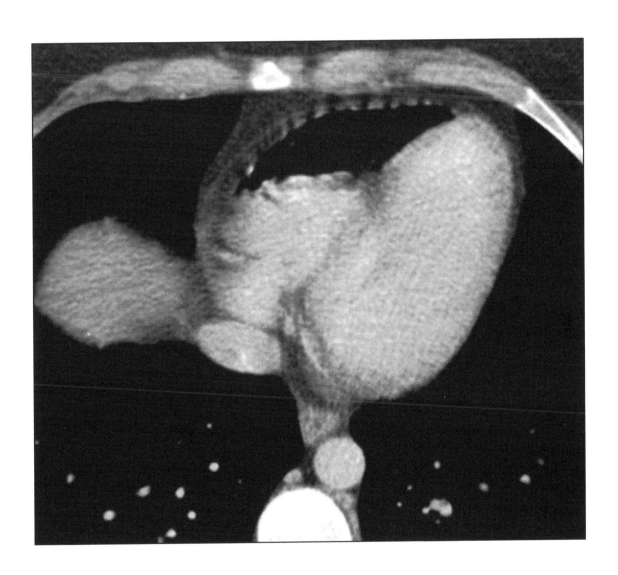

SECTION 1: CARDIAC

Chambers

Right Atrium: Defined by the IVC. The **Crista Terminalis** is a frequently tested normal structure (it's not a clot or a tumor). It is a muscular ridge that runs from the entrance of the superior- to that of the inferior vena cava. Another normal anatomic structure that is frequently shown (usually on IVC gram) is the IVC valve or **Eustachian valve**. It looks like a little flap in the IVC as it hooks up to the atrium. When the tissue of this valve has a more trabeculatated appearance it is called a **Chiari Network**.

Coronary Sinus: The main draining vein of the myocardium. It runs in the AV groove on the posterior surface of the heart and enters the right atrium near the tricuspid valve

Right Ventricle: Defined by the Moderator Band. Has several characteristics that are useful for distinguishing it (and make good test questions).

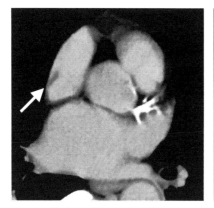
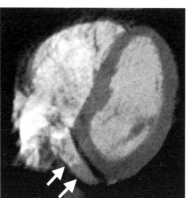
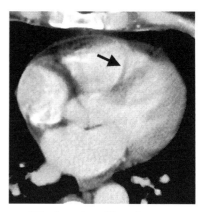

Crista Terminalis
-Not a clot

Coronary Sinus

Moderator Band
-Also not a clot

The tricuspid **papillary muscles insert on the septum** (not the case with the mitral valve). There is no fibrous connection between the AV valve / outflow tract. The pulmonary valve has three cusps, and is separated from the tricuspid valve by a thick muscle known as the crista supraventricularis . This differs from the left ventricular outflow tract, where the mitral and aortic valves lie side by side.

The left sided valves hinge together

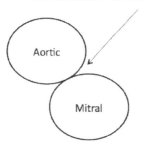

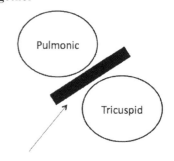

The right sided valves have an infundibulum between them

10

Left Atrium: The most posterior chamber. When you think about multiple choice questions regarding the left atrium, think about the various signs of enlargement.

- *Double Density (direct sign): Superimposed second contour on the right heart, from enlargement of the right side of the left atrium*

- *Splaying of the Carina (indirect sign): Angle over 90 degrees suggests enlargement*

- *Walking Man Sign (indirect sign): Posterior displacement of the left main stem bronchus on lateral radiograph. This creates an upside down "V" shape with the intersection of the right bronchus (looks like a man walking).*

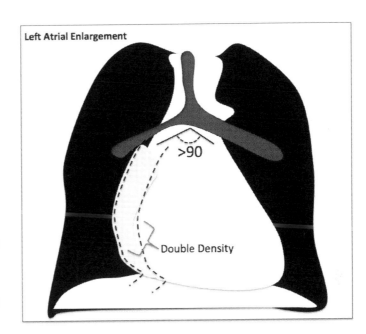

Left Ventricle: The leaflets of the mitral valve are connected to the papillary muscles via cord-like tendons called chordae tendinae. The papillary muscles insert into the lateral and posterior walls as well as the apex of the left ventricle (not the septum, as is the case on the right).

Echogenic Focus in Left Ventricle: Relatively common sonographic observation seen on pre-natal ultrasound. It is a calcified papillary muscle that usually goes away by the third trimester. So who gives a shit? Well they are **associated with an increased incidence of Downs** (13%). Don't get it twisted, having one means nothing other than you should look for other signs of downs (most of the time it's normal).

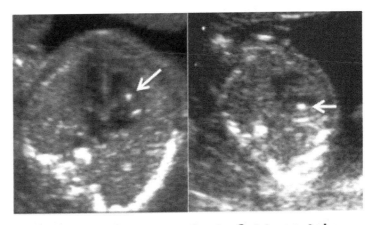

Echogenic Focus in Left Ventricle

Lipomatous Hypertrophy of the Intra-Atrial Septum: This has a very classic look of a dumbbell (bilobed) appearance of fat density in the atrial septum, sparing the fossa ovale. It **spares the fossa ovalis**, creating a dumbbell appearance (*when it doesn't spare it think lipoma*). It's associated with being fat and old. As a point of trivia it can cause supraventricular arrhythmia, although usually does nothing. Additional even more high-yield trivia is that it **can be hot on PET because it's often made of brown fat**.

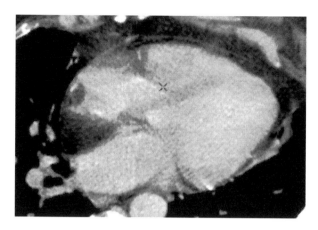

Coronaries

Questions regarding the coronaries will likely come in two flavors: Normal (which will be mostly vocab), and Abnormal (which will only have one or two pathologies).

Normal: There are three coronary cusps; right, left, and non-coronary (posterior). The left main comes off the left cusp, the right main comes off the right cusp.

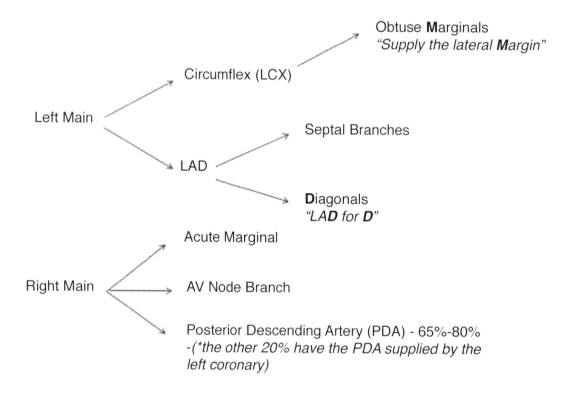

With regard to what perfuses what, the following are high yield factoids:

- RCA perfuses SA node 60%
- RCA perfuses AV node 90%

Typical vascular perfusion territories are a high yield topic.

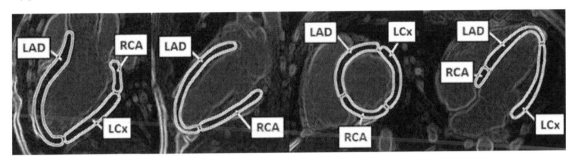

Dominance: Coronary Dominance is determined by **what vessel gives rise to the posterior descending artery and posterior left ventricular branches** (most are **right – 85%**). You can be "co-dominant" if the posterior descending artery arises from the right coronary artery and the posterior left ventricular branches arise from the left circumflex coronary artery

<u>Not Normal</u>: *Anomalies of the Origin, Course, and Termination:*

Malignant Origin: Most Common and Most Serious: **LCA from the Right Coronary Sinus**, coursing between the Aorta and Pulmonary Artery. This guy can get compressed and cause sudden cardiac death.

- Anomalous right off the left cusp --- Repair if symptomatic
- Anomalous left of the right cusp ----Always Repair

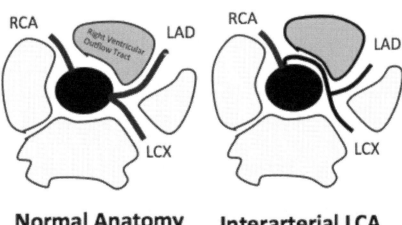

Normal Anatomy   **Interarterial LCA (the bad one)**

ALCAPA: Anomalous Left Coronary from the Pulmonary Artery. There are two types: (a) Infantile type (they die early), and (b) adult (still at risk of sudden death). The multiple choice question is going to be **"STEAL SYNDROME"** – which describes a reversal of flow in the LCA as pressure decreases in the pulmonary circulation.

Myocardial Bridging: This is an intramyocardial course of a coronary artery (usually the LAD). The finding may cause symptoms as the diameter decreases with systole, or may cause an issue for CABG planning. This can be a source of ischemia.

Coronary Artery Aneurysm: By definition this is a vessel with a diameter greater than 1.5x the normal lumen. <u>Most common cause is atherosclerosis.</u> Most common cause in child is Kawasaki (spontaneously resolves in 50%). They can occur from lots of other vasculitides as well. Last important cause is iatrogenic (cardiac cath).

Coronary Fistula: Defined as a connection between a coronary artery and cardiac chamber or great vessels. It's usually the RCA, with drainage into the right cardiac chambers. They are associated / result in coronary aneurysm. *If you see big crazy dilation of the coronaries - think about this.*

Coronary CT

Who is the ideal patient to get a coronary CT? There are two main groups of people getting these. (1) Low risk or atypical chest pain patients. A negative coronary CT will help stop a stress test or cath from occurring. Why do a procedure with risks on someone with GERD? (2) Suspected aberrant coronary anatomy.

What is the ideal heart rate? To reduce motion related artifacts a slow heart rate is preferred. Most books will tell you under 60 beats per min. Beta blockers are used to lower the heart rate to achieve this ideal rate.

Are there contraindications to beta blockers? Yup. Patients with severe asthma, heart block, acute chest pain, or recent snorting of cocaine – should not be given a beta blocker.

Are all heart blocks contraindications to beta blockers ? 2nd and 3rd Degree are contraindications. A 1st degree block is NOT.

What if I can't give the beta blocker? Can he still have the scan? Yes, you just can't use a prospective gating technique. You'll have to use retrospective gating.

What is the difference between prospective and retrospective gating?

–*Prospective:* "Step and Shoot" – R-R interval *data acquisition triggered by R Wave*

- Pro: There is reduced radiation b/c the scanner isn't on the whole time

- Con: No functional imaging

- Trivia: Always axial, not helical

–*Retrospective:* Scans the whole time, then back calculates

- Pro: Can do functional imaging

- Con: Higher radiation (use of low pitch – increases dose)

- Trivia: this is helical

Other than beta blockers, are any other drugs given for coronary CT? Yup. Nitroglycerine is given to dilate the coronaries (so you can see them better).

Are there contraindications to nitroglycerine ? Yup. Hypotension (SBP < 100), severe aortic stenosis, hypertrophic obstructive cardiomyopathy, and Phosphodiesterase (Viagra-Sildenafil) use.

Valvular

Velocity-encoded cine MR imaging (VENC), also known as velocity mapping or phase-contrast imaging, is a technique for quantifying the velocity of flowing blood.

Aortic Stenosis: This may be congenital (bicuspid) or Acquired (Degenerative or Rheumatic Heart). Increased afterload can lead to concentric LV hypertrophy. Peak velocity through the valve can be used to grade the severity. Velocity-encoded cine MR imaging (VENC), which also answers to the name "velocity mapping" or "phase-contrast imaging", is an MRI technique for quantifying the velocity of flowing blood (if anyone would happen to ask). **Dilation of ascending aorta** is due to jet phenomenon related to a stenotic valve. Comes in three flavors: (a) valvular, (b) subvalvular, (c) and supravalvular. Valvular is the most common (90%).

- *When I say "Supra-valvular Aortic Stenosis" you say Williams Syndrome*
- *When I say "Bicuspid Aortic Valve and Coarctation" you say Turners Syndrome*

Bicuspid Aortic Valve: This is very common, some sources will say nearly 2% of the general population. As a result, it becomes the source of significant fuckery with regard to one particular multiple choice question - "what is the most common congenital heart disease?" The answer is probably bicuspid aortic valve, but because it's often asymptomatic and not a problem till later in life when it gets stenotic and causes syncope - I think it messes with peoples math or doesn't get thought of by the question writer. How do you handle this question? Well... if they list bicuspid aortic valve then you have to pick it. If they don't list it then the answer is VSD.

Trivia to know:

- Bicuspid aortic valve (even in absence of stenosis) is independent risk factor for aortic aneurysm

- Association with Cystic Medial Necrosis (CMN).

- Association with Turners Syndrome, and Coarctation

- Association with Polycystic kidney disease.

Aortic Regurgitation: Seen with bicuspid aortic valves, bacterial endocarditis, Marfan's, aortic root dilation from HTN, and aortic dissection. How rapid the regurgitation onsets determines the hemodynamic impact (acute onset doesn't allow for adaptation).

Mitral Stenosis: Rheumatic heart disease is the most common cause. The case could be shown as a CXR with left atrial enlargement (double density sign, splaying of the carina, posterior esophageal displacement).

Mitral Regurgitation: The most common acute causes are endocarditis or papillary muscle / chordal rupture post MI (Step 1 question was "Austin Flint Murmur"). The chronic causes can be primary (myxomatous degeneration) or secondary (dilated cardiomyopathy leading to mitral annular dilation). *Remember the isolated Right Upper Lobe pulmonary edema is associated with mitral regurgitation.*

Pulmonary Stenosis: Just like in the Aortic Valve, comes in three flavors: (a) valvular, (b) subvalvular, (c) and supravalvular. Valvular is the most common, and can lead to ventricular hypertrophy. Associated with **Noonan Syndrome** (male version of turners). **"Peripheral Pulmonary Stenosis" is seen with Alagille syndrome** (kids with absent bile ducts). Williams can give you supra-valvular aortic stenosis (and pulmonic).

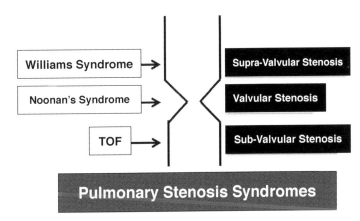

Pulmonary Regurgitation: The most common situation for this is congenital valve disease after valve surgery. The classic scenario is actually TOF patient who has been repaired.

Tricuspid Regurgitation: Most common form of tricuspid disease, due to the relatively weak annulus (compared to the mitral). May occur in the setting **of endocarditis (IV drug use)**, or **carcinoid syndrome** (serotonin degrades the valve). **The most common cause in adults is pulmonary arterial hypertension.** A testable pearl is that TR causes RV dilation (NOT RV Hypertrophy).

Gamesmanship: — Rheumatic heart disease most commonly involves the mitral and aortic valves. Anytime there is multivalve disease, think Rheumatic Fever!

Step 1 Trivia: Rheumatic heart disease is a immune modulated response to Group A-Beta hemolytic strep.

Ebstein Anomaly: Seen in children whose moms used Lithium (most cases are actually sporadic). The tricuspid valve is hypoplastic and the posterior leaf is displaced apically (downward). The result is enlarged RA , decreased RV ("atrialized"), and tricuspid regurgitation. They have the massive "box shaped" heart on CXR.

Tricuspid Atresia: Congenital anomaly that occurs with RV hypoplasia. Almost always has an ASD or PFO. Recognized association with asplenia. Can have a right arch (although you should think Truncus and TOF first). As a point of confusing trivia; tricuspid atresia usually has pulmonary stenosis and therefore will have decreased vascularity. If no PS is present, there will be increased vascularity.

Carcinoid Syndrome: This can result in valvular disease, but only after the tumor has met'd to the liver. The serotonin actually degrades heart valves, **typically both the tricuspid and pulmonic valves.** Left sided valvular disease is super rare since the lungs degrade the vasoactive substances. When you see left sided disease you should think of two scenarios: (1) primary bronchial carcinoid, or (2) right-to-left shunts.

Great Vessels

The most common variant in branching is the "bovine arch" in which the brachiocephalic artery and right common carotid artery arise from a common origin.

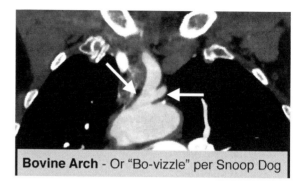

Bovine Arch - Or "Bo-vizzle" per Snoop Dog

The terminology right arch / left arch is described based on the aortic arch's relationship to the trachea.

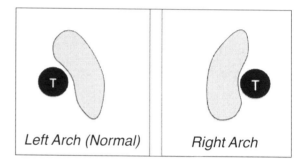

Left Arch (Normal)   *Right Arch*

There are 5 types of right arches, but only two are worth knowing (Aberrant Left, and Mirror Branching).

When I say Right Arch with Mirror Branching, You say congenital heart.

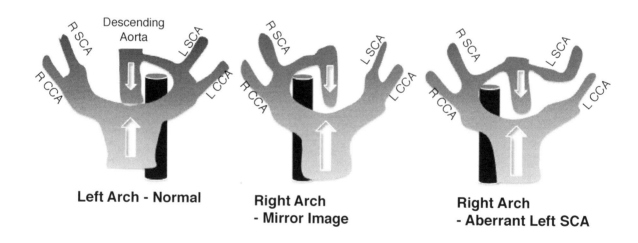

Left Arch - Normal   **Right Arch - Mirror Image**   **Right Arch - Aberrant Left SCA**

Right Arch with Aberrant Left Subclavian: The last branch is the left aberrant subclavian artery. This is a vascular ring because the ligament arteriosum (on the left) complete the "ring" encircling the trachea.

Right Arch with Mirror Branching: Although these are often asymptomatic they are strongly associated with congenital heart disease. Most commonly they are associated with TOF. However, they are most closely associated with Truncus. Obviously, this tricky wording lends itself nicely to a trick question.

- *If there is a mirror image right arch, then 90% will have TOF (6% Truncus).*
- *If the person has Truncus, then they have a mirror image right arch 33% (TOF 25%).*

Left Arch Aberrant Right Subclavian: The most common arch anomaly. Although it is usually asymptomatic it can **sometimes be associated with dysphagia lusoria,** as the RSCA passes posterior to the esophagus. The last branch is the right aberrant subclavian artery. The **origin of the RSCA may be dilated = Diverticulum of Kommerell.**

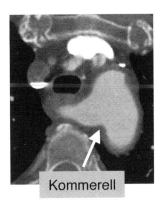

Kommerell

Double Aortic Arch: *The most common vascular ring.* As a point of trivia, <u>symptoms may begin at birth</u> and include tracheal compression and/or difficulty swallowing. The right arch is larger and higher, and the left arch is smaller and lower. Arches are posterior to esophagus and anterior to trachea (encircling them both).

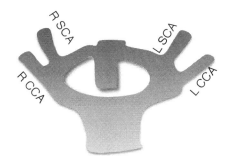

Subclavian Steal Syndrome/Phenomenon: So there is a "Syndrome" and there is a "Phenomenon." The distinction between the two makes for an excellent distractor.

- *SS Phenomenon:* Stenosis and/or occlusion of the proximal subclavian with retrograde flow in the ipsilateral vertebral artery.

- *SS Syndrome:* Stenosis and/or occlusion of the proximal subclavian artery with retrograde flow in the ipsilateral vertebral artery AND associated cerebral ischemic symptoms.

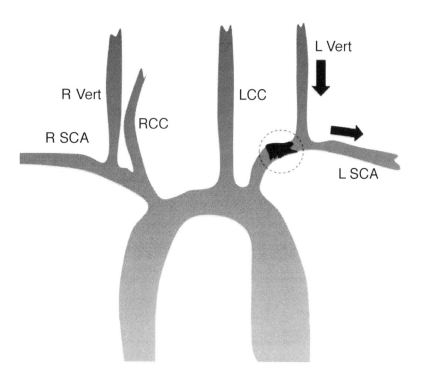

Occlusion proximal to the vertebral in the subclavian can result in retrograde "stolen" flow from the vertebral artery.

If the level of stenosis and/or occlusion is proximal to the vertebral artery, reversal of flow in the vertebral artery can occur, resulting in the theft of blood from the posterior circulation. When the upper limb is exercised, blood is diverted away from the brain to the arm. Cerebral symptoms (dizziness, syncope, etc...) depend on the integrity of collateral intracranial flow (PCOMs).

Subclavian Steal is almost always caused by atherosclerosis (98%), but other very testable causes include Takayasu Arteritis, Radiation, Preductal Aortic Coarctation, and Blalock-Taussig Shunt. In an adult they will show atherosclerosis. If they show a teenager / 20 year old it's gonna be Takayasu. Case books love to show this as an angiogram, and I think that's the most likely way the test will show it. They could also show a CTA or MRA although I'd say that is less likely.

Aortic Aneurysm and Vasculitis: *Will be discussed in the Vascular section.*

Congenital Heart Disease

An extremely high yield and confusing topic which dinosaur Radiologists love to ask questions about on CXR. Obviously, this is stupid since you could only add confusion to a bad situation by suggesting a diagnosis on CXR instead of waiting for ECHO or MRI. Having said that, the next section will attempt to provide a methodology for single answers on CXR cases.

My thoughts on multiple choice questions regarding congenital heart is that they will come in 3 flavors: (A) Aunt Minnie, (B) Differentials with crappy distractors, and (C) Associations / Trivia.

Aunt Minnies / Differentials:

There are a few congenital heart cases that are Aunt Minnies, or easily solvable (most are differential cases). Bottom line is that if they want a single answer they will have to show you either an Aunt Minnie or a differential case, with crappy distractors.

With regard to straight-up Aunt Minnies, I think the usual characters that most third year medical students memorize are fair game.

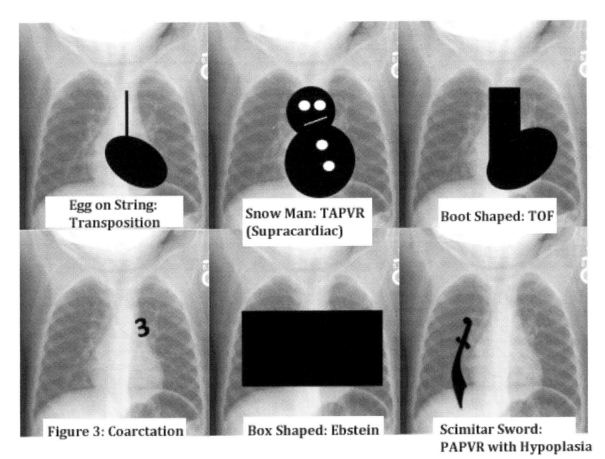

Egg on String: Transposition

Snow Man: TAPVR (Supracardiac)

Boot Shaped: TOF

Figure 3: Coarctation

Box Shaped: Ebstein

Scimitar Sword: PAPVR with Hypoplasia

The easily solvable ones will be shown as a right arch with the associations of **Truncus (*more closely associated*)** and **TOF** *(more common overall)*. Or, they will show you the big box heart and want Ebsteins (which is an Aunt Minnie). Another classic trick with regard to the big box heart is non-cardiac causes of high output failure (Infantile Hemangioendothelioma and Vein of Galen Malformation). The remaining cyanotic syndromes basically look the same, so the questions must be either (a) crappy distractors (none of the others are cyanotic, etc…), or (b) trivia (which is more likely).

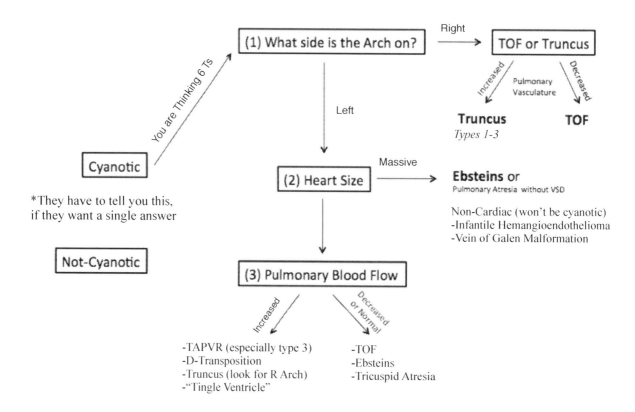

With regard to identifying bad distractors I think the easiest way is the cyanotic vs not cyanotic disorders. They literally must tell you the kid is cyanotic, otherwise there is no way to know.

Cyanotic	Not Cyanotic
TOF	ASD
TAPVR	VSD
Transposition	PDA
Truncus	PAPVR
Tricuspid Atresia	Aortic Coarctation (adult type – post ductal)

There are a few other key differentials that may make it easier to weed out bad distractors, or get "which of the following do NOT" questions.

CHF in Newborn	Survival dependent on admixture: PDA, VSD, PDA - Cyanotics	Small Heart DDx
TAPVR (Infracardiac type "III")	TAPVR (has PFO)	Adrenal Insufficiency (Addisons)
Congenital Aortic or Mitral Stenosis	Transposition	Cachectic State
Left Sided Hypoplastic Heart	TOF (has VSD)	Constrictive Pericarditis
Cor Triatriatum	Tricuspid Atresia (has VSD)	
Infantile (pre-ductal) Coarctation	Hypoplastic Left	

Trivia and Associations:

VSD: The **most common congenital heart disease.** There are several types with Membranous (*just below the aortic valve*) being the most common (70%). **Outlet subtypes (infundibulum) must be repaired** as the right coronary cusp prolapses into the defect. On CXR we are very nonspecific (big heart, increased vasculature, small aortic knob). They could ask or try and show **splaying of the carina** (from big left atrium). About 70% of the small ones close spontaneously.

PDA: The PDA normally closes around 24 hours after birth (functionally), and anatomically around 1 month. A PDA should make you say three things (1) **Prematurity**, (2) **Maternal Rubella,** (3) **Cyanotic Heart Disease**. CXR is nonspecific (big heart, increased pulmonary vasculature, large aortic arch "ductus bump"). You can close it or keep it open with meds.

ASD: Several types with the Secundum being the most common (50-70%). The larger subtype is the Primum, (results from an endocardial cushion defect), is more likely to be symptomatic. Only Secundums may close without treatment (Primum, AV Canal, Sinus Venosus will not). Primums are not amendable to device closure because of proximity to AV valve tissue. On CXR, if it's small it will show nothing, if it's large it will be super nonspecific (big heart, increased vasculature, and small aortic knob). It's more common in female.

- *When I say hand/thumb defects + ASD, you say Holt Oram*
- *When I say ostium primum ASD (or endocardial cushion defect), you say Downs*
- *When I say Sinus Venosus ASD, you say PAPVR*

AV Canal: Also referred to as an endocardial cushion defect. They happen secondary to a deficient development of a portion of the atrial septum, a portion of the inter-ventricular septum, and the AV valves. **Strong association with Downs**. You can't use closure devices on these dudes either. Surgical approach and management is complex and beyond the scope of this text.

Trivia: Of all the congenital heart stuff with Downs patients - AV Canal is the most common

Unroofed Coronary Sinus: This is a rare ASD which occurs secondary to a fenestrated (as in the cartoon) or totally unroofed coronary sinus. The most important clinical is that you can get paradoxical emboli and chronic right heart volume overload.

Trivia: STRONG association with a persistent left SVC.

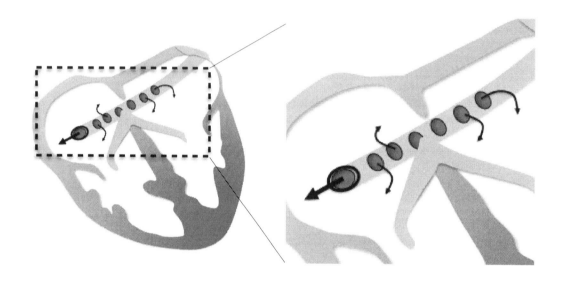

PAPVR: Partial anomalous pulmonary venous return, is defined as one (or more) of the four pulmonary veins draining into the right atrium. It is often of mild or no physiologic consequence. It is often **associated with ASDs (secondum and sinus venosus types)**.

- *When I say Right Sided PAPVR, you say Sinus Venosus ASD*

    - *RUL: SVC association with sinus venosus type ASD*

- *When I say Right Sided PAPVR + Pulmonary Hypoplasia, you say Scimitar Syndrome*

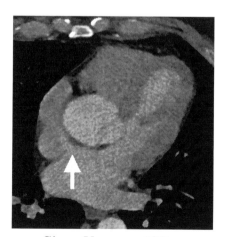

Sinus Venosus ASD

24

TAPVR: A cyanotic heart disease characterized by all of the pulmonary venous system draining to the right side of the heart. A large PFO or less commonly ASD is required for survival (this is a high yield and testable point). There are 3 types, but only two are likely to be tested (cardiac type II just doesn't have good testable features). All 3 types will cause increased pulmonary vasculature, but type 3 is famous for a full on pulmonary edema look in the newborn.

- Type 1: Supracardiac:

    o Most Common Type

    o Veins drain above the heart, **gives a snowman appearance**.

- Type 2: Cardiac

    o Second Most Common Type

- Type 3: Infracardiac

    o Veins drain below the diaphragm (hepatic veins or IVC)

    o **Obstruction on the way back through diaphragm is common and causes a full on pulmonary edema look**

Key Points on TAPVR:

- Supracardiac Type = Snowman

- Infracardiac Type = Pulmonary Edema in Newborn

- Large PFO (or ASD) needed to survive

- Asplenia – 50% of asplenia patients have congenital heart issues, of those nearly 100% include TAPVR, (85% have additional endocardial cushion defects).

Transposition: This is the most common cause of cyanosis during the first 24 hours. It is seen most commonly in infants of diabetic mothers. The basic idea is that aorta arises from the right ventricle and the pulmonary trunk from the left ventricle (*ventriculararterial discordance*).

Which one is the Right Ventricle ? You have to find the moderator band (that defines the RV)

Just like TAPVR survival depends of an ASD, VSD, or PDA (*most commonly VSD*). There are two flavors: D & L. The D type only has a PDA connecting the two systems. Where as the **L** type is "Lucky" enough to be compatible with **L**ife.

D-Transposition: Classic radiographic appearance is the "egg on a string". Occurs from discordance between the ventricles and the vessels. The intra-atrial baffle (Mustard or Senning procedure) is performed to fix them

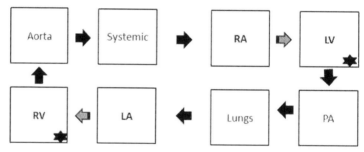

In D-Transposition, the ductus may be the only connection between the two systems, which would otherwise be separate (and not compatible with life)

L-Transposition: The L type is "Lucky" enough to be congenitally corrected. This occurs from a "double discordance" where the atrium hooks up with the wrong ventricle and the ventricle hooks up with the wrong vessels.

In L-Transposition of the great vessels - there is an inversion of the ventricles, leading to a "congenital correction." No PDA is needed.

A **corrected D-transposition** has a very characteristic appearance, lending itself to an Aunt Minnie-type question.

The PA is draped overtop the Aorta, which occurs after a surgeon has performed to *"LeCompte Maneuver"* -- sounds French so must be high yield.

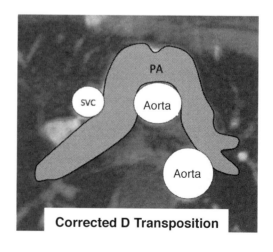

Corrected D Transposition

Tetralogy of Fallot (TOF): The *most common cyanotic heart disease.* Describes 4 major findings; (1) VSD, (2) RVOT Obstruction – often from valvular obstruction, (3) Overriding Aorta, (4) RV hypertrophy (develops after birth). The degree of severity in symptoms is related to how bad the RVOT obstruction is. If it's mild you might even have a "pink tet" that presents in early adulthood. This is called a pentaology of Fallot if there is an ASD. Very likely to have a right arch.

Surgically it's usually fixed with primary repair. The various shunt procedures (Blalock-Taussig being the most famous) is only done if the kid is inoperable or to bridge until primary repair.

Trivia: The most common complication following surgery is pulmonary regurgitation.

Truncus Arteriosus: Cyanotic anomaly where there is a single trunk supplying both the pulmonary and systemic circulation, not of a separate aorta and a pulmonary trunk . It almost always has a VSD, and is closely associated with right arch. **Associated with CATCH-22** genetics (DiGeorge Syndrome).

—

Coarctation: Narrowing of the aortic lumen. This comes in two flavors:

   (1) Infantile (Pre-ductal) – these guys can have pulmonary edema

   (2) Adult (Ductal)

Things to know:

- Strong Association with **Turners Syndrome** (15-20%).

- **Bicuspid Aortic valve** is the most common associated defect (80%).

- They have more **berry aneurysms.**

- **Figure 3 sign** (appearance of CXR).

- *Rib Notching: most often involves 4th - 8th ribs. It does NOT involve the 1st and 2nd because those are fed by the costocervical trunk.*

—

Hypoplastic Left Heart: Left ventricle and aorta are hypoplastic. They present with pulmonary edema. **Must have an ASD** or large PFO. They also typically have a large PDA to put blood in their arch. Strongly associated with aortic coarctation and endocardial fibroelastosis.

Cor Triatriatum Sinistrum: This is a very rare situation where you have an **abnormal pulmonary vein draining into the left atrium** (*sinistrum meaning left*) with an unnecessary fibromuscular membrane that causes a sub division of the left atrium. This **creates the appearance of a tri-atrium heart**. This can be a cause of unexplained pulmonary hypertension in the peds setting. Basically it acts like mitral stenosis, and can cause **pulmonary edema**. The outcomes are often bad (fatal within two years), depending on surgical intervention and associated badness.

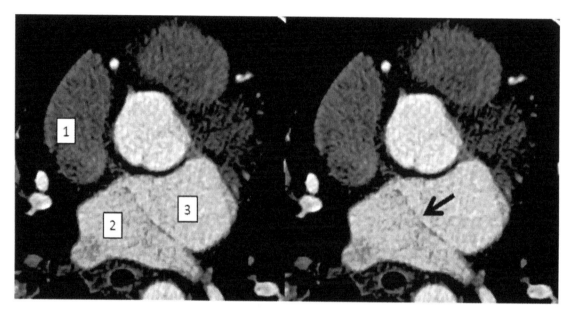

Cor Triatriatum Sinistrum

Ischemic Heart Disease

Imaging regarding ischemic heart disease is going to fall into two modalities; cardiac MR, and Nuclear. Cardiac MRI currently offers the most complete evaluation of ischemic heart disease.

Myocardial infarction typically is initiated by rupture of an unstable coronary atherosclerotic plaque, leading to abrupt arterial occlusion. The **wave front of necrosis always starts subendocardial and progresses to the subepicardium.** The ischemic necrosis will affect not just the myocardium but also blood vessels. The destruction of small capillaries will not allow contrast to the area of injury. This is termed "microvascular obstruction" and manifests as islands of dark signal in an ocean of delayed enhancement. The presence of microvascular obstruction is an independent predictor of death and adverse LV remodeling.

Testable Vocab:

- *Stunned Myocardium:* After an Acute Injury (ischemia or reperfusion injury), dysfunction of myocardium persists even after restoration of blood flow (can last days to weeks). A perfusion study will be normal, but the contractility is crap.

- *Hibernating Myocardium:* This is a more chronic process, and the result of severe CAD causing chronic hypoperfusion. You will have areas of **decreased perfusion and decreased contractility** even when resting. Don't get it twisted, **this is not an infarct. On a FDG PET, this tissue will take up tracer more intensely than normal myocardium, and will also demonstrate redistribution of thallium**. This is reversible with revascularization.

- *Scar:* This is dead myocardium. It will not squeeze normally, so you'll have abnormal wall motion. It's <u>not a zombie</u>. It will NOT come back to life with revascularization.

Stunned	Hibernating	Infract / Scar
Wall Motion Abnormal	Wall Motion Abnormal	Wall Motion Abnormal
Normal Perfusion (Thallium or Sestamibi)	Abnormal Fixed Perfusion	Abnormal Fixed Perfusion
	Will Redistribute with Delayed Thallium and will take up FDG	Will NOT Redistribute with Delayed Thallium, will NOT take up FDG
Associated with acute MI	Associated with chronic high grade CAD	Associated the chronic prior MI

Delayed imaging: It works for two reasons: (1) Increased volume of contrast material distribution in acute myocardial infarction (and inflammatory conditions) (2) Scarred myocardium washes out more slowly. It is **done using an inversion recovery technique** to null normal myocardium, followed by a gradient echo. T1 shortening from the Gd looks bright ("Bright is Dead").

Why stress imaging is done: Because coronary arteries can auto-regulate, a stenosis of 85% can be asymptomatic in a resting state. So demand is increased (by exercise or drugs) making a 45% stenosis significant. An inotropic stress agent (dobutamine) is used for wall motion, and a vasodilator (adenosine) is used for perfusion analysis.

MRI in Acute MI: Cardiac MRI can be done in the first 24 hours post MI (if the patient is stable). Late gadolinium enhancement will reflect size and distribution of necrosis. Characteristic pattern is a **zone of enhancement that extends from the subendocardium toward the epicardium in a vascular distribution**. Microvascular obstruction will present as islands of dark signal in the enhanced tissue (as described above), and this represents an acute and subacute finding . **Microvascular obstruction is NOT seen in chronic disease** as these areas will all turn to scar eventually. In the acute setting (1 week) injured myocardium will have increased T2 signal, which can be used to estimate the area at risk *(T2 Bright – Enhanced = Salvageable Tissue)*.

Acute vs Chronic MI:

- *Both have delayed enhancement*
- *If the infarct was transmural and chronic you may have thinned myocardium*
- *Acute will have normal thickness (chronic can too but shouldn't for the purposes of MC tests.*
- *T2 signal from edema may be increased in the acute setting*
- *You won't see Mircovascular Obstruction in Chronic*
- *Acute is T2 bright (edema), Chronic is T2 Dark (scar)*

How do you diagnose Myocardial Infarction with Contrast Enhanced MR?
(1) Delayed Enhancement follows a vascular distribution, (2) The enhancement extends from the endocardium to the epicardium

Microvascular Obstruction: Islands of dark tissue in an ocean of late Gd enhancement. These indicate microvascular obliteration in the setting of an acute infarct. The Gd is unable to get to these regions even after the restoration of epicardial blood flow. Microvascular obstruction is a **poor prognostic finding**, associated with lack of functional recovery.

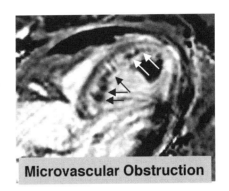

Microvascular Obstruction

Key Point: It's **NOT seen in chronic infarct.**

Trivia: Microvascular obstruction is best seen on first pass imaging (25 seconds)

Ventricular Aneurysm: This is rare (5%), but can occur as the result of MI. The question is always true vs false:

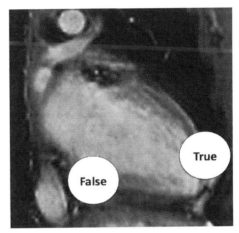

False Aneurysms are Usually Posterior Lateral
True Aneurysms are Usually Anterior Lateral

- *True:* Mouth is wider than body. Myocardium is intact. Usually anterior-lateral wall.

- *False:* Mouth is narrow compared to body. Myocardium is NOT intact (pericardial adhesions contain the rupture). Usually posterior-lateral wall. Higher risk of rupture.

Viability - You can grade this based on % of transmural thickness involved in the infarct.

- <25%: likely to improve with PCI
- 25-50%: may improve
- 50-100%: unlikely to recover function

What is the timing on the bad sequelae of an MI?

Dressler Syndrome	4-6 weeks
Papillary Muscle Rupture	2-7 Days
Ventricular Pseudoaneurysm	3-7 Days
Ventricular Aneurysm	Months – Requires remodeling and thinning.
Myocardial Rupture	Within 3 Days (50% of the time)

Non-Ischemic Disease

Dilated Cardiomyopathy: Defined as dilatation with an end diastolic diameter greater than 55mm, with a decreased EF. Can be idiopathic, ischemic, or from a whole list of other random crap (Alcohol, Doxorubicin, <u>Cyclosporine</u>, Chagas, etc…). The ischemic variety may show subendocardial enhancement. The **idiopathic variety will show** either no enhancement or **linear mid-myocardial enhancement**. There is often an association with mitral regurgitation due to dilation of the mitral ring.

Restrictive Cardiomyopathy: Basically anything that causes a decrease in diastolic function. Can be the result of myocardium replaced by fibrotic tissue (endocardial fibroelastosis), infiltration of the myocardium (Amyloidosis), or damage by iron (hemochromatosis). **The most common cause is actually amyloid.**

> Restrictive = Myocardial Process
> Constrictive = Pericardial

- *Amyloidosis:* Deposits in the myocardium causes abnormal diastolic function with biatrial enlargement, concentric thickening of the left ventricle and reduced systolic function of usually both ventricles. Seen in 50% of cases of systemic amyloid. Has a terrible prognosis. You can sometimes see late Gd enhancement over the entire subendocardial circumference.

  Amyloid Classic Scenario: A **long TI is needed** (like 350 milliseconds, normal would be like 200). TI will be so long that the blood pool may be darker than the myocardium. **Buzzword "difficult to suppress myocardium"**.

- *Eosinophilic Cardiomyopathy (Loeffler)* : **Bilateral Ventricular thrombus** is the classic phrase / buzzword. You will need a long TI to show the thrombus.

Constrictive Pericarditis: Historically this used to be TB or Viral. Now the most common cause is iatrogenic secondary to CABG or radiation. On CT the pericardium is too thick (>0.4cm), and if it's calcified that is diagnostic. Calcification is usually largest over the AV groove. "Sigmoidization" is seen on SSFP cine imaging: The ventricular septum moves toward the left ventricle in a wavy pattern during early diastole (**"Diastolic Bounce"**). This "bounce" will be most pronounced during inspiration - indicating ventricular interdependence.

This vs That: Constrictive vs Restrictive Cardiomyopathy:

- *Pericardium is usually thickened in constrictive*
- *Diastolic septal bounce is seen in constrictive (Sigmoidization of the septum).*

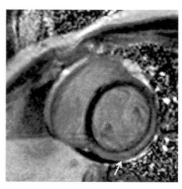

Myocarditis: Inflammation of the heart can come from lots of causes (*often viral i.e. Coxsackie virus*). The late Gd enhancement follows a non-vascular distribution preferring the **lateral free wall**. The **pattern will be epicardial or mid wall (NOT subendocardial)**.

Myocarditis
-Mid Wall Late Gd Enhancement

Sarcoidosis: Cardiac involvement is seen in 5% of Sarcoidosis cases, and is associated with an increased risk of death. Signal in both T2 and early Gd (as well as late Gd) will be increased. Late Gd pattern may be middle and epicardial in a non-coronary distribution. **Focal wall thickening from edema can mimic hypertrophic cardiomyopathy. It often involves the septum.** The RV and papillaries are RARELY affected.

Takotsubo Cardiomyopathy – A takotsubo is a Japanese Octopus trap, which looks like a pot with a narrow mouth and large round base. The octopus will go into the pot, but then can't turn around and get out. A condition with Chest pain and EKG changes seen in post menopausal women after they either break up with their boyfriend , win the lottery, or some other stressful event has been described with the shape of the ventricle looking like a takotsubo. There is **transient akinesia or dyskinesia of the left ventricular apex without coronary stenosis. Ballooning of the left ventricular apex is a buzzword.** No delayed enhancement.

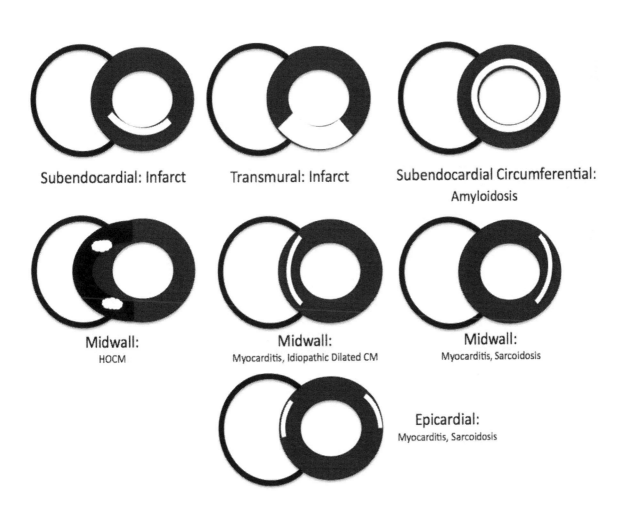

Subendocardial: Infarct

Transmural: Infarct

Subendocardial Circumferential:
Amyloidosis

Midwall:
HOCM

Midwall:
Myocarditis, Idiopathic Dilated CM

Midwall:
Myocarditis, Sarcoidosis

Epicardial:
Myocarditis, Sarcoidosis

Genetic Conditions

Arrhythmogenic Right Ventricular Cardiomyopathy (ARVC): Characterized by fibrofatty degeneration of the RV leading to arrhythmia and sudden death. Features include dilated RV with reduced function, **fibrofatty replacement of the myocardium**, and normal LV. People use this major/minor criteria system that includes a bunch of EKG changes that no radiologist could possibly understand (if they are stupid enough to ask just say left bundle branch block). Watch out for the use of fat sat to demonstrate the fat in the RV wall.

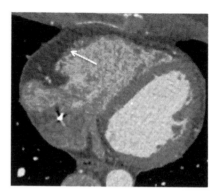

ARVC - Dilated RV, with Fat in the Wall

Hypertrophic Cardiomyopathy: Abnormal hypertrophy (from disarray of myofibrils) of the myocardium that compromises diastole. There are multiple types but the one they are going to show is asymmetric hypertrophy of the intraventricular septum. The condition is a cause of sudden death. There is a subgroup which is associated with LVOT obstruction ("hypertrophic obstructive cardiomyopathy"). Venturi forces may pull the anterior leaflet of the mitral valve into the LVOT (**SAM** – Systolic Anterior Motion of the Mitral Valve). Patchy midwall **delayed enhancement of the hypertrophied muscle** may be seen, as **is an independent risk factor for sudden death.**

Noncompaction: Left ventricular noncompaction is a uncommon congenital cardiomyopathy that is the result of loosely packed myocardium. The left ventricle has a spongy appearance with increased trabeculations and deep intertrabecular recesses. As you might expect these guys get heart failure at a young age. Diagnosis is based of a ratio of non compacted end-diastolic myocardium to compacted end-diastolic myocardium of more than 2.3:1.

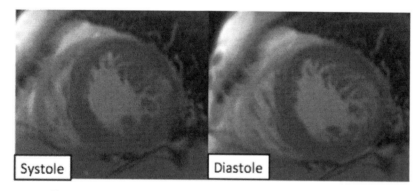

Systole Diastole

Noncompaction - *Spongy LV, with No Myocardial Thickening*

Muscular Dystrophy – Becker (mild one) and Duchenne (severe one) are X-linked neuromuscular conditions. They have biventricular replacement of myocardium with connective tissue and fat (delayed Gd enhancement in the midwall). They often have dilated cardiomyopathy. Just think **kid with dilated heart and midwall enhancement.**

Tumors

Mets: Thirty times more common than a primary malignancy. The **pericardium is the most common site** affected (by far). The most common manifestation is a pericardial effusion (second most common is a pericardial lymph node). Melanoma may involve the myocardium.

Trivia: Most common met to the heart is lunger cancer (pericardium and epicardium)

Angiosarcoma: Most common primary malignant tumor of the heart in adults. They like the RA and tend to involve the pericardium. They often cause right sided failure and/or tamponade. They are bulky and heterogenous. Buzzword is "sun-ray" appearance which describes enhancement appearance of the diffuse subtype as it grows along the perivascular spaces associated with the epicardial vessels.

Left Atrial Myxoma: Most common primary cardiac tumor in adults (rare in children). They are associated with MEN syndromes, and Blue Nevi (Carney Complex). They are most often **attached to the interatrial septum**. They may be calcified. They may prolapse through the mitral valve. They **will enhance with Gd** (important discriminator from a thrombus).

> **Tumor vs Thrombus:**
>
> Cardiac MRI is the way to tell.
>
> - Tumor will enhance
> - Thrombus will NOT enhance.

Rhabdomyoma: Most common fetal cardiac tumor. It is a hamartoma. They prefer the **left ventricle**. Associated with **tuberous sclerosis**. Most tumors will regress spontaneously (those NOT associated with TS are actually less likely to regress).

Fibroma: Second most common cardiac tumor in childhood. They like the IV septum, and are dark / dark on T1/T2. They enhance very brightly on perfusion and late Gd.

Fibroelastoma: Most common neoplasm to involve the **cardiac valves** (80% aortic or mitral). They are highly mobile on SSFP Cine. Systemic emboli are common (especially if they are on the left side).

Pericardial Disease

The pericardium is composed of two layers (visceral and parietal), with about 50cc of fluid normally between the layers.

Pericardial Effusion: Basically more than 50cc between the pericardial layers. This can be from lots and lots of causes – renal failure (uremia) is probably the most common. For the purpose of multiple choice tests you should think about Lupus, and Dressler Syndrome (inflammatory effusion post MI). On CXR they could show this 3 ways: (1) Normal Heart on Comparison, Now Really Big Heart (2) Giant Water Bottle Heart, (3) Lateral CXR with two lucent lines (epicardial and pericardial fat) and a central opaque line (pericardial fluid) – the so called "**oreo cookie sign.**"

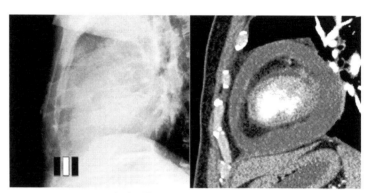

Pericardial Effusion : "Oreo Cookie Sign"

Cardiac Tamponade: Pericardial effusion can cause elevated pressure in the pericardium and result in compromised filling of the cardiac chambers (atria first, then ventricles). This can occur with as little as 100cc of fluid, as the **rate of accumulation is the key factor** (chronic slow filling gives the pericardium a chance to stretch). The question is likely related to **short-axis imaging during deep inspiration showing flattening or inversion of the intraventricular septum toward the LV**, a consequence of augmented RV filing. Another indirect sign that can be shown on CT is reflux of contrast into the IVC and azygos system.

Pericardial Cysts: Totally benign incidental finding. Usually seen on the right cardiophrenic sulcus. They do not communicate with the pericardium. Rarely they can get infected or hemorrhage. **They will show you an ROI measuring water density along the right cardiophrenic sulcus, and this will be the answer**.

Congenital / Acquired Absence: Even though you can have total absence of the pericardium - the most common situation is **partial absence of the pericardium over the left atrium and adjacent pulmonary artery**. When the left pericardium is absent the heart shifts towards the left. They could show you a CT or MRI with the heart contacting the left chest wall, and want you to infer partial absence. Another piece of trivia is that cardiac herniation and volvulus can occur in patients who undergo extrapleural pneumonectomy (herniation can only occur if the lung has also been removed).

Trivia: The left atrial appendage is the most at risk to become strangulated.

Cardiac Surgeries:

Palliative Surgery for the Hypoplastic Left Heart: Surgery for Hypoplasts is not curative, and is instead designed to extend the life (prolong the suffering) of the child. It is done in a 3 stage process, to protect the lungs and avoid right heart overload:

(1) Norwood or Sano – within days of birth

(2) Glenn – at 3- 6 months

(3) Fontan at 1 ½ to 5 years

Norwood: The goal of the surgery is to create an unobstructed outflow tract from the systemic ventricle. So the tiny native aorta is anastomosed to the pulmonary trunk, and the arch is augmentented with a graft (or by other methods). The ASD is enlarged to create non restrictive atrial flow. A Blaylock-Taussig Shunt (see below) is used between the right Subclavian and right PA. The ductus is removed as well to prevent over shunting to the lungs. Apparently, when this goes bad it's usually from issues related to damage of the coronary arteries or **over shunting of blood to the lungs (causing pulmonary edema)**. As a point of trivia, sometimes the thymus is partially removed to get access.

Norwood Procedure

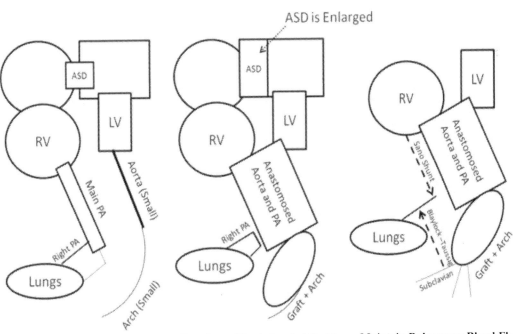

Left Sided Hypoplastic Heart

Creation of Unobstructed Outflow
-Creation of "Neo-Aorta"
-Enlarge ASD for Non-Restrictive Flow

Maintain Pulmonary Blood Flow
-With Either (a) BT Shunt or (b) Sano Shunt

Sano: Same as the Norwood, but instead of using a Blaylock-Taussig shunt a conduit is made connecting the right ventricle to the pulmonary artery. The disadvantage of the BT Shunt undergoes a steal phenomenon (diverted to low pressure pulmonary system).

Classic Glenn: Shunt between the SVC and right pulmonary artery (end-to-end), with the additional step of sewing the proximal end of the Right PA closed with the goal of reducing right ventricular work, by diverting all venous return straight to the lung (right lung).

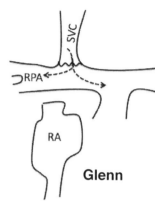

Bi-Directional Glenn: Shunt between the SVC and the right pulmonary artery (**end-to-side**). The RPA is left open, letting blood flow to both lungs. This procedure can be used to address right sided heart problems in general, and is also step two in the palliative hypoplastic series. If it's being used as step two the previously placed Blaylock Taussig Shunt or Sano shunt will come down as the Glenn will be doing its job of putting blood in the lungs.

Fontan Operation: Used for Hypoplastic Hearts. The old school Fontan consisted of a classic Glenn (SVC to RPA), closure of the ASD, and then placing a shunt between the Right atrium to the Left PA. The idea is to let blood return from systemic circulation to the lungs by passive flow (no pump), and turn the right ventricle (the only one the kid has) into a functional left ventricle. There are numerous complications including right atriomegaly with resulting arrhythmias, and plastic bronchitis (they cough up "casts of the bronchus" that look like plastic).

Other Surgeries:

Classic Blalock Taussig Shunt: Originally developed for use with TOF. **Shunt is created between the Subclavian artery and the pulmonary artery**. It is constructed on the **opposite side** of the arch. It's apparently technically difficult and often distorts the anatomy of the pulmonary artery.

High Yield Point:
Glenn = Vein to Artery *(SVC to Pulmonary Artery)*
Blalock Taussig = Artery to Artery *(Subclavian Artery to Pulmonary Artery)*

Modified Blalock Taussig Shunt: This is a gortex shunt between the Subclavian artery and pulmonary artery, and is performed on the **SAME SIDE as the arch**. It's easier to do than the original.

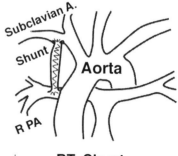

Pulmonary Artery Banding: Done to reduce pulmonary artery pressure (goal is 1/3 of systemic pressure). Most common indication is CHF in infancy with anticipated delayed repair. The **single ventricle is the most common lesion requiring banding**.

Atrial Switch: Mustard and Senning procedures are used to correct transposition of the great arteries by creating a baffle within the atria in order to switch back the blood flow at the level of in-flow. The result is the right ventricle becomes the systemic ventricle, and the left ventricle pumps to the lungs. This is usually done in the first year of life.

- **Senning:** Baffle is created from the right atrial wall and atrial septal tissue WITHOUT use of extrinsic material

- **Mustard:** Involves the resection of the atrial septum and creation of a baffle using pericardium (or synthetic material).

Rastelli Operation: This is the most commonly used operation for transposition, pulmonary outflow obstruction, and VSD. The procedure involves the placement of a baffle within the right ventricle diverting flow from the VSD to the aorta (essentially using the VSD as part of the LVOT. The pulmonary valve is oversewn and the conduit is inserted between the RV and the PA. The primary advantage of this procedure is the left ventricle becomes the system ventricle. The primary limitation of this procedure is that the child will be committed to multiple additional surgeries because the conduit wears out and must be replaced.

Jatene Procedure: This is another arterial switch method that involves transection of the aorta and pulmonary arteries about the valve sinuses , including the removal of the coronaries. The great arteries are switched and the coronaries are sewn into the new aorta (formerly the PA). Apparently this is very technically difficult, but the advantage is there is no conduit to go bad, and the LV is the systemic ventricle.

Ross Procedure: Performed for Diseased Aortic Valves in Children. Replaces the aortic valve with the patient's pulmonary valve and replaces the pulmonary valve with a cryopreserved pulmonary valve homograft. Follow-up studies have shown interval growth of the aortic valve graft in children and infants.

Bentall Procedure: Operation involving composite graft replacement of the aortic valve, aortic root and ascending aorta, with re-implantation of the coronary arteries into the graft. This operation is used to treat combined aortic valve and ascending aorta disease, including lesions associated with Marfan syndrome

Heart Transplant Types

Orthotopic heart transplants all of the heart is removed, except the circular part of the left atrium (the part with the pulmonary veins). The donor heart is trimmed to fit into the left atrium.

Heterotopic heart transplants the recipient heart remains in place, and the donor heart is added on top. This basically creates a double heart. The advantages of this are (1) it gives the native heart a chance to recover , and (2) gives you a backup if the donor is rejected.

SECTION 2: THORACIC

Anatomy

Anatomy is always high yield.

The Lateral CXR "The Radiologists View"

Right Ribs vs Left Ribs on Lateral CXR: By convention, lateral CXRs are taken in the left lateral position (left side against the x-ray film/cassette). Therefore, the left ribs will not be magnified (**rib ribs will be magnified**). **Right ribs also project more posteriorly**. Another strategy is to follow the diaphragm over the stomach bubble (usually left sided).

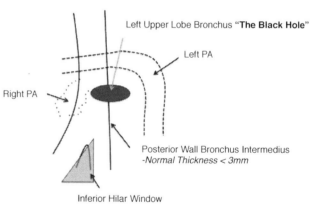

Normal Hilum on Lateral: If you put your finger in the "Dark Hole" – which is the left upper lobe bronchus, in front of it will be the right PA, and overtop of it will be the left PA. The posterior wall of the bronchus intermedius runs through the black hole, and can be thickened by edema.

This is the right hilar anatomy on the frontal view. Of course it never looks that nice in the real world. Ben Felson used to say the right interlobar artery reminded him of a woman's leg... but then again most things did.

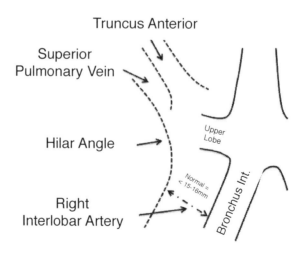

Retrotracheal Triangle **(Raider Triangle).**

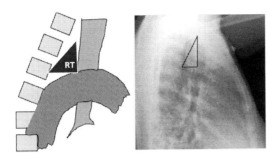

Raider (Retrotracheal) Triangle

This is a triangle which sits on the aortic arch and is bordered anteriorly by the back wall of the trachea, and posteriorly by the upper thoracic vertebral bodies. Many things can obliterate this, but for the purpose of multiple choice tests an opacity in the Raider Triangle is an **Aberrant right subclavian artery**.

Heart Valves on CXR: This is high yield. I like to use a two intersecting line method on both the frontal and lateral chest to answer this kinds of questions.

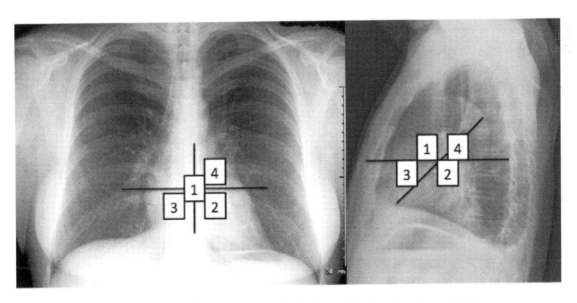

1) Aortic Valve, 2) Mitral Valve, 3) Tricuspid Valve 4) Pulmonic Valve

A few other sneaky tricks include, knowing that the pointy parts of the mechanical valves (*Carpentier-Edwards aortic valve*) point out (towards the direction of blood flow). Know that the mitral valve is larger than the aortic valve (so if you see two metallic rings, the larger is the mitral). Know that a pacemaker wire going through a valve makes it the tricupsid valve (lead terminates in the right ventricle). Know the Pulmonic valve is the most superior in location.

Fissures and Atelectasis:

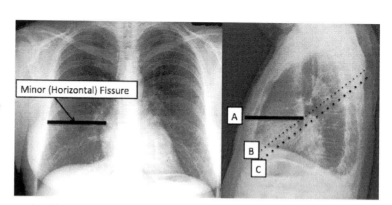

Notice the right major fissure is anterior to the left.

A = Horizontal (Minor) Fissure, B = Right Major, C = Left Major

The classic patterns of atelectasis:

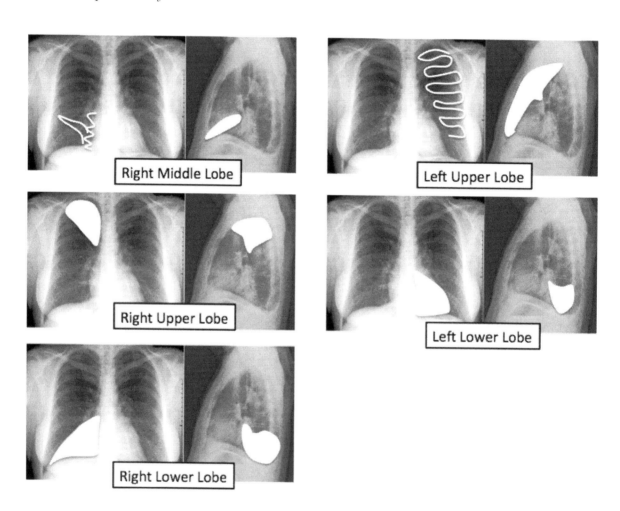

Right Middle Lobe

Left Upper Lobe

Right Upper Lobe

Left Lower Lobe

Right Lower Lobe

A few pearls to point out:

*Right Upper Lobe Collapse = Be aware of the "**Golden S**" type of collapse which infers a central mass.*

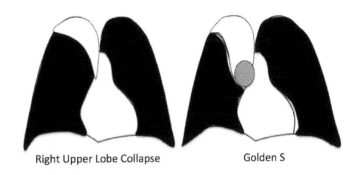

Right Upper Lobe Collapse   Golden S

The "Flat Waist Sign" of Left Lower Lobe Collapse. *For some reason academic Radiologists are obsessed with the name of this sign.*

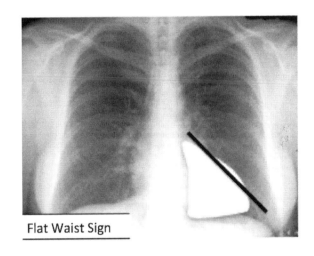

Flat Waist Sign

Luftsichel Sign: *The is seen in the case of left upper lobe collapse, where you get hyperinflation of the superior segment of the left lower lobe. This inflated segment takes the shape of a sickle (made of air).*

Luft = Air.

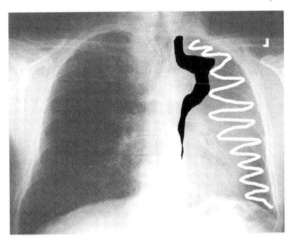

Luftsichel Sign

Segmental Anatomy – The tertiary bronchi are grouped into bronchopulmonary segments. There are 10 segments on the right (3 upper, 2 middle, and 5 lower). On the left there are only 8 segments (4 in the upper lobe / lingula, and 4 in the lower lobe).

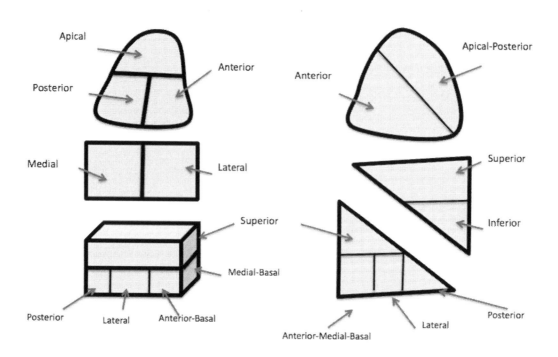

Mediastinum

Anatomy: The mediastinum is classically divided into 4 sections, superior, anterior, middle, and posterior. The borders of these areas make good trivia questions.

Borders:

- *Superior* – The inferior border is the oblique plane from the sternal-manubrial junction.

- *Anterior* – The posterior border is the pericardium

- *Middle* - The heart, pericardium, and bifurcation of the trachea are all included. On lateral CXR, people sometimes say posterior to the trachea, and anterior to the vertebral bodies (or 1cm posterior to the vertebral bodies).

- *Posterior* – From the back of the heart to the spine. Contains the esophagus, thoracic duct, and descending aorta.

Mass localization Questions:

This was a known thing done on the old oral boards, so the idea is not new. They show you a mass on a frontal radiograph and tell you to localize it (anterior, middle, posterior, or pulmonary). Here are the common tactics you can use to get this right.

Cervicothoracic Sign – This takes advantage of the posterior junction line, which demonstrates that *things above the clavicles are in the posterior mediastinum.*

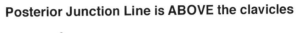
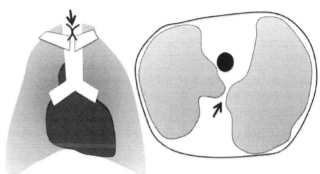

Hilum Overlay Sign: Mass at the level of the hilum arising from the hilum will obliterate the silhouette of the pulmonary vessels. If you can see the edge of the vessels through the mass, then the mass is not in the hilum (so it is either anterior or posterior).

Pulmonary vs Mediastinal Origin: The easiest trick is if they show you air bronchograms. Only a pulmonary mass will have air bronchograms. The harder trick is the angle with the lung. The mass will make an acute angle with the lung if it's within the lung. The mass will make an obtuse margin with the lung if it's in the mediastinum.

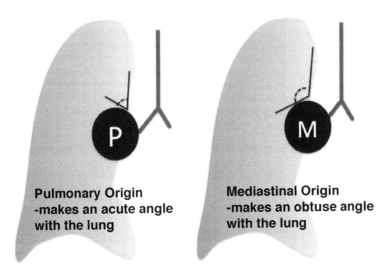

Pulmonary Origin
-makes an acute angle
with the lung

Mediastinal Origin
-makes an obtuse angle
with the lung

Varient Anatomy:

Azygos Lobe – These things happen when the azygos vein is displaced laterally during development. The result is a deep fissure in the right upper lobe. It's not actually an accessory lobe but rather a variant of the right upper lobe. If they show you one, the question is most likely going to be, *"how many layers of pleura?"* The answer is 4.

Pig Bronchus/ Tracheal Bronchus: A tracheal bronchus is a bronchus that comes right off the trachea (prior to bifurcation into right and left mainstem). You can call it a pig bronchus if the entire right upper lobe is supplied by this bronchus. It usually means nothing clinically, but occasionally people can get some air trapping or recurrent infections from impaired ventilation.

Pulmonary Veins: Pulmonary vein anatomy is highly variable. You typically have 4 total (2 right – upper and lower, 2 left – upper and lower). The **most common anatomic variation is a separate vein draining the right middle lobe** (seen 30% of the time). Who cares??? Two people (1) People who write multiple choice tests, (2) Electrophysiologists prior to ablations.

Proximal Interruption of the Pulmonary Artery: Basically you have congenital absence of the right (or left PA) with the more distal pulmonary vasculature present. It's also called unilateral absence of the PA, but that is confusing because the distal pulmonary vasculature is present.

How it's shown:
- Classically with volume loss of one hemi-thorax (could be on CXR or CT), then a contrast CT shot through the heart with only one PA. Normally, you might think one PA is just volume averaging - but once you've been shown volume loss on one side your suspicion for this should be raised.

Trivia to know:
- It's seen on the opposite side of the aortic arch (Absent right PA with left sided aortic arch, Absent left PA with right sided aortic arch).
- Associated with PDA
- Interrupted left PA is associated with TOF, and Trunchus

Pneumonia

Bacterial Infection		
Strep Pneumo	Lobar Consolidation	Favors lower lobes. Can be severe in sickle cell patients post splenectomy. The **most common cause of pneumonia in AIDS patient**.
Staph A.	**Bronchopenumoia** – patchy opacities	Often bilateral, and can make abscess. Can be spread via the blood in endocarditis patients
Anthrax	Hemorrhagic lymphadenitis, mediastinitis, and hemothorax	Classic Look: **Mediastinal widening** with pleural effusion in the setting of bio-terrorism
Klebsiella	Buzzword: "**Bulging Fissure**" from exuberant inflammation. More likely to have pleural effusions, empyema, and cavity than conventional pneumonia.	Alcoholic and Nursing Home Patients. Step 1 Buzzword was "currant jelly sputum"
H. Flu	Usually bronchitis, sometimes bilateral lower lobe bronchopneumonia	Seen in **COPDers**, and people without a spleen
Pseudomonas	Patchy opacities, with abscess formation	ICUers on a ventilator (also CF and Primary Ciliary Dyskinesia). Pleural effusions are common, but usually small
Legionella	Peripheral and sublobar airspace opacity	Seen in **COPDers**, and around crappy air conditioners. Only cavitates in immunosuppressed patients. X-ray tends to lag behind resolution of symptoms.
Aspiration	Anerobes, with airspace opacities. They can cavitate, and abscess is not uncommon	Posterior lobes if supine when aspirating, Basal Lower lobes in upright aspiration May favor the right side, just like an ET tube. The most common complication is empyema (which can get a bronchopleural fistula).
Actinomycosis	Airspace in peripheral lower lobes. Can be aggressive and cause rib osteomyelitis/ invade adjacent chest wall.	Classic story is dental procedure gone bad, leading to mandible osteo, leading to aspiration.
Mycoplasma	Fine reticular pattern on CXR, Patchy airspace opacity with tree-in-bud	

Immunocompromised

Post Bone Marrow Transplant: You see pulmonary infections in nearly 50% of people after bone marrow transplant, and this is often listed as the most common cause of death in this population. The findings are segregated into: early neutropenic, early, and late – and often tested as such.

Post Bone Marrow Transplant Graft vs Host	
Acute (20-100 Days)	Chronic (> 100 days)
Favors extrapulmonary systems (skin, liver, GI tract)	Lymphocytic Infiltration of the airways and obliterative bronchiolitis.

Post Bone Marrow Transplant (Pulmonary Findings)		
Early Neutropenic (0-30 days)	Early (30-90)	Late > 90
Pulmonary Edema, Hemorrhage, Drug Induced Lung Injury	PCP, CMV	Bronchiolitis Obliterans, Cryptogenic Organizing Pneumonia
Fungal Pneumonia (invasive aspergillosis)		

AIDS Related Pulmonary Infection:

Questions related to AIDS and pulmonary infection are typically written is one of two ways (1) with regard to the CD4 count, and (2) by showing you a very characteristic infection.

Infections in AIDS by CD4	
> 200	Bacterial Infections, TB
< 200	PCP, Atypical Mycobacterial
< 100	CMV, Disseminated Fungal, Mycobacterial

CT Pattern – With AIDS	
Focal Airspace Opacity	Bacterial Infection (**Strep Pneumonia**) **is the most common**. DDx should include TB if low CD4. If it's a chronic opacity think Lymphoma or Kaposi.
Multi-Focal Airspace Opacity	Bacterial, or Fungal
Ground Glass	This is gonna be **PCP** (if that's not a choice it could be CMV if CD4 is < 100).

PCP: This is the most classic AIDS infection. This is the one they are most likely to show you. **Ground glass opacity** is the dominant finding, and is seen bilaterally in the perihilar regions with sparing of the lung periphery. Cysts, which are usually thin walled, can occur in the ground glass opacities about 30% of the time.

AIDS High Yield Trivia / Buzzwords:
- *Most common airspace opacity = Strep Pneumonia*
- *If they show you a CT with ground glass = PCP*
- *"Flame Shaped" Perihilar opacity = Kaposi Sarcoma*
- *Persistent Opacities = Lymphoma*
- *Lung Cysts = LIP*
- *Lungs Cysts + Ground Glass + Pneumothorax = PCP*
- *Hypervascular Lymph Nodes = Castlemans or Kaposi*

TB

You can think about TB as either (a) Primary, (b) Primary Progressive, (c) Latent or (d) Post Primary / Reactivation.

- **Primary:** Essentially you inhaled the bug, and it causes necrosis. Your body attacks and forms a granuloma (Ghon Focus). You can end up with nodal expansion (which is bulky in kids, and less common in adults), this can calcify and you get a "Ranke Complex." The bulky nodes can actually cause compression leading to atelectasis (which is often lobar). If the node ruptures you can end up with either (a) endobronchial spread or (b) hematogenous spread – depending on if the rupture is into the bronchus or a vessel. This hematogenous spread manifests as a miliary pattern. **Cavitation in the primary setting is NOT common.** Effusions can be seen but are more common in adults (uncommon in kids).

- **Primary Progressive**: This term refers to local progression of parenchymal disease with the **development of cavitation** (at the initial site of infection / or hematogenous spread). This primary progression is uncommon – with the main risk factor being **HIV**. Other risk factors are all the things that make you immunosuppressed – transplant patients, people on steroids. The ones you might not think about is jejunoileal bypass, subtotal gastrectomy, and silicosis. This form is **similar in course to post primary disease**.

- **Latent:** This is a positive PPD, with a negative CXR, and no symptoms. If you got the TB vaccine, you are considered latent if your PPD converts by the US health care system/industry. This scenario buys you 9 months of INH and maybe some nice drug induced hepatitis.

- **Post Primary (reactivation):** This happens about 5% of the time, and describes an endogenous reactivation of a latent infection. The classic location is in the apical and posterior upper lobe and superior lower lobe (more oxygen, less lymphatics). In primary infection you tend to have healing. In post primary infection you tend to have progression. The **development of a cavity** is the thing to look for when you want to call this. Arteries near the cavity can get all pseudoaneursym'd up – "Rasmussen Aneurysm" they call it – in the setting of a TB cavity.

Immune Reconstitution Inflammatory Syndrome: The story will be patient with TB and AIDS started on highly active anti-retroviral therapy (HAART) now doing worse. The therapy is steroids.

Pleural Involvement with TB: This can occur at any time at the initial infection. In primary TB the development of a pleural effusion can be seen around 3-6 months after infection – as a hypersensitivity response. This pleural fluid is usually culture negative (usually in this case is like 60%). You have to actually biopsy the pleura to increase your diagnostic yield. You don't see pleural effusions as much with post primary disease, but when you do, the fluid is usually culture positive.

High Yield Factoids Regarding TB:
- Primary = No Cavity, Post Primary / Primary Progressive = Cavity
- Ghon Lesion = Calcified TB Granuloma ; sequela of primary TB
- Ranke Complex = Calcified TB Granuloma + Calcified Hilar Node ; Healed primary TB
- Bulky Hilar and Paratracheal Adenopathy = Kids
- Location for Reactivation TB = Posterior / Apical upper lobes, Superior Lower Lobes
- Miliary Spread when? – Hematogenous dissemination (usually in the setting of reactivation), but can be in primary progressive TB as well
- Reactive TB Pattern (Cavitation) seen in HIV patient when the CD4 is > 200
- Primary Progressive Pattern (Adenopathy, Consolidation, Miliary Spread) in HIV is CD4 < 200
- TB does NOT usually cause a lobar pattern in HIV

Non Tuberculous Mycobacteria: Not all mycobacterium is TB. The two non-TB forms worth knowing are mycobacterium avium-intracellulare complex (MAC) and Mycobacterium Kansasii. I find that grouping these things into 4 buckets is most useful for understanding and remembering them.

- **Cavitary** ("Classic") – This one is usually caused by MAC. It favors an old white man with COPD (or other chronic lung disease), and it looks like reactivation TB. So you have an upper lobe cavitary lesion with adjacent nodules (suggesting endobronchial spread).

- **Bronchiectatic** ("Non-Classic") – This is the so called "**Lady Windermere**" disease (everyone knows it's just not lady-like to cough). They often do not cough, and are asymptomatic. This favors an old white lady. You see tree-in-bud opacities and cylindric bronchiectasis in the right middle lobe and lingula.

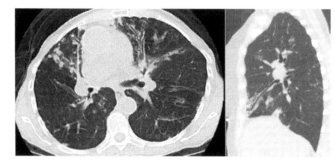

Lady Windermere - MAC
-Bronchiectasis with tree-in-bud funk in the right middle lobe and lingula

- **HIV Patients** – You see this with low CD4s (< 100). The idea is that it's a GI infection disseminated in the blood. You get a big spleen and liver. It frequently is mixed with other pulmonary infections (PCP, etc…) given the low CD4 – so the lungs can look like anything. Mediastinal lymphadenopathy is the most common manifestation.

- **Hypersensitivity Pneumonitis** – This is the so called "**hot-tub lung**." Where you get aerosolized bugs (which exist in natural sea water and in fresh water). The lungs look like ill-defined, **ground glass centrilobular nodules**.

Non Tuberculous Mycobacteria - Rapid Review		
Cavitary Type	Old White Male Smoker	Looks like reactivation TB
Non-Classic *(Lady Windermere)*	Old Lady	Middle Lobe and Lingula, bronchiectasis and tree in bud.
HIV	Low CD4 (< 100)	Mediastinal Lymphadenopathy
Hypersensitivity *(Hot Tub Lung)*	History of hot tub use	Ground glass centrilobular nodules

Fungal

Aspergillus: So this can cause a variable appearance and the trivia surrounding that variability comes in three flavors: (1) normal immune, (2) immune depressed, or (3) Hyper-immune.

- *Normal Immune:* This is the situation when aspergillus makes a fungus ball "Aspergilloma" in an existing cavity. The way this is asked is pretty much always the same. They will show you a fungus ball, and they want you to call it invasive. Don't fall for that. This is not the same thing as invasive. They can be totally normal people who have a cavity from trauma, or prior infection ect...

- *Immune Suppressed (AIDS, or Transplant Patient):* This is when you get your **invasive aspergillus**. This is going to be shown one of two ways. (1) A **halo sign** – consolidative nodule/mass with a ground glass halo. The halo of ground glass is actually the invasive component. (2) **Air Crescent sign** – a thin crescent of air within the consolidative mass. This actually represents healing, as the necrotic lung separates from the parenchyma. The timing is usually about 2-3 weeks after treatment. Lastly, they could show you some peripheral wedge shaped infarcts in the setting of some halo signs.

- *Hyper-Immune:* This is your asthmatic with **ABPA**. Allergic Brocho-Pulmonary Aspergillosis. This is "Always" seen in patients with **long standing asthma** (sometimes CF). You classically have upper lobe central saccular bronchiectasis with mucoid impaction (finger-in-glove).

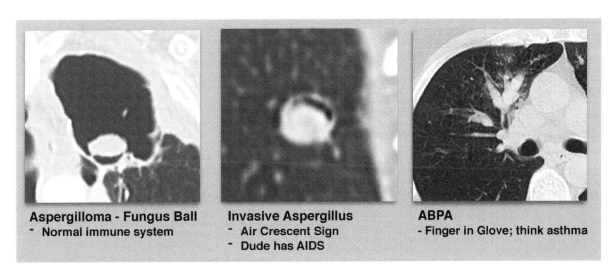

Aspergilloma - Fungus Ball
- Normal immune system

Invasive Aspergillus
- Air Crescent Sign
- Dude has AIDS

ABPA
- Finger in Glove; think asthma

Mucormycosis – This aggressive fungal infection almost always occurs in impaired patients (AIDS, Steroids, Bad Diabetics Etc..). You usually think about mucor eating some diabetic's face off, but it can also occur in the lungs. Think about this when you have <u>invasion of the mediastinum, pleura, and chest wall.</u>

Viral

- **CMV** – This can be seen in two classic scenarios: (1) Reactivation of the latent virus after prolonged immunosuppression (post bone marrow transplant), and (2) Infusing of the CMV positive marrow or in other blood products. The timing for bone marrow patients is "early" between 30-90 days. The radiographic appearance is multiple nodules, ground glass or consolidative.

Random Viral Trivia		
Measles	Multifocal ground glass opacities with small nodular opacities	Pneumonia can be before or after the skin lesions. Complications higher in pregnant and immunocompromised
Influenza	Coalescent lower lobe opacity. Pleural effusion is rare.	
SARS	Lower lobe predominant ground glass opacities	
Varicella	Multiple peripheral nodular opacities. They form small round calcific lung nodules in the healed version.	About 1/6th with skin findings will get a pneumonia. It's usually in kids. When you see it they are usually immunocompromised (have AIDS or lymphoma).
Ebstein Barr	Uncommonly affects the lung. Can cause lymph node enlargement	Most common radiographic abnormality is a big spleen.

Septic Emboli

There are a variety of ways you can throw infectious material into the lungs via the bloodstream (pulmonary arteries). Some common sources would include; infected tricupsid valves, infection in the body, infected catheters, infected teeth…etc…

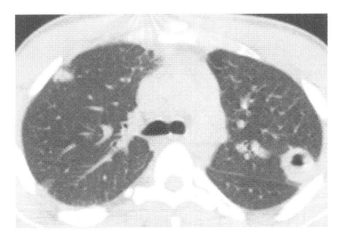

Septic Emboli - Multiple round opacities, one with cavitation

Things to know about Septic Emboli:
- It's lower lobe predominant (more blood flow)
- You get peripheral nodular densities and wedge shaped densities (can infarct).
- They can **cavitate**, and likely will be cavitated if they show you a CT image.
- The **feeding vessel sign** – nodule with a big vessel going into it can be shown (also seen with hematogenous mets).
- Empyema and pneumothorax are both known complications.

CAVITY Mnemonic For Lung Cavity:

C – **C**ancer (usually squamous cell)
A – **A**uto-immune (Wegeners, Rheumatoid / Caplan Syndrome)
V – **V**ascular – Septic Emboli / Bland Emboli
I – **I**nfection - TB
T – **T**rauma - Pneumatoceles
Y – **Y**oung – "Congenital" – CCAMs, Sequestrations

Lemierre Syndrome: This is an eponym referring to **jugular vein thrombosis with septic emboli** classically seen after an oropharyngeal infection or recent ENT surgery.

Classic Lemierre Question:
> *Q: What is the bacterial agent responsible in the majority of cases?*
> *A: "**Fusobacterium Necrophorum**."*

Lung Cancer

Screening: Recently, the US preventive services task force has approved lung cancer screening with low dose CT for asymptomatic adults aged 55-80 who have a 30 pack-year history and currently smoke (or have quit within the past 15 years). Obviously this is going to be a huge cash cow for radiology not just in the CT, but for the numerous incidental follow ups. Follow up recommendations are still being developed (so they won't be on the exam). The old Fleischner society stuff might be, with the most likely questions being that *Fleischner Society Recommendations do NOT apply to patient's with known cancers.*

Solitary Pulmonary Nodule: A SPN is defined as a round or oval lesion measuring less than 3cm in diameter (more than 3cm = mass). Technically to be "solitary" it needs to be surrounded by lung parenchyma, with no associated adenopathy, or pleural effusion.

There are 4 classic "benign calcification" patterns: solid, laminated, central, and popcorn. Anything else is considered suspicious. Eccentric patterns are considered the most suspicious. Some notable (testable) exceptions include when you see popcorn and central calcifications in the setting of a GI cancer. Solid calcifications can be bad in the setting of osteosarcoma.

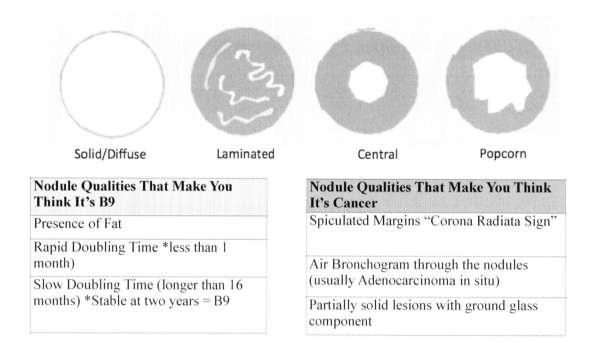

| Solid/Diffuse | Laminated | Central | Popcorn |

Nodule Qualities That Make You Think It's B9	Nodule Qualities That Make You Think It's Cancer
Presence of Fat	Spiculated Margins "Corona Radiata Sign"
Rapid Doubling Time *less than 1 month)	Air Bronchogram through the nodules (usually Adenocarcinoma in situ)
Slow Doubling Time (longer than 16 months) *Stable at two years = B9	Partially solid lesions with ground glass component

Solid and Ground Glass Components: A **part solid lesion with a ground glass component is the most suspicious morphology you can have**. Non-solids (only ground glass) is intermediate. Totally solid is actually the least likely morphology to be cancer.

PET for SPN: You can use PET for SPNs larger than 1cm. Lung Cancer is supposed to be HOT (SUV > 2.5). Having said that, infectious and granulomatous nodules can also be hot. If you are dealing with a ground glass nodule it's more likely to be:

COLD = Cancer,   HOT = Infection.

Lung Cancer Risk factors include; being over 30 (under 30 is super rare), exposures to bad stuff (arsenic, nickel, asbestos, chromium, beryllium, radon), having lung fibrosis, COPD (even if you didn't smoke), and family history.

Types: There 4 types of lung cancer.

- **Squamous:** Usually centrally located, and strongly associated with smoking. Cavitation is common, and is the most likely question. The prognosis is relatively good, as this subtype likes to met late. You can get ectopic PTH production.

- **Small Cell:** Usually central (common near the main or lobar bronchi). You may only have central lymphadenopathy with this one. It has a terrible prognosis, and is basically a death sentence. Paraneoplatic syndromes with SIADH and ACTH can occur.

> **Lambert Eaton:** Paraneoplastic Syndrome seen with patient's having Small Cell Lung Cancer. They get proximal weakness from abnormal release of acetylcholine at the neuromuscular junction. The clinical presentation often comes before the cancer diagnosis.

- **Large Cell:** Usually peripheral and large (> 4cm). Prognosis sucks.

- **Adenocarcinoma:** It's usually peripheral (75%) often in the upper lobes. It's the most common subtype overall and the **most common subtype to present as a solitary pulmonary nodule**. This guy has a known association with lung fibrosis.

BAC (Subtype of Adenocarcinoma): This has recently undergone a name change. Why change its name? Well it's a simple reason. Academic Radiologists need to be on committees to get promoted. Committees need an excuse to go on vacation ("International Meetings" they call them). Name changes happen...

- **Atypical Adenomatous Hyperplasia of Lung (AAH):** This is a precursor of adenocarcinoma of the lung.

- **Adenocarcinoma in situ (ACIS):** These are < 3cm. This in itself has multiple subtypes. The most common of these is the non-mucinous one.

- **Minimally Invasive Adenocarcinoma (MIA):** These are also < 3cm. The distinction is that there is < 5mm of stromal invasion (> 5mm will be called a lepidic predominant adeoncarcinoma).

    o *Things to know:*
      - It's usually ground glass
      - It's classically COLD on PET
      - "Fried Egg" – Ground glass halo around nodule
      - "Pseudocavitation" bubble like lucencies

Key Concept: The larger the solid component of the "part solid" nodule gets the more likely it is to be malignant. In other words, **partially solid nodules are more likely to be cancer than ground glass nodules.**

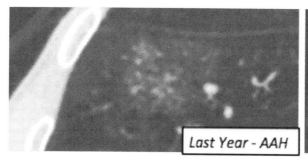
Last Year - AAH

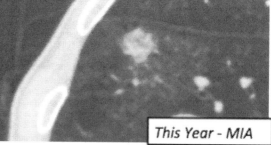
This Year - MIA

Staging:

Lung cancer staging is different for small cell vs non-small cell (NSCLC) . NSCLC staging is much more testable. *The big thing to know about lung cancer staging is that **stage 3B is unresectable.*** So what makes something stage 3B?

Stage 3B implies N3 or T4 disease

Another piece of trivia I think lends well to multiple choice, is the difference in multi-centric locations of tumors. Two in the same lobe is a T3, Two in different ipsilateral lobes is T4, and Two in different lungs is an M1a.

Stage 3B (NOT resectable)
Supraclavicular , Scalene or Contralateral Mediastinal or Hilar Adenopathy
Tumor in the same lung but different lobes from the primary mass
Malignant Pleural Effusion

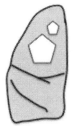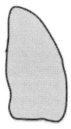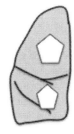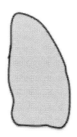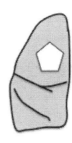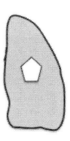

Stage T3 *(two in same lobe)*   Stage T4 *(two in different lobes)*   Stage M1a *(two in different lungs)*

Treatment: Treatment for lung cancer is either surgery, radiotherapy, chemotherapy, thermal ablation (RFA/MWA) in isolation or combination, depending on the stage. **Stage 3B being non-operable as the big testable point.**

Radiation Changes: - The appearance of radiation pneumonitis is variable and based on the volume of lung involved, how much/long radiation was given, and if chemotherapy was administered as well.

Radiation Changes	
Early *(within 1-3 months)*	**Late**
Homogenous or patchy ground glass opacities.	Dense consolidation, traction bronchiectasis, and volume loss.

Bronchopleural Fistula – This is an uncommon complication of pneumonectomy, that has a characteristic look and therefore easy to test. So normally after a pneumonectomy the space will fill with fluid. If you see it filling with air than this is the dead give away. You can confirm the diagnosis with a xenon nuclear medicine ventilation study, which will show xenon in the pneumonectomy space. The major risk factor is ischemia to the bronchi (disrupted blood supply from aggressive lymph node dissection, or using a long bronchial stump).

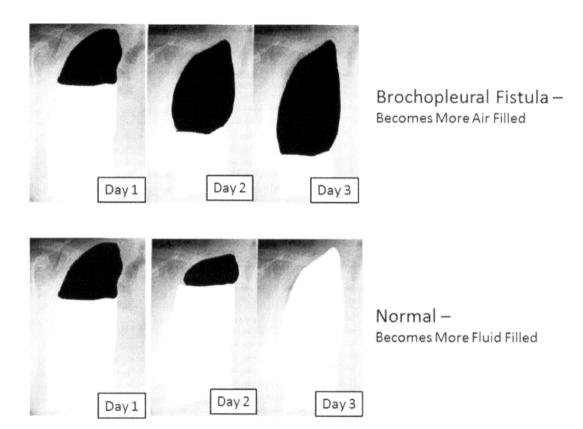

Brochopleural Fistula –
Becomes More Air Filled

Normal –
Becomes More Fluid Filled

Other Tumors:

Mets – Metastatic disease to the lungs can be thought of in 3 categories; direct invasion, hematogenous, lymphangitic:

- **Direct Invasion:** This is seen with cancer of the mediastinum, pleura, or chest wall. The most common situation is an esophageal carcinoma, lymphoma, or malignant germ cell tumor. More rarely you are going to have mets to the pleura then invading the lung. Even more rarely you can have malignant mesothelioma, which can invade the lung. It should be obvious.

- **Hematogenous Mets:** The most common manifestation of hematogenous mets to the lung is the pulmonary nodule (usually multiple, in a **random distribution**, and **favoring the lower lobes** which have greater blood volume). The nodules tend to be smoother than the primary neoplasm. The main culprits are breast, kidney, thyroid, colon, and head & neck squamous cells. Obviously the squamous mets can cavitate. "**Cannonball Mets" are classically from renal cell or choriocarcinoma** (testicle).

> **Feeding Vessel Sign:** A prominent pulmonary vessel heading into a nodule. This supposedly means it's from a hematogenous origin. It's nonspecific – but if you see it the answer is (1) mets , or (2) septic emboli.

- **Lymphangetic Carcinomatosis (LC):** The most common cause of unilateral LC is actually bronchogenic carcinoma lung cancer invading the lymphatics. The most common extrathroacic culprits are breast, stomach, pancreas, and prostate. The finding is nodular thickening of the interlobular septa and subpleural interstitium. Unlike interstitial fibrosis, this thickening classically does NOT distort the pulmonary lobule.

Carcinoid: Carcinoid can be classified either based on location; (a) peripheral pulmonary, and (b) bronchial – or by histologic type (a) typical and (b) atypical. The typical carcinoids are slow growing and locally invasive (only met to nodes about 10% of the time). There is no association with smoking. These typical carcinoids typically **appear centrally within a bronchus** (only 1% are in the trachea). As they occur endobronchially, they **often cause obstructive symptoms**. They can also cause hemoptysis because they are highly vascular. An octreotide scan can be used to localize a carcinoid tumor. The pulmonary tumors can cause a carcinoid syndrome with flushing etc… The valvular degradation that occurs tends to be on the left side (mitral and aortic), as opposed to the GI carcinoid syndrome which affects the right side (tricuspid and pulmonic). The atypical carcinoids are more rare, seen in older patients, and more likely to be a mass.

Adenoid Cystic (Cylindroma) – This is the most common bronchial gland tumor. It is NOT associated with smoking. They are usually in the main or lobar bronchus.

Carcinoid	More common in bronchus, Rare in Trachea
Adenoid Cystic	Occurs in Bronchus, 20:1 more common than carcinoid in the Trachea.

Lymphoma – There are basically 4 flavors of pulmonary lymphoma; primary, secondary, AIDS related, or PTLD. Radiographic patterns are variable and can be lymphangitic spread (uncommon), parahilar airspace opacities, and/or mediastinal adenopathy.

- **Primary:** This is rare, and usually non-Hodgkin in subtype. You define it as the lack of extrathoracic involvement for 3 months. Almost always (80%) of the time we are talking about a low grade MALToma.

- **Secondary:** Here we are talking about pulmonary involvement of a systemic lymphoma. This is much much much more common than primary lung lymphoma. The thing to see is that NHL is much more common, but if you have HL it is more likely to involve the lungs. With HL you gets nodes and parenchyma, in NHL you might just get parenchyma.

Secondary NHL	Secondary HL
80-90% of lymphoma cases	10-20% of lymphoma cases
45% have intrathoracic disease at presentation	85% have intrathoracic disease at presentation
25% have pulmonary parenchymal disease	40% have pulmonary parenchymal disease
Pulmonary involvement frequently occurs in the absence of mediastinal disease	Lung involvement almost always associated with intrathoracic lymph node enlargement

- **PTLD:** This is seen after solid organ or stem cell transplant. **This usually occurs within a year of transplant** (late presentations > 1 year have a more aggressive course). This is a B-Cell lymphoma, with a relationship with EB Virus. You can have both nodal and extra nodal disease. The typical look is well defined pulmonary nodules / mass, patchy airspace consolidation, halo sign, and interlobular septal thickening.

- **AIDS related pulmonary lymphoma (ARL)** - This is the second most common lung tumor in AIDS patients (Kaposi's is first). Almost exclusively a high grade NHL. There is a relationship with EBV. It is seen in patients with a **CD4 < 100**. The presentation is still variable with multiple peripheral nodules ranging from 1cm-5cm being considered the most common manifestation. Extranodal locations (CNS, bone marrow, lung, liver, bowel) is common. **AIDS patient with lung nodules, pleural effusion, and lymphadenopathy = Lymphoma.**

Kaposi Sarcoma: This is the most common lung tumor is AIDS patients (Lymphoma is number two). The tracheobronchial mucosa and perihilar lung are favored. The buzzword is "flame shaped." A bloody pleural effusion is common (50%).

Kaposi Sarcoma	Lymphoma
Thallium ^{201} Positive	Thallium ^{201} Positive
Gallium ^{67} Negative	Gallium ^{67} Positive

Things to know about KS:
- *Most common lung tumor in AIDS (requires CD4 < 200)*
- *Most common hepatic neoplasm in AIDS*
- *Buzzword = Flame Shaped Opacities*
- *Slow Growth, with asymptomatic patients (despite lungs looking terrible)*
- *Thallium Positive, Gallium Negative*

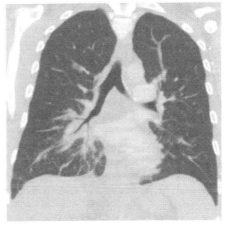

Kaposi Sarcoma
– "Flame Shaped" Hilar Opacities

Hamartoma – this is an Aunt Minnie because it will have **macroscopic fat and "popcorn" calcifications.** It is the most common benign lung mass. It's usually incidental, but can cause problems if it's endobronchial (rare – like 2%).

Technically the fat is only seen in 60%, but for sure if the exam shows it, it will have fat. These **can be hot on PET**, they are still benign.

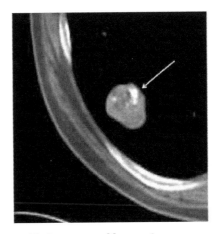

Pulmonary Hamartoma
- Popcorn Calcifications
- Fat Density

Congenital:

Bronchial Atresia – This most commonly involves the apical-posterior segment of the left upper lobe. The usual look is a blind ending bronchus , filled with mucus ("**finger in glove**"), with the **distal lung hyper-inflated** – from collateral drift and air trapping.

AVM - They can occur sporadically. For the purpose of multiple choice when you see them think about HHT (Hereditary Hemorrhagic Telangiectasia / Osler Weber Rendu). Pulmonary AVMs are most commonly found in the lower lobes (more blood flow), and can be a source of right to left shunt (**worry about stroke and brain abscess**). The rule of **treating once the afferent vessel is 3mm** is based on some tiny little abstract and not powered at all. Having said that, it's quoted all the time, and a frequent source of trivia that is easily tested.

Persistent Left SVC - This is the most common congenital venous anomaly of the chest. It usually only matters when the medicine guys drop a line in it on the floor and it causes a confusing post CXR (line is in a left paramedian location). It usually **drains into the coronary sinus**. In a minority of cases (like 5%) it will drain into the left atrium, and cause right to left shunt physiology (very mild though). This is typically shown on an axial CT at the level of the AP window, or with a pacemaker (or line) going into the right heart from the left.

Swyer-James - This is the classic **unilateral lucent lung**. It typically occurs after a viral lung infection in childhood resulting in **post infectious obliterative bronchiolitis** (from constrictive bronchiolitis). The *size of the affected lobe is smaller* than a normal lobe (it's not hyperexpanded).

Poland – Unilateral absence of a pectoral muscle. It can cause a unilateral hyperlucent chest. They can have limb issues (small weird arms / hands).

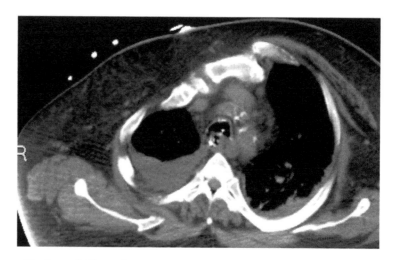

Poland Syndrome – Absent Pectoral on Right

Sequestration These are grouped into intralobar and extralobar with the distinction being which has a pleural covering. You can NOT tell the difference radiographically. The practical difference is age of presentation; intralobar presents in adolescence or adulthood with recurrent pneumonias, extralobar presents in infancy with respiratory compromise.

Intralobar: Much more common (75%). Presents in adolescence or adulthood as recurrent pneumonias (bacteria migrate in from pores of Kohn). **Most commonly in the left lower lobe posterior segment** (2/3s). Uncommon in the upper lobes. In contradistinction from extralobar sequestration, it is rarely associated with other developmental abnormalities.

Extralobar: Less common of the two (25%). Presents in infancy with respiratory compromise (primarily because of the associated anomalies - *Congenital cystic adenomatoid malformation (CCAM), congenital diaphragmatic hernia, vertebral anomalies, congenital heart disease, pulmonary Hypoplasia)*. It rarely gets infected since it has its own pleural covering.

Intralobar	Extralobar
More Common	Less Common
Presents in Adolescence	Presents in Infancy
Recurrent Infections	Associated Congenital Anomalies
No Pleural Cover	Has it's own pleural cover
Pulmonary Venous Drainage	Systemic Venous Drainage

CCAM - As the name suggests it's a malformation of adenomatoid stuff that replaces normal lung. Most of the time it only affects one lobe. There is no lobar preference (unlike CLE which favors the left upper lobe). There are cystic and solid types (type 1 cystic, type 3 solid, type 2 in the middle). There is a crop of knuckle heads who want to call these things CPAMs and have 5 types, which I'm sure is evidence based and will really make an impact in the way these things are treated. CCAMs communicate with the airway, and therefore fill with air. Most of these things (like 90%) will spontaneously decrease in size in the third trimester. The treatment *(at least in the US)* is to cut these things out, because of the iddy bitty theoretical risk of malignant transformation *(pleuropulmonary blastoma, rhabdomyosarcoma)*.

Q: *What if you see a systemic arterial feeder (one coming off the aorta) going to the CCAM ?*
A: Then it's not a CCAM, it's a Sequestration. — sneaky

Diseases Primarily Involving the Interstitial Lung

Cystic Lung Disease:

Pulmonary Langerhans Cell Histiocytosis (LCH) – This cystic lung disease classically effects **smokers, who are young (20s-30s).** The disease starts out with centrilobular nodules with an upper lobe predominance. These nodules eventually cavitate into cysts which are thin walled to start, and then some become more thick walled. Late in the disease you are primarily seeing cysts. The buzzword is **bizarre shaped**, which occurs when 2 or more cysts merge together. In about half the cases this spontaneously resolves (especially if you stop smoking). Another piece of trivia is the LCH spares the costophrenic angles.

> **What Spares the Costophrenic Angles???**
> *LCH and Hypersensitivity Pneumonitis*

Lymphangiomyomatosis (LAM) – This cystic lung disease can occur in **child bearing aged women** or in association with **tuberous sclerosis (a trick is to show the kidneys with multiple AMLs first)**. The cysts are **thinned walled** with a uniform distribution. There is an **association with chylothorax** (which is HIGH YIELD Trivia). The pathophysiology is that it is estrogen dependent (why it strongly favors women). This is usually progressive despite attempts at hormonal therapy (tamoxifen).

LCH	LAM
Cysts and Nodules	Cysts (no nodules)
Smoker	Women, Pts with Tuberous Sclerosis
Upper and Mid Lungs	Diffuse
Thicker Cysts (Bizarre)	Thin Round Cysts

LCH	Bizarre Shape	Thick Wall
LAM	Round	Thin Wall
BHD	Oval	Thin Wall

Birt Hogg Dube (BHD) – This is a **total zebra**. This cystic lung disease has **thin walled "oval" shaped cysts.** There is an association with renal findings (bilateral oncocytomas, and chromophobe RCCs). They also have a bunch of gross skin stuff.

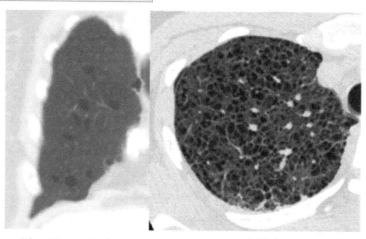

Birt-Hogg-Dube
– Oval Cysts

LAM
– Multiple Thin Walled Round Cysts

Lymphocytic Interstitial Pneumonitis (LIP) – This is a benign lymphoproliferative disorder, with infiltration of the lungs. It has an association with autoimmune diseases (**SLE, RA, Sjogrens**). **The big one to know is Sjogrens which is concomitant in 25% of LIP cases**. The other one to know is **HIV** – which is the LIP in a younger patient *(children, – LIP in HIV positive adults is rare)*. There is also an association with Castlemans. The appearance of LIP varies depending on the underlying cause. **The cystic lung disease is usually thin walled, "deep within the lung parenchyma," and seen predominantly with Sjogrens**. The dominant feature described as ground glass or nodules is seen more in the other causes and is far beyond the scope of the exam.

When I say LIP... You say Sjogrens & HIV
When I say LIP in a kid... You say HIV

Pneumocystis Pneumonia (PCP) – This is the most common opportunistic infection in AIDS. The typical buzzword is **ground glass appearance, predominantly in the hilar and mid lung zones**. Pneumatoceles are present in 30% of cases. In patients receiving aerosolized prophylaxis, a cystic form is more common, which **may have bilateral thin walled upper lung predominant cysts. Gallium ^{67} scan will show diffuse uptake** (Thallium will be negative).

When I say AIDS + Ground Glass Lungs.... You say PCP

Emphysema- The textbook definition is "permanent enlargement of the airspaces distal to the terminal bronchioles accompanied by destruction of the alveolar wall without clear fibrosis." What you need to know are (1) the CXR findings and (2) the different types.

- CXR Findings: Until it's really really bad, CXR doesn't have direct signs, but instead has indirect signs. **Flattening of the hemidiaphrams** is regarded as the most reliable sign. The AP diameter increases. The retrosternal clear space becomes larger. There is a paucity of, or pruning of the blood vessels.

- Types:

    o *Centri-lobular*: By far the **most common type**. Common in asymptomatic elderly patients. It has an apical to basal gradient – **favoring the upper zones** of each lobe. It appears as focal lucencies, located centrally within the secondary pulmonary lobule, often with a central dot representing the central bronchovascular bundle. This **central dot sign is a buzzword**. This is the **type of emphysema dominant in smokers.**

    o *Pan-lobular:* In contradistinction to centrilobular this one favors the lower lobes. It also has a more uniform distribution across parts of the secondary pulmonary lobule. The association is with **alpha 1 antitrypsin**. A piece of trivia is the **"Ritalin Lung"** from IV Ritalin use can also cause a pan-lobular appearance ("Ritalin keeps you from 'trypsn' out"). *If they show this it will be in the coronal view on CT to demonstrate the **lower lobe predominance**.* Patient's will present in their 60s and 70s (unless they smoke – then they present in their 30s). **Smoking accelerates the process.**

    o *Para-septal*: This one is found adjacent to the pleura and septal lines with a peripheral distribution within the secondary pulmonary lobule. The affected lung is almost always sub-pleural, and demonstrates small focal lucencies up to 10mm in size. This looks like honeycombing but is less than 3 bubbles thick.

- Trivia:

    o Saber Sheath Trachea – Diffuse coronal narrowing of the trachea, sparing the extrathroacic potion. This is said to be pathognomonic for COPD.
    o If the Main PA is larger than the Aorta COPD patient have a worse outcome (pulmonary HTN can be caused by emphysema).
    o Surgery to remove bad lung "volume reduction" is sometimes done

Vanishing Lung Syndrome: This is an idiopathic cause of giant bullous emphysema, resulting from avascular necrosis of the lung parenchyma and hyperinflation. It favors the bilateral upper lobes, and is **defined as bullous disease occupying at least one-third of a hemithorax**. The most common demographic is a young man. About 20% of these guys have alpha-1 antitrypsin deficiency.

Compensatory Emphysema (Postpneumonectomy Syndrome): There is no obstructive process here. Instead you have hyperexpansion of one lung to compensate for the absence of the other one.

Honeycomb Lung- When I say honeycombing you should say UIP. However, this is seen with a variety of causes of end stage fibrotic lung processes. The cysts are tightly clustered (2-3 rows thick) and subpleural. The walls are often thick.

PneumocoI nioses

As a general rule, these are inhaled so they tend to be upper lobe predominant. You can have centilobular nodules (which makes sense for inhalation), or often perilymphatic nodules – which makes a little less sense, but is critical to remember * especially with silicosis and CWP.

Asbestos Exposure: The term "Asbestosis" refers to the changes of pulmonary fibrosis – NOT actual exposure to the disease. The look is very **similar to UIP**, with the presence of **parietal pleural thickening** being the "most important feature" to distinguish between IPF and Asbestosis. Obviously, the history of working in a ship yard or finding asbestos bodies in a bronchoalveolar lavage is helpful.

Things to know about Asbestos:
- *"Asbestosis" = the lung fibrosis associated with exposure, NOT actual exposure*
- *Interstitial pattern looks like UIP + parietal pleural thickening*
- *There is a 20 year latency between initial exposure and development of lung cancer or pleural mesothelioma*
- *There is an association with extraplulmonary cancer including: Peritoneal mesothelioma, GI cancer, Renal Cancer, Laryngeal Cancer, and Leukemia*
- *Benign pleural effusions are the "earliest pleural based phenomenon" associated with exposure – still with a lag time of around 5 years*

Benign Asbestosis Related Changes: Pleural effusion is the earliest and most common. Pleural plaques may develop around 20-30 years, with calcifications occurring around 40 years. These plaques tend to spare the apices and Costophrenic angles. *Round atelectasis – which is associated with pleural findings is sometimes called the "asbestos pseudotumor."*

Malignant Mesothelioma – The most common cancer of the pleura. About 80% of them have had asbestos exposure, and development is NOT dose dependent. The lag time is around 30-40 years from exposure. The **buzzword pleural rind** is worth knowing. The tendency is for direct invasion. **Extension into the fissure is highly suggestive.**

Silicosis: This is seen in miners, and quarry workers. You can have simple silicosis, which is going to be multiple nodular opacities favoring the upper lobes, with egg shell calcifications of the hilar nodes. You also get perilymphatic nodules. The complicated type is called **progressive massive fibrosis (PMF). This is the formation of large masses in the upper lobes with radiating strands.** You can see this with both silicosis and coal workers pneumoconiosis (something similar also can happen with Talcosis). These masses can sometimes cavitate – but you should always raise the suspicion of TB when you see this (especially in the setting of silicosis).

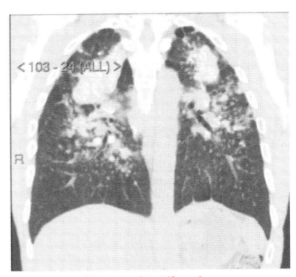

Progressive Massive Fibrosis
- Large Apical Masses with Radiating Strands

Silicotuberculosis: Silicosis actually raises your risk of TB by about 3 fold. If you see *cavitation in the setting of silicosis you have to think about TB.*

MRI : Cancer vs PMF	
Cancer = T2 Bright	PMF = T2 Dark

Coal Workers Pneumoconiosis: This is the result of exposure to "washed coal." Just like silicosis there are simple and complicated forms. There is also an increased risk of TB (just like silicosis). The simple form was multiple nodular opacities, with calcifications showing a central nodular dot. The small nodule pattern tends to have a perilymphatic distribution. The complicated form gives you a progressive massive fibrosis that is similar to that seen in silicosis.

Additional Inhalational Diseases - Not Worthy of a Full Discussion		
Berryliosis	Metal used in aircraft and space industries	Generalized granulomatous disease with hilar adenopathy and upper lobe predominant reticular opacities.
Silo Filler's Disease	Nitrogen Dioxide	Pulmonary Edema Pattern. Recovery is typically within 5 weeks.
Talcosis	Filler in tablets, sometimes injected (along with drugs) in IV drug users.	Hyperdense micronodules, with conglomerate masses (similar to PMF). Ground glass opacities

ILDs

Everyone seems to be afraid of interstitial lung diseases. The concept is actually not that complicated, it's just complicated relative to the rest of chest radiology (which overall isn't that complicated). The trick is to ask yourself two main questions: (1) Acute or Chronic ? – as this narrows the differential considerably, and (2) What is the primary finding ? – as this will narrow the differential further. Now, since we are training for the artificial scenario of a multiple choice test (and not the view box), I'll try and keep the focus on superficial trivia, and associations. Remember when you are reading to continue to ask yourself "how can this material be written into a question?"

Vocab: Like most of radiology, the bulk of understanding the pathology is knowing the right words to use (plus, a big vocabulary makes you sound smart).

- **Consolidation** = Density that obscures underlying vessels
- **Ground Glass Opacity** = Density that does **NOT** obscure underlying vessels
- **Secondary Pulmonary Lobule** = The basic unit of pulmonary structure and function. It is the smallest part of the lung that is surrounded by connective tissue. In the middle runs a terminal bronchial with an accompanying artery. Around the periphery runs the vein and lymphatics.

Anatomy of the Secondary Pulmonary Lobule

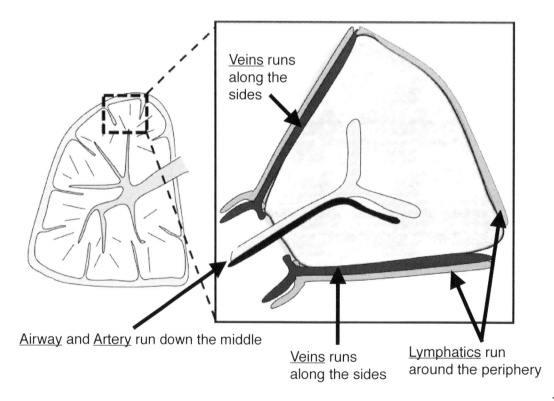

Veins runs along the sides

Airway and Artery run down the middle

Veins runs along the sides

Lymphatics run around the periphery

Nodule Vocabulary (Random, Perilymphatic, Centrilobular)

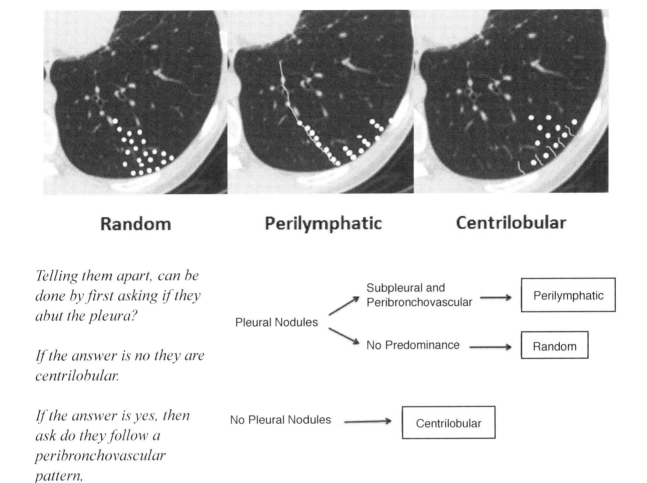

Random   **Perilymphatic**   **Centrilobular**

Telling them apart, can be done by first asking if they abut the pleura?

If the answer is no they are centrilobular.

If the answer is yes, then ask do they follow a peribronchovascular pattern,

Pleural Nodules → Subpleural and Peribronchovascular → Perilymphatic

Pleural Nodules → No Predominance → Random

No Pleural Nodules → Centrilobular

if the answer is no then they are random, if the answer if yes then they are perilymphatic.

Nodule Pattern	Key DDx
Perilymphatic	•Sarcoid (90%), •Lymphangitic Spread of CA •Silicosis
Random	•Miliary TB •Mets •Fungal
Centrilobular	•Infection •RB-ILD •Hypersensitivity Pneumonitis *(if ground glass)*

Patterns and Pathology

Interlobular Septal Thickening: Reticular abnormality, that outlines the lobules characteristic shape and size (about 2cm). It's usually from **pulmonary edema** (*usually symmetric and smooth*), or **lymphangitic spread of neoplasm** (*often asymmetric and nodular*). **Kerley B Lines are the plain film equivalent.**

Honeycombing: Cystic areas of lung destruction in a subpleural location. This is a hallmark of UIP. Paraseptal emphysema is a mimic, but the distinction is made by how many rows of bubbles.

- *One Row of Bubbles = Paraseptal Emphysema.*
- *Two-Three Rows of Bubbles = Honey combing.*

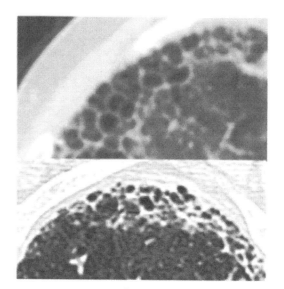

Honeycombing – *Two Examples*

Pathology Time:

Idiopathic Interstitial Pneumonias – These are NOT diseases, but instead lung reactions to lung injury. They occur in a variety of patterns and variable degrees of inflammation and fibrosis. The causes include: idiopathic, collage vascular disease, medications, and inhalation.

For practical purposes the answer is either (a) UIP or (b) Not UIP. Not UIP will get better with steroids. UIP will not. UIP has a dismal prognosis (similar to lung cancer). Not UIP often does ok. The exam will likely not make it this simple, and will instead focus on buzzwords, patterns, and associations (which I will now discuss).

***UIP (Usual Interstitial Pneumonia)* -** This is the <u>*most common*</u> Interstitial Lung Disease. When the cause is idiopathic it is called IPF. On CXR the lung volume is reduced (duh, it's fibrosis). *Reticular pattern in the posterior costophrenic angle is supposedly the first finding on CXR.*

Buzzwords include:
- **Apical to basal gradient** (it's worse in the lower lobes),
- **Traction bronchiectasis**, and honeycombing.
- **Honeycombing** is found 70% of the time, and people expect you to knee jerk UIP when that term is uttered.
- Histologic Buzzword = Heterogenous. ***"The histology was heterogenous"* = UIP.**

It's important to know that basically any end stage lung disease (be it from sarcoid, RA, Scleroderma, or other collagen vascular disease) has a similar look once the disease has ruined the lungs. *Technically honeycombing is uncommon in end stage sarcoid – but the rest of the lung looks jacked up.*

The prognosis is terrible (similar to lung cancer).

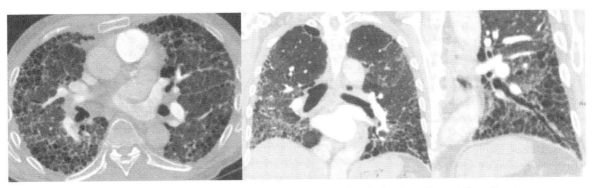

UIP- Honey Combing, Traction Bronchiectasis, Apical to Basal Gradient

NSIP (Nonspecific Interstitial Pneumonia)- Less Common than UIP. Even though the name infers that its non-specific, it's actually is a specific entity. Histologically it is homogenous inflammation or fibrosis (UIP was heterogeneous). It is a common pattern in collagen vascular disease, and drug reactions.

It comes in 2 flavors (cellular or fibrotic):

- Ground Glass Alone = Cellular
- Ground Glass + Reticulation = Cellular or Fibrotic
- Reticulation + Traction Bronchiectasis = Fibrotic NSIP
- Honeycombing – uncommon and usually minimal in extent

The disease has a lower lobe, posterior, peripheral predominance with sparing of the immediate subpleural lung seen in up to 50% of cases. This finding of **immediate subpleural sparing is said to be highly suggestive**. Ground glass is the NSIP equivalent of honeycombing.

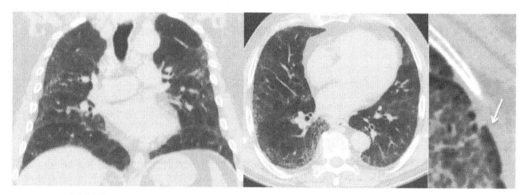

NSIP - *Peripheral Ground Glass with Subpleural Sparing*

UIP	NSIP
Apical to Basal Gradient	Gradient is less obvious (but still more in lower lobes)
Heterogenous Histology	Homogenous Histology
Honeycombing	Ground Glass
Traction Bronchiectasis	Micronodules

Trivia:
- *NSIP is the most common Interstitial Lung Disease in Scleroderma*

RB-ILD and DIP : I'm going to discuss these two together because some people feel they are a spectrum. For sure they are **both smoking related diseases**.

- RB-ILD – Apical Centrilobular ground glass nodules
- DIP – More diffuse GGO, with patchy or subpleural distribution

RB-ILD: Respiratory Brochiolitis + Symptoms = RB-ILD. This tends to be more upper lobe predominant (note that DIP tends to be more lower lobe predominant). Localized centrilobular ground glass nodules. The pathology tends to involve the entire cross section of lung.

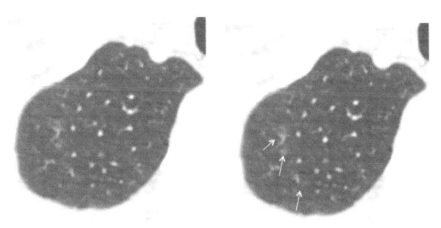

RB-ILD- Apical Centrilobular ground glass nodules + Smoking History

DIP: Thought of as the end spectrum of RB-ILD. Peripheral lower lobe predominant ground glass, with small cystic spaces.

Sarcoid: This is a multi-system disease that creates "non-caseating granulomas." The classic age is between 20-40. Along those lines, if the header to the question describes an African American female in her 20s-30s the answer is probably sarcoid. The lungs are by far the most common organ affected (90%).

Misc Trivia to know:
- Elevated angiotensin-converting enzyme (ACE)
- Hypercalcemia

Mediastinal lymph nodes are seen in 60-90% of times (classically in a 1-2-3 pattern of bilateral hila and right paratracheal). They have **perilymphatic nodules**, with an **upper lobe predominance**. Late changes include, upper lobe fibrosis, and traction bronchiectasis (honey combing is rare). Aspergillomas are common in the cavities of patient's with end stage sarcoid.

- *1-2-3 Sign - bilateral hila and right paratracheal*
- *Lambda Sign – same as 1-2-3, but on Gallium Scan*
- *CT Galaxy Sign – upper lobe masses (conglomerate of nodules) with satellite nodules*

CXR can be used to "Stage" Sarcoid

Stage 0 = Normal
Stage 1 = Hilar / Mediastinal Nodes Only
Stage 2 = Nodes + Parenchyma Disease
Stage 3 = Parenchymal Disease
Stage 4 = End Stage (Fibrosis)

CHF – Congestive heart failure occurs because of cardiac failure, fluid overload, high resistance in the circulation, or some combination of the three.   There are three phases of CHF, and these lend themselves to testable trivia.

Stages of CHF		
Stage 1 " Redistribution"	Wedge Pressure 13-18	Cephalization of vessels, Big heart, Big Vascular Pedicle
Stage 2 " Interstitial Edema"	Wedge Pressure 18-25	Kerley Lines, Peribronchial Cuffing, Less distinct contour of Central Vessels
Stage 3 "Alveolar Edema"	Wedge Pressure > 25	Airspace "fluffy" opacity, Pleural effusion

Right Heart Failure – This is less common than left heart failure, which ironically is the most common cause. Left heart failure causes pulmonary venous HTN which causes pulmonary artery HTN, which causes right heart failure. Some other less common causes of right heart failure include chronic PE, and right sided valve issues (tricuspid regurg). The imaging features of right heart failure include dilation of the azygos vein, dilation of the right atrium, dilation of the SVC, ascites, big liver, and contrast reflux into the hepatic veins on CTPA.

Lung Transplant Complications – Lung transplants are done for end-stage pulmonary disease (fibrosis, COPD, etc..). The complications lend themselves easily to multiple choice test questions, and are therefore high yield. The best way to think about the complications is based on time.

Immediate Complications (< 24 hours)	
Donor-Recipient Size Mismatch	Mismatch up to 25% is ok. You can have a compressed lung (by the hyperexpanded emphysematous lung). Imaging is usually atelectasis.
Hyperacute Rejection	Secondary to HLA and ABO antigens. It's rapid and often fatal. Imaging shows massive homogenous infiltration
Early Complications (24 hours – 1 week)	
Reperfusion Injury	Peaks at day 4 as a non-cardiogenic edema related to ischemia-reprofusion. Typically improves by day 7.
Air Leak / Persistent Pneumothorax	Defined as a continuous leak for more than 7 days.
Intermediate Complication (8 days – 2 months)	
Acute Rejection	Ground Glass opacities and intralobular septal thickening. (No ground glass = no rejection). Improves with steroids.
Bronchial Anastomotic Complications	Leaks occur in the first month, stenosis can develop later (2-4 months).
Late Complications (2-4 months)	
CMV Infection	**The most common opportunistic infection.** Ground glass, tree-in-bud. Rare before 2 weeks.
Later Complications (> 4 months)	
Chronic Rejection	Bronchiolitis Obliterans; **Affects 50% at 5 years**. Brochiectasis, bronchial wall thickening, air trapping.
Cryptogenic Organizing Pneumonia	Occurs with chronic rejection (but more commonly with acute rejection). Responds to steroids.
PTLD	Typically seen within the first year. EBV in 90%.
Upper Lobe Fibrosis	Associated with chronic rejection

Chronic Rejection / Bronchiolitis Obliterans Syndrome: This is the major late complication, that affects at least half of the transplants at 5 years (most commonly at 6 months). The term bronchiolitis obliterans is often used interchangeably with chronic rejection. The findings on CT include bronchiectasis, bronchial wall thickening, air trapping, and interlobular septal thickening. Just think **air trapping on expiration seen at or after 6 months = chronic rejection.**

Recurrence of Primary Disease after Transplant: For the purpose of multiple choice tests know that sarcoidosis is the **most common recurrent primary disease (around 35%).** Lots of other things can recur.

Lung Cancer after Transplant: Just remember that that native lung is still diseased, and can get cancer. The highest rate is with pulmonary fibrosis, and the most common risk factor is heavy tobacco use.

—

Alveolar Lung Disease:

Pulmonary Alveolar Proteinosis (PAP): For the purpose of multiple choice, this is an Aunt Minnie - always shown as crazy paving lung (interlobular septal thickening, with ground glass). This can be primary (90%), or secondary (10%). The secondary causes worth knowing are cancer or inhalation (silico-proteinosis).

Trivia Worth Knowing:
- They are at increased risk of **Nocardia infections**, and can be nocardia brain abscess.
- **Smoking is strongly associated with the disease**.
- When seen in children (presenting before age 1) there is a known association with alymphoplasia.
- Can progress to pulmonary fibrosis (30%).
- Treatment is bronchoalveolar lavage

Crazy Paving – Interlobular septal thickening and ground glass. This isn't always PAP, in fact in real life that it is usually NOT PAP. There is a differential that includes common things like edema, hemorrhage, BAC, Acute Interstitial Pneumonia. **Just know that for the purpose of multiple choice test the answer is almost always PAP.**

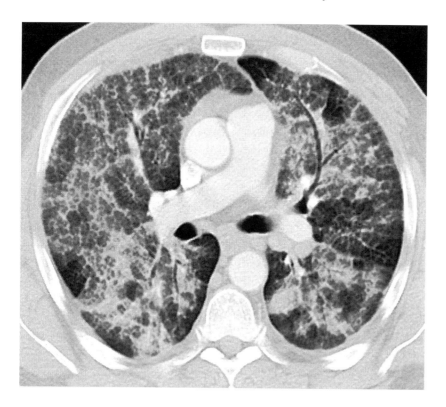

Lipoid Pneumonia – There are actually two types; endogenous and exogenous.

- **Exogenous:** A certain percentage of elderly people become absolutely obsessed with their bowel movements. If you did Family Medicine addressing this psychopathology would steal a certain amount of hours out of your life per week. Lipoid pneumonia is seen in **old people who like to drink/aspirate mineral oil** (as a laxative). It can also be seen with the aspiration of vegetable oil or other animal oils. The look on plain film is an area of lung opacification that is chronic or slowly increases with time. The look on CT is a dead give away and the most likely way this will be shown is with **low attenuation / fat density in the consolidation**. Having said that this is also in the crazy paving differential.

- *Acute Exogenous Lipoid Pneumonia* – This is seen is children who accidentally poison themselves with hydrocarbons, or idiots trying to perform fire-eating or flame blowing.

- **Endogenous** – This is actually more common than the exogenous type, and results from post obstructive processes (cancer) causing the building up of lipid laden macrophages.

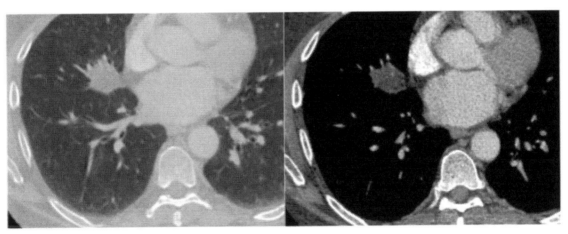

Lipoid Pneumonia – *Fat Density in the consolidation*

> ### *Gamesmanship: "Why are you showing me the lung on that window?"*
>
> Obviously pulmonary pathology is best shown on a lung window. So anytime the test writer is showing you a pulmonary pathology on a non-lung window that should cue you to think about some different things.
>
> (1): Is the findings in the mediastinum or ribs?
> (2): If it's clearly a lung findings then what window are they using?
> - Soft tissue window is classically used to show fat in a lesion - think hamartoma, or lipoid pneumonia.
> - Bone window might be used to show a diffuse process such as pulmonary microlithiasis.

Organizing Pneumonia *(cryptogenic when cause not known "COP")*

This used to be called BOOP, which was a lot more fun to say. There are lots of different causes; idiopathic, infection, drugs (amiodarone), collagen vascular disease, fumes etc… These guys respond well to steroids, and have an excellent prognosis.

Patchy air space consolidation or GGO (90%), in a **peripheral** or peri-bronchial distribution. Opacities tend to be irregular in shape. Findings of fibrosis are typically absent.

Reverse Halo (Atoll) Sign is the classic sign: Consolidation around a ground glass center

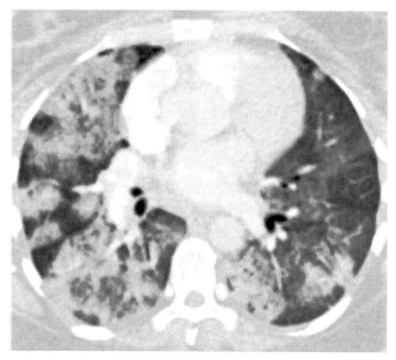

Cryptogenic Organizing Pneumonia –
-Reverse Halo Sign

Chronic Eosinophilic Pneumonia: Can be idiopathic or associated with a known antigen. Peripheral eosinophilia (blood test) is usually present. An asthma history is found in about 50% of cases. It looks exactly look COP. When you say COP you should say this one too (some people think it's the same disease as COP).

CT Findings: Peripheral GGO or consolidation. Upper lobes tend to be favored.

Hypersensitivity Pneumonitis: This is actually common. It's caused by inhaled organic antigens. It has acute, subacute, and chronic stages. Most of the time it's imaged in the subacute stage.

- **Subacute:** Patchy ground glass opacities. Ill-defined Centrilobular ground glass nodules (80%). Often has mosaic perfusion, and air trapping.

- **Chronic:** *Looks like UIP + Air trapping*. You are gonna have traction bronchiectasis and air trapping. A **buzzword is "headcheese"** because it's a mix of everything (Ground Glass, Consolidation, Air-Trapping, and Normal Lung)

Halo Signs

Reverse Halo (Atol)
-Central ground glass with rim of consolidation

Halo
-Nodule with ground glass around it
-Represents hemorrhage / invasion into surrounding tissues

DDx:
- **COP (Classic)**
- Fungal Pneumonia
- TB
- Wegeners
- Pulmonary Infarct

DDx:
- **Invasive Aspergilosis (Classic)**
- Other Fungus
- Hemorrhagic Mets
- Wegeners

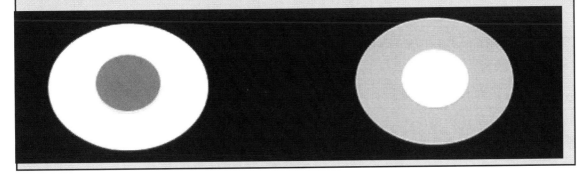

Airways

Trachea: The basic anatomy of the trachea is a bunch of anterior horseshoes of cartilage, with a posterior floppy membrane. This membrane can bow inward on expiratory CT (and this is normal). The transverse diameter should be no more than 2.5 cm (same as the transverse diameter of an adjacent vertebral body).

Tracheal Disease Game plan: Three big questions to ask yourself. (1) Does it involve the posterior membrane ? (2) is it focal or diffuse ? and (3) is there calcification ?

Relapsing Polychondritis: Spare the posterior membrane. Diffuse thickening of the trachea. No calcifications. Characterized by recurrent episodes of cartilage inflammation, and recurrent pneumonia.

Post Intubation Stenosis: Focal Subglottic **circumferential** stenosis, with an hourglass configuration.

Wegener's: Circumferential thickening, which can be **focal or long segment**. No calcifications. Subglottic involvement is common.

Tracheobronchopathia Osteochondroplastica (TBO): Spares the posterior membrane. You have development of **cartilaginous and osseous nodules** within the submucosa of the tracheal and bronchial walls.

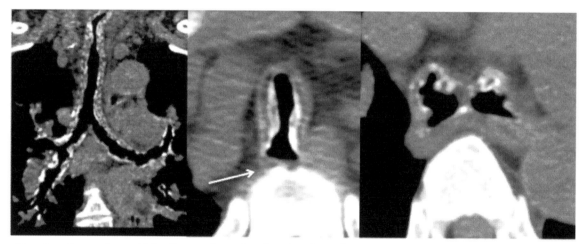

Tracheobronchopathia Osteochondroplastica (TBO) – Spares Posterior Membrane (arrow).

Amyloidosis: Irregular focal or short segment thickening, which can involve the posterior membrane. Calcifications are common.

Spares the Posterior Membrane		Does NOT Spare the Posterior Membrane	
Relapsing Polychondritis	Recurrent episodes of cartilage inflammation (ears, nose, joints, laryngeal and thyroid cartilage). Recurrent pneumonia is the most common cause of death.	Amyloid	Often confined to the trachea and main bronchi. Calcifications are common.
Tracheobronchopathia Osteochondroplastica (TBO):	Development of cartilaginous and osseous nodules. Typically occurs in men older than 50.	Wegeners	C-ANCA +, Sub-glottic trachea is the most common location.

Saber Sheath Trachea: Defined as a coronal diameter of less than two thirds the sagittal diameter.

I say "saber sheath trachea," you say <u>COPD.</u>

Trivia: The main bronchi will be normal in size. The tracheal wall will be normal in thickness.

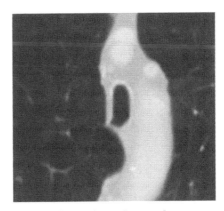

Saber Sheath Trachea

Tracheal tumors – Tumors of the trachea are not common in the real world.

Tracheal Tumors	
Squamous Cell	**Most Common.** Associated with smoking, Often multifocal (10%), favors the **lower trachea** / proximal bronchus
Adenoid Cystic	2nd Most common. Favors the **upper trachea**, and prefers the posterior lateral trachea. Has a **variable look** – can be a thickening, a mass, or a nodule.
Mets	Usually via direct extension (lung, thyroid, esophagus)
Squamous Cell Papilloma	**Most common benign** tumor. When it's **a single papilloma think smoking**. When it's **multiple papillomas think HPV**.

Cystic fibrosis - The sodium pump doesn't work and they end up with thick secretions and poor pulmonary clearance. The real damage is done by recurrent infections.

Things to know:
* *Bronchiectasis (begins as cylindrical and progresses to varicoid)*
* *It has an apical predominance (lower lobes are less affected)*
* *Hyperinflation*
* *Pulmonary Arterial Hypertension-*
* *Mucus plugging (finger in glove)*

Primary Ciliary Dyskinesia: Those little hairs in your lungs that clear secretions don't work. You end up with bilateral lower lobe bronchiectasis (remember that CF is mainly upper lobe). Other things these kids get is chronic sinusitis (prominent from an early age), and impaired fertility (sperm can't swim, girls get ectopics). They have chronic mastoid effusions, and conductive hearing loss is common. An important testable fact is that only **50% of the primary ciliary dyskinesia patients have Kartagener's Syndrome.**

Kartagener Syndrome: Primary Ciliary Dsykinesia + Situs Inversus.

CF	Primary Ciliary Dyskinesia
Abnormal Mucus, Cilia cannot move it	Normal Mucus, Cilia don't work
Normal Sperm, Absent Vas Deferens	Abnormal Sperm (they can't swim), Normal Vas Deferens
Upper lobe bronchiectasis	Lower lobe bronchiectasis

 Williams Campbell Syndrome – Huge zebra that is manifests as congenital cystic bronchiectasis from a deficiency of cartilage in the 4th-6th order bronchi.

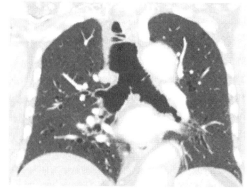

Mounier-Kuhn (Tracheobronchomegaly) – There is a massive dilatation of the trachea (> 3cm). It's not well understood, and really the only thing that does this.

Mounier-Kuhn— Big Fucking Trachea

Small Airways Disease

Bronchiolitis – This is an inflammation of the small airways. It can be infectious (like the viral patterns you see in kids) or inflammatory like RB-ILD in smokers, or asthma in kids.

Air Trapping - When you see areas of lung that are more lucent than others - you are likely dealing with air trapping. Technically, air trapping can only be called on an expiration study as hypoperfusion in the setting of pulmonary arterial hypertension can look similar. Having said that for the purpose of multiple choice test taking I want you to think (1) bronchiolitis obliterans in the setting of a lung transplant, or (2) small airway disease - asthma / bronchiolitis.

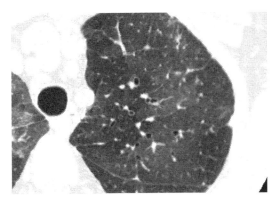

Air Trapping
— The poster boy for small airway disease

Tree in Bud – This is a nonspecific finding that can make you think small airway disease. It's caused by dilation and impaction of the centrilobular airways. Because the centrilobular airways are centered 5-10mm from the pleural surface, that's where they will be. It's usually associated with centrilobular nodules.

Follicular Bronchiolitis – This is an inflammatory process seen in rheumatoid arthritis or Sjogrens. It's not well understood and related to some lymphoid hyperplasia. It looks like centrilobular ground glass nodules with scattered areas of bronchial dilation.

Constrictive Bronchiolitis – This is another inflammatory process that can be seen secondary to viral illness, transplant patients, drug reactions, or inhalation injury. It occurs secondary to mononuclear cells which form granulation tissue and plug the airway. You see air trapping on expiatory imaging. This is supposedly the cause of Swyer-Jame's hyperlucent lung.

Small Airway Disease	
Infectious Bronchiolitis	Tree-in-bud
RB-ILD	Smokers. Centrilobular ground glass nodules (upper lobe predominant)
Sub-acute Hypersensitivity Pneumonitis	Inhaling dust / other misc garbage. Centrilobular Ground glass nodules
Follicular Bronchiolitis	RA and Sjogrens. Centrilobular ground glass nodules
Constrictive Bronchiolitis	Viral, Drugs, Transplant, Inhalation. Air-Trapping.

Aspiration Pneumonia – Stroked-out old people and drunks love to aspirate. The testable trivia is to know the typical location of aspiration; posterior segment of upper lobes and superior segment of lower lobes if supine when aspirating, bilateral basal lower lobes in upright aspiration. May favor the right side, just like an ET tube.

The most common complication is infection which can manifest as an empyema (which can then get a broncho-pleural fistula).

Aspiration Patterns (depends on what you aspirated)	
Aspiration of Gastric Acid "Mendelson's Syndrome"	Gives you an airspace opacity, if massive can look like pulmonary edema
Aspiration of water or neutralized gastric contents	"Fleeting Opacity" that resolves in hours
Aspiration of Bugs (often mouth bugs)	Gives you a real pneumonia, can get para-pneumonic effusion, empyema, or even broncho-pleural fistula.
Aspiration of Oil (often mineral oil)	Lipoid Pneumonia. Will be low density

Pulmonary manifestations of systemic disease

Collagen vascular disease – Interstitial lung diseases are common in patients with collagen vascular diseases. I've tried to hit the high points of testable trivia.

Collagen Vascular Disease Pulmonary Manifestations		
Lupus	More **pleural effusions and pericardiac effusions** than with other connective tissue disease	Fibrosis is uncommon. Can get a "shrinking lung."
Rheumatoid Arthritis	Looks like UIP and COP. Lower lobes are favored.	Reticulations with or without honeycombing, and consolidative opacities which are organizing pneumonia
Scleroderma	**NSIP** > UIP ; lower lobe predominant findings.	Look for the dilated fluid filled esophagus.
Sjogrens	**LIP**	Extensive ground glass attenuation with scattered thin walled cysts.
Ankylosing Spondylitis	**Upper lobe** **fibrobullous disease**	Usually unilateral first, then progresses to bilateral.

Caplan Syndrome = Rheumatoid Arthritis + Upper Lobe Predominant Lung Nodules. These nodules can cavitate, and there may also be a pleural effusion.

"Shrinking Lung" – This is a progressive loss of lung volume in both lungs seen in patients with **Lupus** ("S"hrinking "L"ung for "SLe"). The etiology is either diaphragm dysfunction or pleuritic chest pain.

Trivia: Most common manifestation of SLE in Chest = Pleuritis with/without pleural effusion.

Hepatopulmonary syndrome – This is seen in liver patients with the classic history of *"shortness of breath when sitting up."* The opposite of what you think about with a CHF patient. The reason it happens is that they develop distal vascular dilation in the lung bases (subpleural telangiectasia), with dilated subpleural vessels that don't taper and instead extend to the pleural surface. When the dude sits up, these things engorge and shunt blood – making him/her short of breath. A Tc MAA scan will show shunting with tracer in the brain (outside the lungs). They have to either tell you the patient is cirrhotic, show you a cirrhotic liver, or give you that classic history if they want you to get this.

Wegener Granulomatosis - The classic triad is upper tract, lung, and kidneys (although this triad is actually rare). The lungs are actually the most common organ involved (95%). There is a highly variable look. The most common presentation is also probably the most likely to be tested; **nodules with cavitation**. The nodules tend to be random in distribution with about half of them cavitating. They can also show you ground glass changes which may represent hemorrhage.

Goodpasture Syndrome – Another autoimmune pulmonary renal syndrome. It favors young men. It's a super nonspecific look with bilateral coalescent airspace opacities that look a lot like edema (but are hemorrhage). They resolve quickly (within 2 weeks). If they are having recurrent bleeding episodes then they can get fibrosis. Pulmonary hemosiderosis can occur from recurrent episodes of bleeding as well, with iron deposition manifesting as small ill defined nodules.

Pleura, diaphragm and chest wall

Plaque – If they show you a pleural plaque they probably want you to say asbestos related disease. Remember the plaque doesn't show up fro like 20-30 years after exposure. Remember that the pleural plaque of asbestosis typically spares the Costophrenic angles.

Pleural Calcifications (other than asbestos)
• Old Hemothorax,
• Old Infection,
• TB,
• Extraskeletal Osteosarcoma

Mesothelioma – The most common cancer of the pleura. About 80% of them have had asbestos exposure, and development is NOT dose dependent. The lag time is around 30-40 years from exposure. The **buzzword pleural rind** is worth knowing. The tendency is for direct invasion. **Extension into the fissure is highly suggestive.**

Fibrous tumors of the pleura – This is usually a solitary tumor arising from the visceral pleura. The key is to know that they are **NOT associated with asbestos**, smoking, or other environmental pollutants. They can get very large, and be a source of chest pain (although 50% are incidentally found). The second high yield testable fact is the association with **hypoglycemia and hypertrophic osteoarthropathy.**

Metastases – Here is the high yield trivia on this. As a general rule the subtype of adenocarcinoma is the most likely to met to the pleura. Lung cancer is the most common primary, with breast and lymphoma at 2nd and 3rd. Remember that a **pleural effusion is the most common manifestation** of mets to the pleura.

Lipoma – This is the most common benign soft tissue tumor of the pleura. The patients sometimes feel the "urge to cough." They will not cause rib erosion. They "never" turn in a sarcoma. The differential consideration is extra-pleural fat, but it is usually bilateral and symmetric.

Effusion – Some random factoids on pleural effusions that could be potentially testable. There has to be around 175cc of fluid to be seen on the frontal view (around 75cc can be seen on the lateral). Remember that medicine docs group these into transudate and exudate based on protein concentrations (Lights criteria). You are going to get elastic / compressive atelectasis of the adjacent lung.

Subpulmonic Effusion – A pleural effusion can accumulate between the lung base and the diaphragm. These are more common on the right, with "ski-slopping" or **lateralization of the diaphragmatic peak**. A lateral decubitus will sort it out in the real world.

Empyema – Basically this is an infected pleural effusion. It can occur with a simple pneumonia but is seen more in people with AIDS. Usually these are more asymmetric than a normal pleural effusion. Other features include; enhancement of the pleura, obvious septations, or gas.

Empyema vs Pulmonary Abscess	
Empyema	**Pulmonary Abscess**
Lentiform	Round
Split Pleural Sign (thickening and separation of the visceral and parietal pleura)	Claw Sign (acute angle with pleura)
Treated with chest tube	NOT treated with chest tube (risk of brochopleural fistula).

Empyema Necessitans – This is the fancy Latin word for when the empyema eats through the chest wall and into the soft tissues. It's classically seen with **TB** (70%), with the second most common cause being actinomyces.

Diaphragmatic Hernia – These can be acquired via trauma, or congenital. The congenital ones are most common in the back left (Bochdalek), with anterior small and right being less common (Morgagni). The traumatic ones are also more common on the left (liver is a buffer).

Paralysis – This is a high yield topic because you can use fluoro to help make the diagnosis. Obviously the dinosaurs that write these tests love to ask about fluoro (since that was the only thing they did in residency). Diaphragmatic paralysis is actually idiopathic 70% of the time, although when you see it on multiple choice tests they want you to **think about phrenic nerve compression from a lung cancer**. Normally the right diaphragm is higher, so if you see an elevated left diaphragm this should be a consideration.

On a fluoroscopic sniff test you are looking for paradoxical movement (going up on inspiration – instead of down).

Mediastinal masses

Superior Mediastinal Masses: *These are often lumped into anterior mediastinal masses – as extension often occurs upward.*

- **"Superior Sulcus Tumor"** – Notice I didn't call it a Pancoast tumor. To be a "Pancoast" tumor you need to have "Pancoast syndrome" , which is shoulder pain, C8-T2 radicular pain, and Horner Syndrome. The superior sulcus tumor can cause these but doesn't have to. The most common tumor to do this is a squamous cell lung cancer (or bronchogenic adenocarcinoma – depending on what you read). Non-Small cell tumors may be a safer way to say it.

> *The Classic Question:*
> ***When is the superior sulcus (pancoast) tumor unresectable?***
>
> 1. *Brachial Plexus involvement above T1 (C8 or higher)*
> 2. *Diaphragm Paralysis (infers involvement of C3-4-5)*
> 3. *Greater than 50% vertebral body*
> 4. *Distal Nodes or Mets... etc..*

Anterior Mediastinal Masses:

- **Thymus:** The thymus can do a bunch of sneaky things. It can rebound from stress or chemotherapy and look huge. It can get cysts, cancer, carcinoid, etc…

  > **Rebound vs Residual Lymphoma**
  >
  > (1) PET might help - both are hot, but lymphoma is hotter.
  > (2) MRI - Thymic Rebound should drop out on in-out of phase imaging (it has fat in it). Lymphoma will not drop out.

  - **Rebound** – Discussed in detail in the Peds chapter. After stress or chemotherapy the thing can blow up 1.5 times the normal size and simulate a mass. Can be hot on PET.

  - **Thymic Cyst** – Can be congenital or acquired. **Acquired is classic after thoracotomy, chemotherapy, or HIV**. They can be unilocular or multilocular. T2 bright is gonna seal the deal for you.

  - **Thymoma** – So this is kind of a spectrum ranging from non-invasive thymoma, to invasive thymoma, to thymic carcinoma. Calcification makes you think it's more aggressive. The thymic carcinomas tend to eat up the mediastinal fat and adjacent structures. The average age is around 50, and they are rare under 20. These guys can "drop met" into the pleural and retroperitoneum, so you have to image the abdomen.

    - **High Yield Trivia:** *Thymoma associations: Myasthenia Gravis, Pure Red Cell Aplasia, Hypogammaglobinemia.*

  - **Thymolipoma** – I only mention this zebra because it has a characteristic look. It's got a bunch of fat in it. Think "fatty mass with interspersed soft tissue."

- **Germ Cell Tumor – Almost always Teratoma (75%)**

  - **Mediastinal Teratoma** – This is the most common extragonadal germ cell tumor. They occur in kids (below age 1) and adults (20s-30s). They are benign, but carry a small malignant transformation risk. Mature subtypes are equal in Men and Women, but immature subtypes are exclusively seen in men (which should be easy to remember). There is an **association with mature teratomas and Klinefelter Syndrome.** The imaging features include a **cystic appearance (90%), and fat.** They can have calcifications including teeth – which is a dead give away.

- **Thyroid** – *Thyroid cancer and goiter are described in detail in the endocrine chapter.*

- **Lymphoma** - *this is discussed in detail in the cancer section of this chapter.*

- **Pericardial Cyst** – This is uncommon and benign. **The classic location is the right anterior cardiophrenic angle.** This classic location is the most likely question.

Middle Mediastinal Masses

- **Fibrosing Mediastinitis** – This is a proliferation of fibrous tissue that occurs within the mediastinum. It's **classically caused by histoplasmosis** (but the most common cause is actually idiopathic). Other causes include TB, radiation, and Sarcoid. It's a **soft tissue mass with calcifications** that infiltrates the normal fat planes. It has been **known to cause superior vena cava syndrome.** It's associated with retroperitoneal fibrosis when idiopathic.

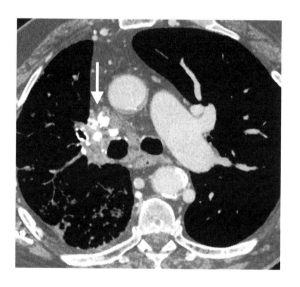

- **Bronchogenic Cyst** – These congenital lesions are usually within the mediastinum (most commonly found in the subcarinal space) or less commonly intraparenchymal. For the purpose of the exam , they are going to be in the subcarinal region, causing obliteration of the azygoesophageal line on a CXR, and being waterish density on CT.

- **Lymphadenopathy** - Could be mets, could be infection, could be reactive.

- **Mediastinal Lipomatosis** – Excess unencapsulated fat seen in patients with iatrogenic steroid use, Cushings, and just plain old obesity.

Posterior Mediastinal Masses:

- **Neurogenic** – The most common posterior mediastinal mass is one of neurogenic origin. This includes schwannomas, neurofibromas, and malignant peripheral nerve sheath tumors.

- **Bone Marrow** - Extramedullary hematopoiesis (EMH) is a response to failure of the bone marrow to respond to EPO. Classic conditions include CML, Polycythemia vera, myelofibrosis, sickle cell, and thalassemia.

Pulmonary arteries

Pulmonary Embolism: This is a significant cause of mortality in hospitalized patients. The gold standard is catheter angiography, although this is invasive and carries risks. As a result tests like the D-Dimer (which has an almost 100% negative predictive value), and the DVT lower extremity ultrasound were developed. Now, the CTPA as the primary tool.

Historical "High-Yield" Signs of PE on a CXR	
Westermark Sign	Regional Oligemia
Fleishner Sign	Enlarged Pulmonary Artery
Hampton's Hump	Peripheral Wedge Shaped opacity
Pleural Effusion	Obviously not specific, but seen in 30% of PEs.

Differentiating acute vs chronic PE is a high yield tool.

Acute vs Chronic PE	
Acute	**Chronic**
Central	Peripheral
Venous Dilation	Shrunken Veins with collateral vessels
Perivenous soft tissue edema	Calcifications within the thrombi, and within the venous walls

Pulmonary infarct mimics – A pulmonary infarct is a wedge shaped opacity, that is going to "melt" (resolve slowly), and sometimes can cavitate. Obviously a cavitary lesion throws up lots of flags and makes people say TB, or cancer. When it's an opacity in the lung and the patient doesn't have a fever sometimes people think cancer – plenty of pulmonary infarcts have been biopsied.

Pulmonary Artery Aneurysm / Pseudoanuersym – Think about three things for multiple choice; (1) **Iatrogenic from swan ganz catheter *most common** (2) Behcets, (3) Chronic PE. When they want to lead swan ganz they may say something like "patient in the ICU." The buzzwords for Behcets are: "Turkish descent", and "mouth and genital ulcers."

- **Hughes-Stovin Syndrome:** This is a zebra cause of pulmonary artery aneurysm that is similar (and maybe the same thing) as Behcets. It is characterized by recurrent thrombophlebitis and pulmonary artery aneurysm formation and rupture.

- **Rasmussen Aneurysm:** This has a cool name, which instantly makes it high yield for testing. This is a pulmonary artery **pseudoaneurysm secondary to pulmonary TB**. It usually involves the upper lobes in the setting of reactivation TB.

- **Tetrology of Fallot Repair Gone South:** So another possible testable scenario is the patch aneurysm, from the RVOT repair.

Pulmonary Hypertension – Pulmonary arterial pressures over 25 are going to meet the diagnosis. I prefer to use the "outdated" primary and secondary way of thinking about this.

Primary: The idiopathic type is very very uncommon, seen in a small group of young women in their 20s.

Secondary: This is by far the majority, and there are a few causes you need to know: Chronic PE , Right Heart Failure/ Strain, Lung Parenchymal Problems- (This would include emphysema, and various causes of fibrosis). COPDers with a pulmonary artery bigger than the aorta (A/PA ratio) have increased mortality (says the NEJM).

Imaging Signs of Pulmonary HTN: The big pulmonary artery (> 29mm), or larger than the aorta. Mural calcifications of central pulmonary arteries (seen in Eisenmenger phenomenon). Right ventricular dilation and hypertrophy. Centrilobular ground-glass nodules.

Pulmonary Veno-Occlusive Disease: Uncommon variant of primary pulmonary hypertension, that affects the post capillary pulmonary vasculature. For **gamesmanship PAH + Normal Wedge**, you should think this. The normal wedge pressure differentiates it from other post capillary causes; such as left atrial myxoma, mitral stenosis, and pulmonary vein stenosis

Trauma:

Diaphragmatic Injury – There is a lot of testable trivia regarding diaphragmatic injury and therefore it is probably the most high yield subject with regard to trauma:

Things to know:
- Left side is involved 3 times more than the right (liver is a buffer)
- Most ruptures are "radial", longer than 10cm, and occur in the posterior lateral portion
- **Collar Sign** – This is sometimes called the hour glass sign, is a waist-like appearance of the herniated organ through the injured diaphragm
- **Dependent Viscera Sign** – This is an absence of interposition of the lungs between the chest wall and upper abdominal organs (liver on right, stomach on left).

Tracheo-Bronchial Injury: Airway injury is actually pretty uncommon. When it does occur it's usually within 2cm of the carina. **Injury close to the carina is going to cause a pneumomediastinum rather than a pneumothorax** – that is a testable fact. When you get a tracheal laceration, it most commonly occurs at the junction of the cartilaginous and membranous portions of the trachea.

Macklin Effect: This is probably the most common cause of pneumomediastinum in trauma patients (and most people haven't head of it). The idea is that you get alveolar rupture from blunt trauma, and the air dissects along bronchovascular sheaths into the mediastinum.

Boerhaave Syndrome: You probably remember this from step 1. The physical exam buzzword was "Hammonds Crunch." Basically you have a ruptured esophageal wall from vomiting, resulting in pneumomediastinum / medianstinitis.

Flail Chest: This is 3 or more segmental (more than one fracture in a rib) fractures, or more than 5 adjacent rib fractures. The physical exam buzzword is "paradoxical motion with breathing."

Pneumothorax: Obviously you don't want to miss the tension pneumothorax. The thing they could ask is "inversion or flattering of the ipsilateral diaphragm."

Malpositioned Chest Tubes: Sometimes the ED will ram them into the parenchyma. This is more likely to occur in the setting of background lung disease or pleural adhesions. You'll see blood around the tube. Bronchopleural fistula may occur as a sequela. The placement of a tube in a fissure is sorta controversially bad (might be ok).

Hemothorax: If you see pleural fluid in the setting of trauma, it's probably blood. The only way I can see them asking this is a density question; a good density would be **35-70 H.U.**

Extrapleural Hematoma: This is a little tricky, and they could show you a picture of it. If you have an injury to the chest wall that damages the parietal pleura then you get a hemothorax. If you have an injury to the chest wall, but your parietal pleural is still intact you get an extrapleural hematoma. The **classic history is "persistent fluid collection after pleural drain/tube placement."** The **buzzword / sign is displaced extrapleural fat**. There is a paper out there that suggests a biconvex appearance is more likely arterial and should be watched for rapid expansion. This may be practically useful, but is unlikely to be asked. Just know the classic history, and displaced extrapleural fat sign.

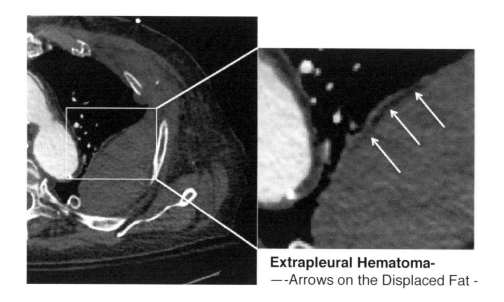

Extrapleural Hematoma-
—-Arrows on the Displaced Fat -

Pulmonary Contusion: This is the most common lung injury from blunt trauma. Basically you are dealing with alveolar hemorrhage without alveolar disruption. The typical look is non-segmental ill defined areas of consolidation with **sub pleural sparing**. Contusion should appear within 6 hours, and disappear within 72 hours (if it lasts longer it's probably aspiration, pneumonia, or a laceration).

Pulmonary Laceration: So a tear in the lung will end up looking like a pneumatocele. If they show you one it will probably have a **gas –fluid (blood) level** in it. These things can be masked by surrounding hemorrhage early on. The major difference between contusion and laceration is that a laceration **resolves much more slowly** and can even produce a nodule or a mass that persists for months.

Aorta – The aorta is injured **most commonly at the aortic isthmus** (some sources say 90%). The second and third most common locations are the root and at the diaphragm. Some people say the root is actually the most common, but most of these people die prior to making it to the hospital. This is a minority opinion. If asked what is the most common site of traumatic aortic injury the answer is isthmus. It's usually obvious on a candy cane CTA. The main mimic would be a "ductus bump" which is a normal variant. The way to tell (if it isn't obvious) is the presence of secondary signs of trauma (mediastinal hematoma).

Blunt Cardiac Injury: If you have hemopericardium in the setting of trauma, you can suggest this and have the ED correlate with cardiac enzymes and EKG findings.

Fat Embolization Syndrome: This is seen in the setting of a long bone fracture or Intramedullary rod placement. You get fat embolized to the lungs, brain and skin (clinical triad of rash, altered mental status, and shortness of breath). The timing is **1-2 days after the femur fracture**. The lungs will have a ground glass appearance that makes you think **pulmonary edema**. You will not see a filling defect – like a conventional PE. If they don't die, it gets better in 1-3 weeks.

Barotrauma: Positive pressure ventilation can cause alveolar injury, with air dissecting into the mediastinum (causing pneumomediastinum, and pneumothorax). Patients with acute lung injury or COPD have a high risk of barotrauma from positive pressure ventilation. Lungs with pulmonary fibrosis are actually protected because they don't stretch.

Lines / Devices:

Central Lines: The main way to ask questions about central lines is to show them being malpositioned and asking you where they are. An abrupt bend at the tip of the catheter near the cavo-atrial junction should make you think azygos. If it's on the left side of the heart, it's either (1) arterial or (b) in a duplicated SVC.

This is a sneaky trick, related to Central Lines.   They can show you the pseudo lesion / hot quadrate sign (seen with SVC syndrome), and then show you a CXR with a central venous catheter. The idea is that **central lines are a risk factor for SVC occlusion**.

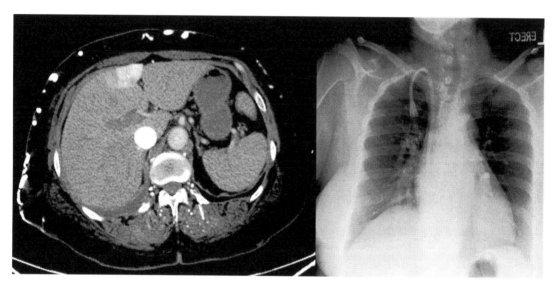

Hot Quadrate Sign from – SVC Obstruction

Endotracheal Tube (ETT) Positioning -   The tip of the ETT should be about 5cm from the carina (halfway between the clavicles and the carina). The tip will go down with the chin tucked, and up with the chin up ("the hose goes, where the nose goes"). Intubation of the right main stem is the most common goof (because of the more shallow angle) – this can lead to left lung collapse. You can sometimes purposefully intubate one lung if you have massive pulmonary hemorrhage (lung biopsy gone bad), to protect the good lung.

Intra-Aortic Balloon Pump (IABP) - This is used in cardiogenic shock to help with "diastolic augmentation," – essentially providing some back pressure so the vessels of the great arch (including the coronaries) enjoy improved perfusion.

For the purpose of multiple choice tests you can ask three things:

(1) *What is the function?* - decrease LV afterload, and increased myocardial perfusion,

(2) *What is the correct location ?* the balloon should be located in the proximal descending aorta, just below the origin of the left subclavian artery (balloon terminates just above the splanchnic vessels),

(3) *Complications ?* – dissection during insertion, obstruction of the left subclavian from malpositioning.

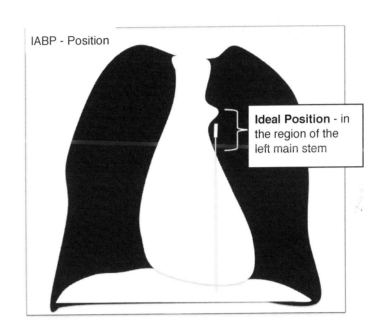

IABP - Position

Ideal Position - in the region of the left main stem

103

SECTION 3: VASCULAR

Anatomy:

Aorta: The thoracic aorta is divided anatomically into four regions; the root, the ascending aorta, the transverse aorta (arch), and the descending aorta. The "root" is the defined as the portion of the aorta extending from the aortic valve annulus to the sino-tubular junction. The diameter of the thoracic aorta is largest at the aortic root and gradually decreases *(average size is 3.6cm at the root, 2.4cm in the distal descending).*

- *Sinuses of Valsalva:* There are 3 out-pouching (right, left, posterior) above the annulus that terminate at the ST Junction. The right and left coronaries come off the right and left sinuses. The posterior cusp is sometimes called the "non-coronary cusp."

- *Isthmus:* The segment of the aorta between the origin of the left Subclavian and the ligamentous arteriosum.

- *Ductus bump:* Just distal to the isthmus is a contour bulge along the lesser curvature, which is a normal structure (not a pseudoaneurysm).

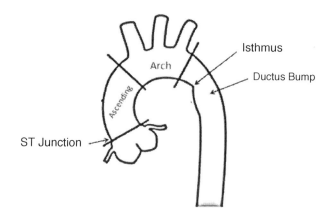

Aortic Arch Variants: There are 4 common variations: Normal (75%), Bovine Arch (15%) – common origin of brachiocephalic artery and left common carotid artery, left common carotid coming off the brachiocephalic proper (10%), and 5% of people the left vertebral artery originates separately from the arch. Branching with regards to right arch, left arch and double arch are discussed in more detail in the cardiac chapter.

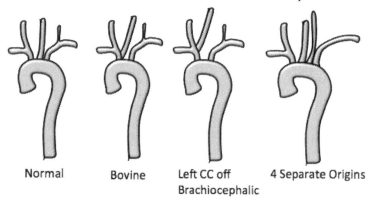

Normal   Bovine   Left CC off Brachiocephalic   4 Separate Origins

Adamkiewicz: The thoracic aorta puts off multiple important feeders including the great anterior medullary artery (Artery of Adamkiewicz) which serves as a dominate feeder of the spinal cord. This thing usually comes off on the **left side (70%) between T8-L1 (90%).**

Mesenteric Branches – The anatomy of the SMA and IMA is high yield, and can be shown on a MIP coronal CT, or Angiogram. I think that knowing the inferior pancreaticoduodenal comes off the SMA first, and that the left colic (from IMA) to the middle colic (from SMA) make up the Arc of Riolan are probably the highest yield facts.

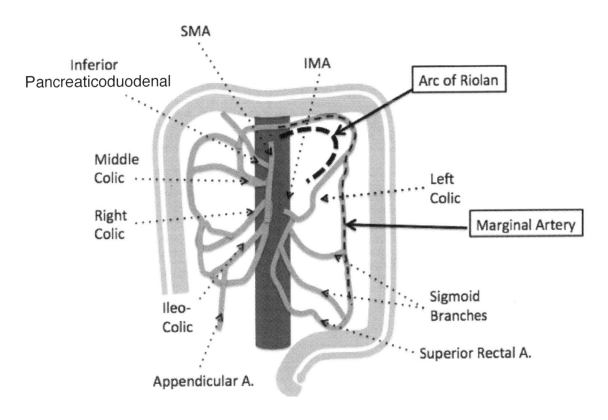

Celiac Branches: – The classic branches of the celiac axis are the common hepatic, left gastric, and the splenic arteries. The "common" hepatic artery becomes the "proper" hepatic artery after the GDA. This "traditional anatomy" is actually only seen in 55% of people.

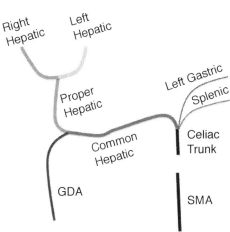

Celiac Anatomy - Remember this can be shown with an angiogram, CTA, or MRA.

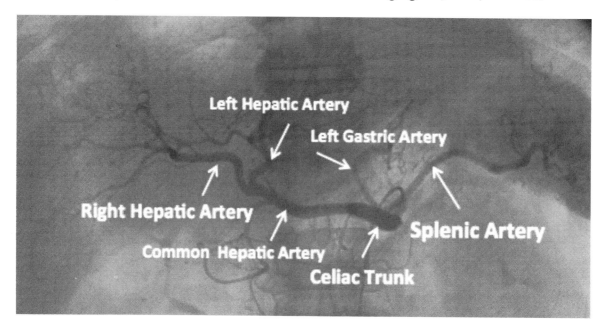

Variant Hepatic Artery Anatomy – The right hepatic artery and left hepatic arteries may be "replaced" (originate from a vessel other than the proper hepatic) or duplicated - which anatomist called "accessory." This distinction of "replaced" vs "accessory" would make a great multiple choice question.

Trivia to know:

- Replaced = Different Origin, usually off the left gastric or SMA

- Accessory = Duplication of the Vessel, with the spare coming off the left gastric or SMA

- If you see a **vessel in the fissure of the ligamentum venosum** (where there is not normally a vessel), it's probably an accessory or **replaced left hepatic artery arising from the left gastric artery**.

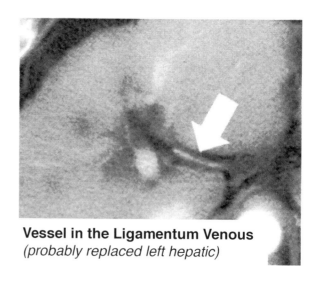

Vessel in the Ligamentum Venous
(probably replaced left hepatic)

- **The proper right hepatic artery is anterior to the right portal vein, whereas the replaced right hepatic artery is posterior to the main portal vein.** This positioning of the replaced right increases the risk of injury in pancreatic surgeries.

Iliac Anatomy: The branches of the internal iliac are high yield, with the most likely question being "which branches are from the posterior or anterior divisions?" A *useful mnemonic is "I Love Sex," Illiolumbar, Lateral Sacral, Superior Gluteal, for the posterior division.*

My trick for remembering that the mnemonic is for posterior and not anterior is to think of that super religious girl I knew in college — *I Like Sex in the butt / posterior.*

I don't think they will actually show a picture, it's way more likely to be a written question.

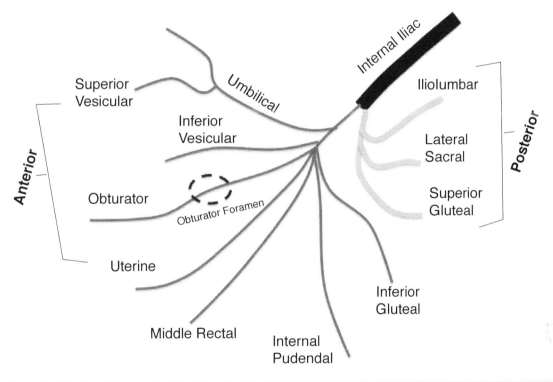

Anterior Division	Posterior Division
Umbilical	Iliolumbar
Superior Vesicular (off umbilical)	Lateral Sacral
Inferior Vescular	Superior Gluteal
Uterine (if you have a uterus)	*Inferior Gluteal *** sometimes*
Middle Rectal	
Internal Pudenal	
Inferior Gluteal	
Obturator	

Trivia: The ovarian arteries arise from the anterior-medial aorta 80-90% of time.

Persistent Sciatic Artery – An anatomic variant, which is a **continuation of the internal iliac**. It passes posterior to the femur in the thigh and then will anastomose with the distal vasculature. Complications worth knowing include aneurysm formation and early atherosclerosis in the vessel. The classic vascular surgery boards question is "external iliac is acutely occluded, but there is still a strong pulse in the foot", the answer is the patient has a persistent sciatic.

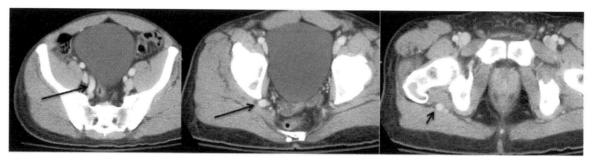

Persistent Sciatic Artery

Mesenteric Arterial Collateral Pathways:

Celiac to SMA: The conventional collateral pathway is Celiac -> Superior Pancreatic Duodenal -> Inferior Pancreatic Duodenal -> GDA.

Arc of Buhler: This is a variant anatomy (seen in like 4% of people), that represents a collateral pathway from the celiac to the SMA. The arch is independent of the GDA and inferior pancreatic arteries. This rare collateral can have an even more rare aneurysm, which occurs in association with stenosis of the celiac axis.

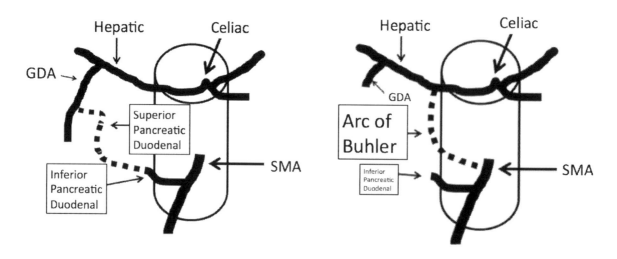

SMA to IMA: The conventional collateral pathway is SMA -> Middle Colic -> Left Branch of the Middle Colic -> Arc of Riolan (as below) -> Left Colic - > IMA.

Arc of Riolan – Also referred to as the meandering mesenteric artery. Classically a **connection between the middle colic of the SMA and the left colic of the IMA.**

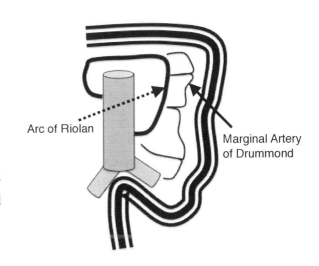

Marginal Artery of Drummond – This is another **SMA to IMA connection**. The anastomosis of the terminal branches of the ileocolic, right colic and middle colic arteries of the SMA, and of the left colic and sigmoid branches of the IMA, form a **continuous arterial circle or arcade along the inner border of the colon.**

IMA to Iliacs: - The conventional collateral pathway is IMA -> Superior Rectal -> Inferior Rectal -> Internal Pudendal -> Anterior branch of internal iliac.

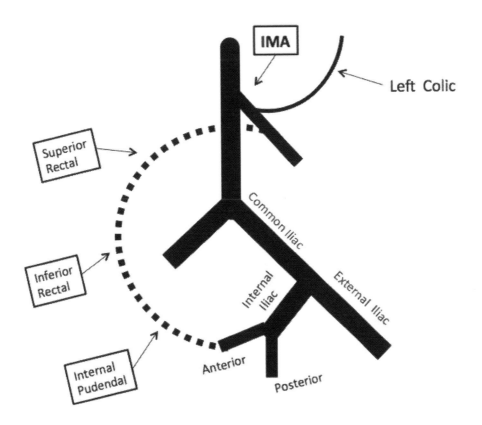

Winslow Pathway – This is a collateral pathway that is seen in the setting of aorto-iliac occlusive disease. The pathway apparently can be inadvertently cut during transverse abdominal surgery. The pathway runs from subclavian arteries -> internal thoracic (mammary) arteries -> superior epigastric arteries -> inferior epigastric arteries -> external iliac arteries.

Corona Mortis – Classically described as a vascular connection between the **obturator and external iliac.** Some authors describe additional anastomotic pathways, but you should basically think of it as any vessel **coursing over the superior pubic rim**, regardless of the anastomotic connection. The "crown of death" is significant because it can (a) be **injured in pelvic trauma** or (b) be **injured during surgery – and is notoriously difficult to ligate.** Some authors report that it causes 6-8% of deaths in pelvic trauma. The last piece of trivia is that it could hypothetically cause a type 2 endoleak.

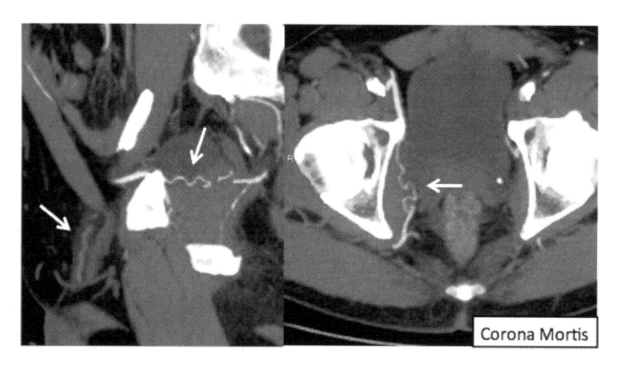

Corona Mortis

Upper Extremity Anatomy:

The scalene muscles make a triangle in the neck. If you have ever had the pleasure of reading a brachial plexus MRI finding this anatomy in a sagittal plane is the best place to start (in my opinion). The relationship to notice (because it's testable) is that the subclavian vein runs anterior to the triangle, and the subclavian artery runs in the triangle (with the brachial plexus).

Trivia to Remember: The subclavian artery runs posterior to the subclavian vein.

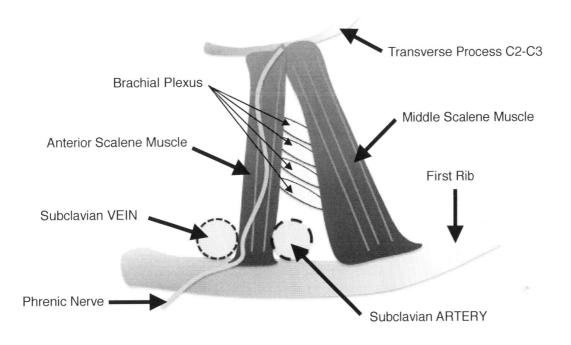

The subclavian artery has several major branches: the vertebral , the internal thoracic, the thyrocervical trunk, the costocervical trunk, and the dorsal scapular.

As the subclavian artery progresses down the arm, anatomists decided to change it's name a few times. This name changing makes for great multiple choice fodder. The highest yield thing you can know with regard to upper extremity vascular anatomy is when stuff becomes stuff:

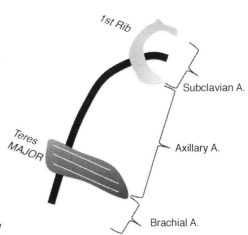

- *Axillary Artery: Begins at the first rib*
- *Brachial Artery: Begins at the lower border of the teres major (major NOT minor!)*
- *Brachial Artery: Bifurcates to the ulnar and radial*

Around the radial head the brachial artery splits into the radial and ulnar arteries. I have three tricks for telling the radial from the ulnar artery apart (in case it's not obvious).

1. The ulnar artery is usually bigger.

2. The ulnar artery usually gives off the common interosseous

3. The ulnar artery supplies the superficial planar arch (usually), and therefore the radial supplies the deep arch (usually).

Normal Variants:

- Anterior Interosseous Branch (Median Artery) persists and supplies the deep palmar arch of the hand.

- **"High Origin of the Radial Artery"** – Radial artery comes off either the axillary or high brachial artery (remember it normally comes off at the level of the radial head).

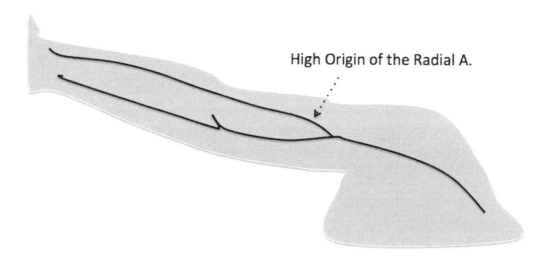

High Origin of the Radial A.

Lower Extremity Anatomy:

Every medical student knows the aorta bifurcates into the right and left common iliac arteries, which subsequently bifurcate into the external and internal iliac arteries. The nomenclature pearl for **the external iliac is that it becomes the common femoral once it gives off the inferior epigastric** *(at the inguinal ligament).*

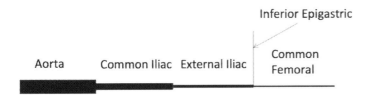

Once the inferior epigastric comes off (level of the inguinal ligament) you are dealing with the common femoral artery(CFA). The CFA divides into the deep femoral (profunda) and superficial femoral. The deep femoral courses lateral and posterior. The superficial femoral passes anterior and medial into the flexor muscle compartment (ADDuctor / Hunter's Canal). At the point the vessel emerges from the canal it is then the popliteal artery. At the level of the distal border of the popliteus muscle the popliteal artery divides into the **anterior tibialis (the first branch)** and the tibial peritoneal trunk. The anterior tibialis courses anterior and lateral, then it <u>transverses the interosseous membrane</u>, running down the front of the anterior tibia and terminating as the dorsalis pedis. The tibial peroneal trunk bifurcates into the posterior tibialis and fibular (peroneal) arteries. A common quiz is "what is the most medial artery in the leg?" , with the answer being the posterior tibial (felt at the medial malleolus). Notice how lateral the AT is - you can imagine it running across the interosseous membrane, just like it's suppose to.

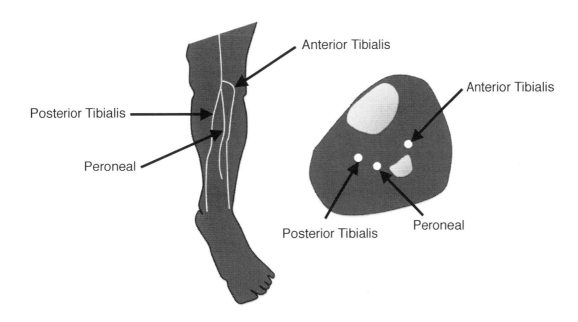

Venous Collaterals:

Gastric Varicies: - As described in more detail in the GI chapter, portal hypertension shunts blood away from the liver and into the systemic venous system. Spontaneous portal-systemic collaterals develop to decompress the system. The thing to know is that **most gastric varcies are formed by the left gastric (coronary vein)** . That is the one they always show big and dilated on an angiogram. Isolated gastric varices are secondary to splenic vein thrombosis. Gastric Varcies (80-85%) drain into the inferior phrenic and then into the left renal vein, forming a gastro-renal shunt.

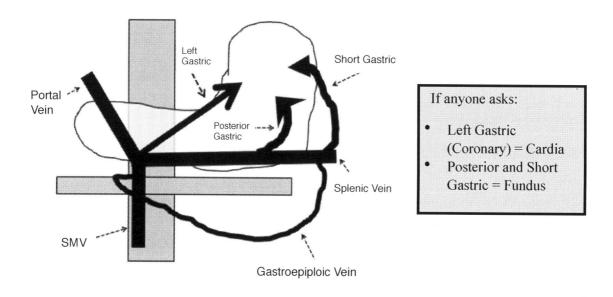

Splenorenal Shunt – Another feature of portal hypertension, this is an abnormal collateral between the splenic vein and renal vein. This is actually a desirable shunt because it is **not associated with GI bleeding**. However, **enlarged shunts are associated with hepatic encephalopathy** (discussed in greater detail in the BRTO section of the IR chapter). A common way to show this is an enlarged left renal vein and dilatation of the inferior vena cava at the level of the left renal vein.

Caval Variants:

Left Sided SVC – The most common congenital venous anomaly in the chest. In a few rare cases these can actually result in a right to left shunt. They are only seen in isolation in 10% of cases (the other 90% it's "duplicated"). The location and appearance is a total **Aunt Minnie**.

Trivia to know:

- Most common associated CHD is the ASD

- Associated with an unroofed coronary sinus

- Nearly always (92% of the time) it drains into the coronary sinus

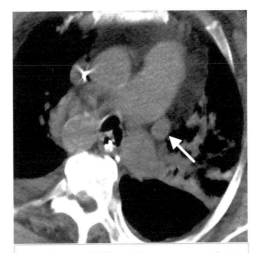

Left Sided SVC - *When you see that son of a bitch right there, that thing can only be one of two things - a lymph node or a duplicated SVC.*

Duplicated SVC – This is usually seen in the scenario of a left sided SVC, with a smaller right SVC also present.

Duplicated IVC - There are two main points worth knowing about this: (1) that the appearance is an **Aunt Minnie**, and (2) it's **associated with Renal stuff**. Renal associations include horse shoe and crossed fused ectopic kidneys. Also these dudes often have circumaortic renal collars (see below).

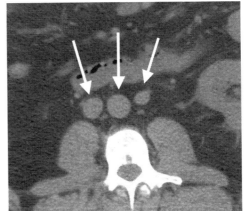

Duplicated IVC *(IVCs are the bread, Aorta is the cheese or peanut butter… or bacon)*

Circumaortic Venous Collar – Very common variant with an additional left renal vein that passes posterior to the aorta. It only matters in two situations (a) renal transplant, (b) IVC filter placement. The classic question is that the **anterior limb is superior**, and the posterior limb is inferior.

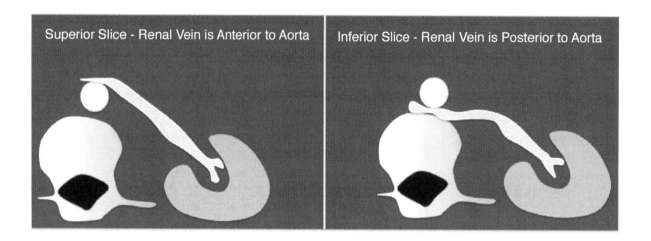

Azygos Continuation – This is also known as absence of the hepatic segment of the IVC. In this case, the hepatic veins drain directly into the right atrium. Often the IVC is duplicated in these patients, with the left IVC terminating in the left renal vein , which then crosses over to join the right IVC.

The first thing you should think when I say azygous continuation is **polysplenia** (reversed IVC/ Aorta is more with asplenia).

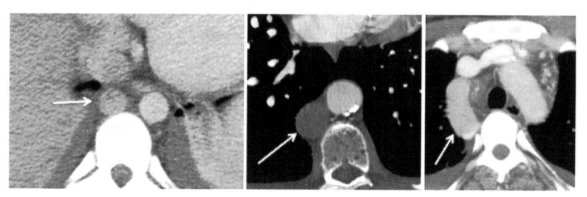

Azygos Continuation – *No IVC in the Liver, Dilated Azygos in the chest*

Pathology

Acute Aortic Syndromes - There are 3 "acute aortic syndromes", aortic dissection, intramural hematoma, and penetrating ulcer.

Aortic Dissection: This is the most common cause of acute aortic syndrome (70%), and is most commonly **caused by hypertension (70%).** This can be described as either acute (< 2 weeks), or chronic.

It can additionally be classified by location:

- Stanford A: account for 75% of dissection and involve the ascending aorta and arch proximal to the take off of the left subclavian. These guys need to be treated surgically.

- Stanford B: occur distal to the take off of the left subclavian and are treated medically unless there are complications (organ ischemia etc...)

Causes: Hypertension is the most frequent predisposing factor for aortic dissection. Other associations include Marfans, Turners (Aortic valve defects), infection, and pregnancy. Cocaine has also been associated in otherwise normotensive patients.

Findings: Displacement of intimal calcifications on Non-contrast. An intimal flap is seen in only 70% of cases. When you do see two lumens, these will spiral around each other. Thrombus is located in the false lumen (which will enhance later and is generally larger than the true lumen).

True vs False Lumen:

True	False
Continuity with undissected portion of aorta	"CobWeb Sign" – slender linear areas of low attenuation
Smaller cross sectional areas (with higher velocity blood)	**Larger** cross section area (slower more turbulent flow)
Surrounded by calcifications (if present)	Beak Sign -
Usually contains the origin of celiac trunk, SMA, and right renal artery	Usually contains the origin of left renal artery
	Surrounds true lumen in Type A Dissection

Intimo-intimal intussusception – Unusual type of dissection. It is produced by circumferential dissection of the intimal layer, which subsequently invaginates (this has been compared to a windsock). The intimal tear usually starts near the coronary orifices.

Floating Viscera Sign: This is a classic angiographic sign of abdominal aortic dissection. It is shown as opacification of abdominal aortic branch vessels during aortography (catheter placed in the aortic true lumen), with the branch vessels—(celiac axis, superior mesenteric artery, and renal arteries) arising out of nowhere. *They appear to be floating*, with little or no antegrade opacification of the aortic true lumen.

Aneurysm with Thrombus vs Dissection with Thrombus in False Lumen:

- *Dissection has spiral shape, Thrombus tend to be circumferential*
- *Mural thrombus has an irregular border, Dissection has a smooth border*
- *Intimal Calcification displacement - favors thrombus in dissection*

Intramural Hematoma: Classically seen in old hypertensives (same as dissection). Spontaneous hemorrhage caused by rupture of the vaso vasorum in the media without an intimal tear. This can be really difficult to distinguish from a thrombosed dissection (it won't spiral the way dissection does). Can proceed to classic dissection.

Trivia:

- It's still classified Type A or Type B
- Mortality Predictors: Ascending Aorta > 5cm, IMH > 2cm, Pericardial Effusion. **Maximum aortic diameter > 5cm is the strongest predictor to dissection.**

Unenhanced CT scan depicts **crescent-shaped areas with high attenuation**. Intimal calcifications may be displaced. MRI will show T2 bright blood in the acute phase, and T1 and T2 bright blood when subacute.

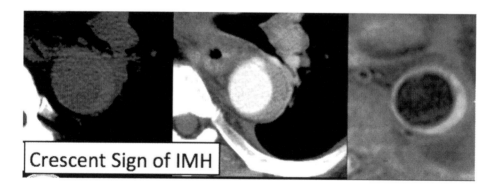

Crescent Sign of IMH

Penetrating Ulcer: This is an ulceration of an atheromatous plaque that has eroded the inner elastic layer of the aortic wall. When it reaches the media it produces a hematoma within the media. These things most often occur in old people with **severe underlying atherosclerosis**. They **can lead to saccular aneurysm**. They are often multiple and therefore difficult to treat. You still use the A &B Stanford classification based on location, with corresponding medical and surgical treatment. Apparently when these guys need surgery for type Bs (symptoms etc…) they do way worse than dissected B's because they actually need surgery and can't get an endograft.

Trivia:

- It's still classified Type A or Type B
- Mortality Predictors: Ascending Aorta > 5cm, IMH > 2cm, Pericardial Effusion. **Maximum aortic diameter > 5cm is the strongest predictor to dissection.**

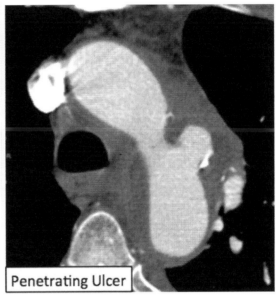

Penetrating Ulcer

What is the highest yield testable trivia regarding Acute Aortic Syndromes?

- *Causes?*
  - Dissection & IMH = Hypertension
  - Penetrating Ulcers = Atherosclerosis

- *Stanford A vs B ?*
  - Locations before of after left subclavian takeoff.
  - A is surgical, B is medical management.

- *IMH progression to dissection?*
  - IMH maximum diameter of 5cm is the strongest predictor for dissection

- *True Lumen vs False Lumen Dissection?*
  - If you aren't sure, the bigger one is probably the false one.

Other Pathology:

Aneurysm vs Pseudo-aneurysm – The distinction between a true and false aneurysm lends its self well to multiple choice testing. A true aneurysm is an enlargement of the lumen of the vessel to 1.5 times its normal diameter. **True = 3 layers are intact.** In a **false (pseudo) aneurysm all 3 layers are NOT intact**, and it is essentially a contained rupture. The risk of actual rupture is obviously higher with false aneurysm. It can sometimes be difficult to tell, but as a general rule fusiform aneurysms are true, and saccular aneurysms might be false. Classic causes of pseudoaneurysm include trauma, cardiologists (groin sticks), infection (mycotic), pancreatitis, and some vasculitides. On ultrasound they could show you the classic ying/yang sign, with "to and fro" flow on pulsed Doppler. The yin/yang sign can be seen in saccular true aneurysms, so you shouldn't call it on that alone (unless that's all they give you). **To and Fro flow within the aneurysm neck + clinical history is the best way to tell them apart**.

SVC Syndrome - Occurs secondary to complete or near complete obstruction of flow in the SVC from external compression (lymphoma, lung cancer) or intravascular obstruction (Central venous catheter, or pacemaker wire with thrombus). A less common but testable cause is fibrosing mediastinitis (just think histoplasmosis). The dude is gonna have face, neck, and bilateral arm swelling.

Traumatic Pseudoaneurysm – Again a pseudoaneurysm is basically a contained rupture. The most common place to see this (in a living patient) is the **aortic isthmus (90%)**. This is supposedly the result of tethering from the ligamentum arteriosum. The second and third most common sites are the ascending aorta and diaphragmatic hiatus - respectively. Ascending aortic injury is actually probably number one, it just kills them in the field so you don't see it. They could show you a CXR with a wide mediastinum, deviation of the NG Tube to the right, depressed left main bronchus, or left apical cap and want you to suspect acute injury.

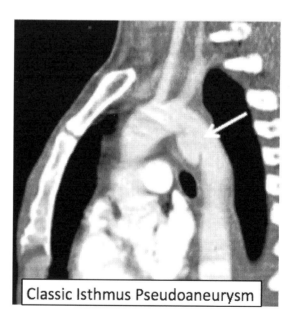

Classic Isthmus Pseudoaneurysm

Ascending Aortic Calcifications - There are only a few causes of ascending aortic calcifications, as atherosclerosis typically spares the ascending aorta. **Takayasu and Syphilis** should come to mind. The real life significance is the clamping of the aorta may be difficult during CABG.

Aneurysm - Defined as enlargement of the artery to 1.5 times its expected diameter (> 4cm of the Ascending and Transverse, > 3.5cm Descending, > 3.0 cm Abdominal). Atherosclerosis is the most common overall cause. Medial degeneration is the most common cause in the ascending aorta. Patients with connective tissue (Marfans, Ehlers Danlos) diseases tend to involve the aortic root. *When I say cystic medial necrosis you should think Marfans.* Aneurysms may develop in any segment of the aorta, but most involve the infra-renal abdominal aorta. This varies based on risk factors, rate of growth, etc… but a general rule is surgical repair for aneurysms at 6cm in the chest (5.5cm with collagen vascular disease) and 5cm in the abdomen.

Sinus of Valsalva Aneurysm – Aneurysms of the valsalva sinus (aortic sinus) are rare in real life, but have been known to show up on multiple choice tests. Factoids worth knowing are that they are more common in Asian Men, and **typically involve the right sinus**. They can be congenital or acquired (infectious). VSD is the most common associated cardiac anomaly. Rupture can lead to cardiac tamponade. Surgical repair with Bentall procedure.

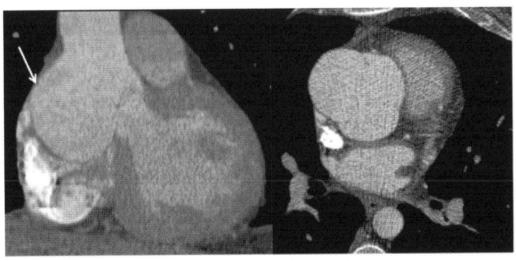

Sinus of Valsalva Aneurysm

AAA pre/ post Endograft

After an aneurysm has been treated with an endograft, things can still go south. There are 5 described types of endoleaks that lend themselves easily to multiple choice questions.

- **Type 1:** Leak at the top (A) or the bottom (B) of the graft. They are typically high pressure and require intervention (or the sac will keep growing).
- **Type 2:** Filling of the sac via a feeder artery. This is the **MOST COMMON** type, and is usually seen after repair of an abdominal aneurysm. The most likely culprits are the IMA or a Lumbar artery. The majority spontaneously resolve, but may require treatment. Typically, you follow the sac size and if it grows you treat it.
- **Type 3:** This is a defect/fracture in the graft. It is usually the result of pieces not overlapping.
- **Type 4:** This is from porosity of the graft. (*"4 is from the Pore"*). It's of historic significance, and doesn't happen with modern grafts.
- **Type 5:** This is endotension. It's not a true leak and maybe due to pulsation of the graft wall. Some people don't believe in these, but I've seen them. They are real.

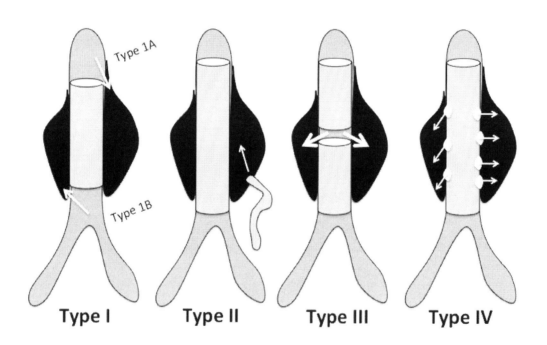

Type I   Type II   Type III   Type IV

Rupture / Impending Rupture- Peri-aortic stranding, rapid enlargement (10mm or more per year), or pain are warning signs of impending rupture. A retroperitoneal hematoma adjacent to an AAA is the most common imaging finding of actual rupture. The most common indicator for elective repair is the maximum diameter of the aneurysm, "Sac Size Matters," with treatment usually around 6cm (5.5cm in patients with collagen vascular disease). A thick circumferential mural thrombus is thought to be protective against rupture. Enlargement of the patent lumen can indicate lysis of thrombus and predispose to rupture.

Findings of Impending Rupture	
Draped Aorta Sign	Posterior wall of the aorta drapes over the vertebral column.
Increased Aneurysm Size	10mm or more increased per year
Focal Discontinuity in Circumferential Wall Calcifications	
Hyperdense Crescent Sign	Well defined peripheral crescent of increased attenuation. One of the most specific manifestations of impending rupture.

Mycotic Aneurysm – These are most often **saccular** and most often **pseudoaneurysms**. They are prone to rupture. They most often occur via hematogenous seeding in the setting of septicemia (**endocarditis**). They can occur from direct seeding via a psoas abscess or vertebral osteomyelitis (but this is less common). **Most occur in the thoracic or supra-renal aorta** (most atherosclerotic aortic aneurysms are infra-renal). Typical findings include saccular shape, lobular contours, peri-aortic inflammation, abscess, and peri-aortic gas. They tend to expand faster than atherosclerotic aneurysms. In general small, asymptomatic, and unruptured

Gamesmanship - If you see a saccular aneurysm of the aorta (especially the abdominal aorta) you have to lead with infection.

NF 1 – One of the more common neurological genetic disorders, which you usually think about causing all the skin stuff (Café au lait spots, and freckling), and bilateral optic gliomas. Although uncommon, vascular findings also occur in this disorder. **Aneurysms and stenosis are also sometimes seen in the aorta and larger arteries**, while dysplastic features are found in smaller vessels. **Renal artery stenosis can occur leading to renovascular hypertension** (found in 5% of children with NF). **The classic look is orificial renal artery stenosis presenting with hypertension in a teenager or child.** The mechanism is actually Dysplasia of the arterial wall itself (less common from peri-arterial neurofibroma).

Marfan Syndrome – Genetic disorder caused by mutations of the fibrillin gene (step 1 question). There are lots of systemic manifestations including ectopic lens, being tall, pectus deformity, scoliosis, long fingers etc… Vascular findings can be grouped into aneurysm, dissection, and pulmonary artery dilation:

- *Aneurysm:* Dilation with Marfans is classically described as **"Annuloaortic ectasia"**, with dilatation of the aortic root. The dilation usually begins with the aortic sinuses, and then progresses into the sinotubular junction , ultimately involving the aortic annulus. **Dilatation of the aortic root leads to aortic valve insufficiency.** Severe aortic regurgitation occurs that may progress to aortic root dissection or rupture. The mechanism for all this nonsense is that disruption of the media elastic fibers causes aortic stiffening, and predisposes to aneurysm and dissection. The buzzword for the Marfans ascending aneurysm is **"tulip bulb."** They are usually repaired earlier than normal aneurysm (typically around 5.5cm).

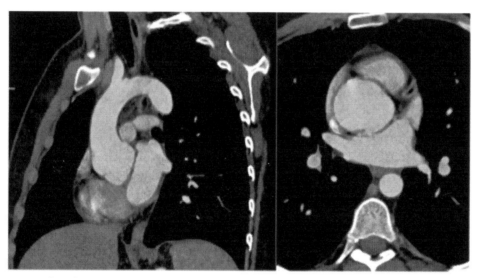

Marfan's - *Annuloaortic Ectasia", with dilatation of the aortic root.*

- *Dissection:* Recurrent dissections are common, and even "triple barreled dissection" can be seen (dissections on both sides of a true channel).

- *Pulmonary Artery Enlargement:* Just like dilation of the aorta, pulmonary artery enlargement favors the root.

Loeys Dietz Syndrome - Just think of this as the really shitty version of Marfans. They have a terrible prognosis, and rupture their aortas all the time. **Vessels are very tortuous** (twisty). They also have crazy wide eyes (hypertelorism).

Ehlers Danlos - This one is a disorder in collagen, with lots of different subtypes. They have the stretchy skin, hypermobile joints, blood vessel fragility with bleeding diatheses. Invasive diagnostic studies such as conventional angiography and **other percutaneous procedures should be avoided** because of the excessive risk of arterial dissection. Imaging characteristics of aortic aneurysms in Ehlers-Danlos syndrome **resemble those in Marfan syndrome, often involving the aortic root.** Aneurysms of the abdominal visceral arteries are common as well.

Syphilitic (Luetic) aneurysm – This is super rare and only seen in patients with untreated tertiary syphilis. There is classically a saccular appearance and involves the ascending aorta as well as the aortic arch aorta. Classic description **"saccular asymmetric aortic aneurysm with involvement of the aortic root branches. "** Often heavily calcified **"tree bark" intimal calcifications**. Coronary artery narrowing (at the ostium) is seen 30% of the time. Aortic valve insufficiency is also common.

Aorto-Enteric Fistula - These come in two flavors: (a) Primary, and (b) Secondary.

- **Primary:** Very, very, very rare. Refers to an A-E fistula without history of instrumentation. They are only seen in the setting of aneurysm and atherosclerosis.

- **Secondary:** Much more common. They are **seen after surgery** with or without stent graft placement.

The question is usually what part of the bowel is involved, and the answer is **3rd and 4th portions of the duodenum**. The second most likely question is A-E fistula vs perigraft infection (without fistula)? The answer to that is unless you see contrast from the aorta into the bowel lumen (usually duodenum), you can't tell. Both of them have ectopic perigraft gas > 4 weeks post repair, both have perigraft fluid and edema, both lose the fat place between the bowel and aorta (tethering of the duodenum to the anterior wall of the aorta), both can have pseudoaneurysm formation.

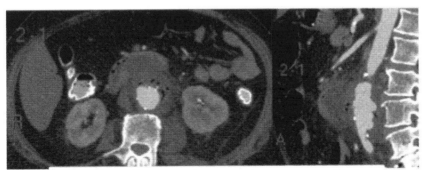

Aorto-Enteric Fistula – *Primary Type*

Inflammatory Aneurysms - Most are **symptomatic**, more common in **young men**, and associated with increased risk of rupture regardless of their size. Unlike patients with atherosclerotic AAA, most with the inflammatory variant have an **elevated ESR**. Their etiology is not well understood but may be related to periaortic retroperitoneal fibrosis or other autoimmune disorders (SLE, Giant Cell, RA). **Smoking is apparently a strong risk factor**, and smoking cessation is the first step in medical therapy. **In 1/3 of cases hydronephrosis or renal failure** is present at the time of diagnosis because the inflammatory process usually involves the ureters. Imaging findings include a thickened wall, inflammatory or fibrotic changes in the periaortic regions. Often there is asymmetrical thickening of the aorta with sparing of the posterior wall (helps differentiate it from vasculitis).

Leriche Syndrome - Refers to complete occlusion of the aorta distal to the renal arteries (most often at the aortic bifurcation). It is often secondary to bad atherosclerosis. There can be large collaterals.

The most likely question is the **triad:**

1- Ass Claudication,
2- Absent/ Decreased femoral pulses,
3- Limp Dick (Impotence)

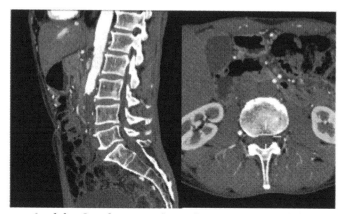

Leriche Syndrome – *Complete occlusion of the aorta distal to the renal arteries*

Mid Aortic Syndrome: - Refers to progressive narrowing of the abdominal aorta and its major branches. Compared to Leriche, this is higher, and longer in segment. It's also a total freaking zebra. It tends to affect children / young adults. This thing is characterized by progressive narrowing of the aorta. It is **NOT secondary to arteritis or atherosclerosis** but instead the result of some intrauterine insult (maybe) with fragmentation of the elastic media.

This also has a triad:

1. **HTN (most common presenting symptom)**,

2. Claudication,

3. Renal failure.

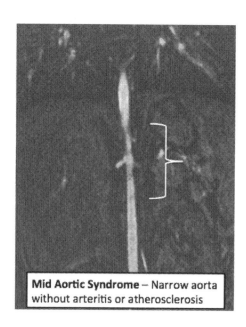

Mid Aortic Syndrome – Narrow aorta without arteritis or atherosclerosis

Aortic Coarctation: This comes in two flavors:

- Infantile (Pre-ductal) – these guys can have pulmonary edema. More typically a long segment. Blood supply to the descending aorta is via the PDA.

- Adult (Ductal) – Not symptomatic until later in childhood. Often presents with differential arm/leg blood pressures. More typically a short segment.

OK, things to know: **Strong Association with Turners Syndrome** (15-20%). **Bicuspid Aortic valve is the most common associated defect (80%)**. They have more berry aneurysms. Figure 3 sign (appearance of CXR). Rib Notching: most often involves 4th - 8th ribs. It does NOT involve the 1st and 2nd because those are fed by the costocervical trunk.

Pseudocoarctation: This is a favorite of multiple choice writers. You will have elongation with narrowing and kinking of the aorta. It really looks like a coarctation, BUT there is **NO pressure gradient, collateral formation, or rib notching -** that is the most likely question. The second most likely question is the area of aneurysmal dilation may occur distal to the areas of narrowing in pseudocoarctation, and they may become progressively dilated and should therefore be followed.

Thoracic Outlet Syndrome – Congenital or acquired compression of the Subclavian vessels (artery and vein), and brachial plexus nerves as they pass through the thoracic inlet. *It is a spectrum: Nerve (95%) >>>>>> Subclavian Vein >> Subclavian Artery*. With symptoms varying depending on what is compressed. **Compression by the anterior scalene muscle is the most common cause**. However, cervical rib, muscular hypertrophy, fibrous bands, pagets, tumor etc… can all cause symptoms. Treatment is usually surgical removal of the rib / muscle. The way they will show this is arms up and arms down angiography (occlusion occurs with arms up).

Paget Schroetter – This is **essentially thoracic outlet syndrome, with development of a venous thrombus in the Subclavian vein**. It's sometimes called "effort thrombosis" because it's associated with athletes (pitchers, weightlifters) who are raising their arms a lot. They will use catheter directed lysis on these dudes, and surgical release of the offending agent as above. Stenting isn't usually done (and can only be done after surgery to avoid getting the stent crushed).

Pulmonary Artery Aneurysm/Pseudoaneurysm – Think about three things for multiple choice; (1) **Iatrogenic from swan ganz catheter *most common** (2) Behcets, (3) Chronic PE. When they want to lead swan ganz they may say something like "patient in the ICU." The buzzwords for Behcets are: "Turkish descent", and "mouth and genital ulcers."

- **Hughes-Stovin Syndrome:** This is a zebra cause of pulmonary artery aneurysm that is similar (and maybe the same thing) as Behcets. It is characterized by recurrent thrombophlebitis and pulmonary artery aneurysm formation and rupture.

- **Rasmussen Aneurysm:** This has a cool name, which instantly makes it high yield for testing. This is a pulmonary artery **pseudoaneurysm secondary to pulmonary TB.** It usually involves the upper lobes in the setting of reactivation TB.

- **Tetrology of Fallot Repair Gone South:** So another possible testable scenario is the patch aneurysm, from the RVOT repair.

Splenic Artery Aneurysm: The most common visceral arterial aneurysm. They can be true or false. The true ones are associated with HTN, portal HTN, cirrhosis, liver transplant, and **pregnancy. More common in pregnancy, and more likely to rupture in pregnancy.** In contrast to normal aneurysms **atherosclerosis is NOT considered the underlying cause.** Most are located in the distal artery. False aneurysms are associated with pancreatitis. An important mimic is the islet cell pancreatic tumor (which is hypervascular). Don't be a dumb ass and try and biopsy the aneurysm. If you are forced to choose *which ones to treat* I guess I'd go with: anything over 2cm, any false one, and anyone in a women planning on getting pregnant.

Median Arcuate Ligament Syndrome (Dunbar Syndrome) : This is compression of the celiac artery by the median arcuate ligament (fibrous band that connects the diaphragm). Most people actually have some degree of compression, but it's not a syndrome until there are symptoms (abdominal pain, weight loss). Typical age is 20-40 years old. The buzzword is **"hooked appearance."** It's classically shown on angiography and they will want you to know that it gets **worse with expiration.** It can actually lead to the development of pancreaticoduodenal collaterals and aneurysm formation. It's treated surgically.

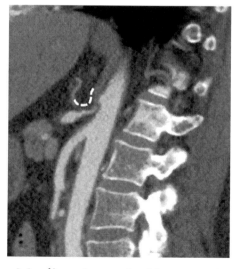

Median Arcuate Ligament

Mesenteric Ischemia: – This can be broadly classified as acute or chronic.

Chronic: Significant Stenosis of 2 out of 3 main mesenteric vessels + symptoms ("food fear"), LUQ pain after eating, pain out of proportion to exam). Some practical pearls are that you can have bad disease and no symptoms if you have good collaterals. Alternatively if you have bad one-vessel disease you can have symptoms if you have crappy collaterals. Remember that the *splenic flexure is the most common* because it's the watershed of the SMA and IMA.

Acute: This comes from 4 main causes. Arterial, Venous, Hypovolemic, and Strangulation.

- **Arterial:** Occlusive emboli (usually more distal, at branch points), or Thrombus (usually closer to the ostium). Vasculitis can also cause it. The SMA is most commonly affected. Arterial typically has a **thinner wall** (no arterial inflow), and is **NOT typically dilated**. After reperfusion the bowel wall will become thick, with target appearance.

- **Venous: Dilation with wall thickening** *(8-9mm, with < 5mm being normal)* is more common. Fat stranding and ascites are especially common findings in venous occlusion.

- **NonOcclusive**: Seen in patients in shock or on pressors. This is the most difficult to diagnose on CT. The involved segments are often thickened. Enhancement is variable. *Look for delayed filling of the portal vein at 70 seconds.*

- **Strangulation:** This is almost always secondary to a closed loop obstruction. This is basically a mixed arterial and venous picture, with **congested dilated bowel**. Hemorrhage may be seen in the bowel wall. The lumen is often fluid filed.

Mesenteric Ischemia			
Arterial	**Venous**	**Strangulation**	**Nonocclusive**
Thin Bowel Wall (thick after reperfusion)	Thick Bowel Wall	Thick Bowel Wall	Thick Bowel Wall
Diminished Enhancement	Variable	Variable	Variable
Bowel Not Dilated	Moderate Dilation	Severe Dilation (and fluid filled)	Bowel Not Dilated
Mesentery Not Hazy (until it infarcts)	Hazy with Ascites	Hazy with Ascites, and "whirl sign" with closed loop.	Mesentery Not Hazy (until it infarcts)

This is my general algorithm if I see angry bowel:

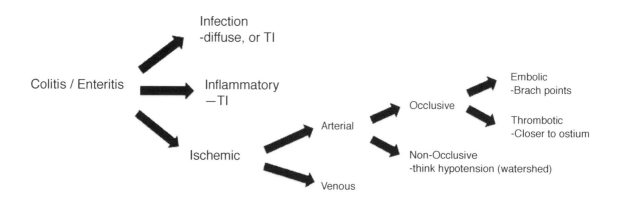

Colonic Angiodysplasia – This is the second most common cause of colonic arterial bleeding (diverticulosis being number one). This is primarily **right sided** with angiography demonstrating a cluster of small arteries during the arterial phase (along the antimesenteric border of the colon), with *early opacification of dilated draining veins* that persists late into the venous phase. There is an **association with aortic stenosis which carries the eponym Heyde Syndrome** (which instantly makes it high yield for multiple choice).

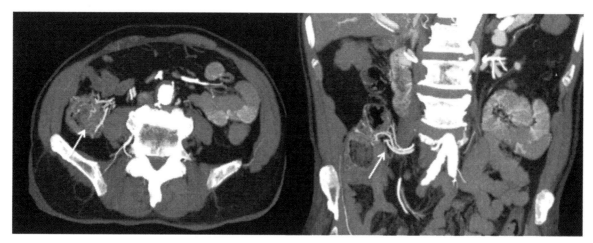

Colonic Angiodysplasia

Osler Weber Rendu (Hereditary Hemorrhagic Telangiectasia) – This is an AD multi-system disorder characterized by multiple AVMs. On step 1 they used to show you the tongue / mouth with the telangiectasis and a history of recurrent bloody nose. Now, they will likely show multiple hepatic AVMs or multiple pulmonary AVMs. Extensive shunting in the liver can actually cause biliary necrosis, and bile leak. They can have high output cardiac failure. ***Most die from stroke, or brain abscess.***

Gamesmanship "Next Step" - If the syndrome is suspected these guys need CT of the Lung & Liver (with contrast), plus a Brain MR / MRA

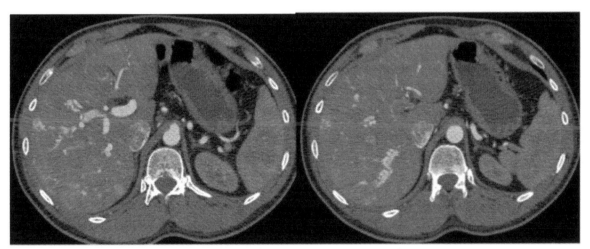

Osler Weber Rendu *(Hereditary Hemorrhagic Telangiectasia)*

Renal Artery Stenosis – Narrowing of the renal artery most commonly occurs secondary to atherosclerosis (75%). This type of narrowing is usually near the ostium, and can be stented. FMD is the second most common cause and typically has a beaded appearance sparing the ostium (should not be stented). Additional more rare causes include PAN, Takayasu, NF-1, and Radiation.

FMD (Fibromuscular Dysplasia) – A nonatherosclerotic vascular disease, primarily affecting the renal arteries of young white women.

Things to know:

- Renovascular HTN in Young Women = FMD

- Renal arteries are the most commonly involved (carotid #2, iliac #3)

- There are 3 types, but just remember medial is the most common (95%)

- They are predisposed to spontaneous dissection

- Buzzword = String of Beads

- Treatment = Angioplasty WITHOUT stenting.

Nutcracker Syndrome – Smashing of the left renal vein as it slides under the SMA, with resulting abdominal pain(left flank) and hematuria. The left renal vein gets smashed a lot, but it's not a syndrome without symptoms. Since the left gonadal vein drains into the left renal vein, it can also cause left testicle pain in men, and LLQ pain in women.

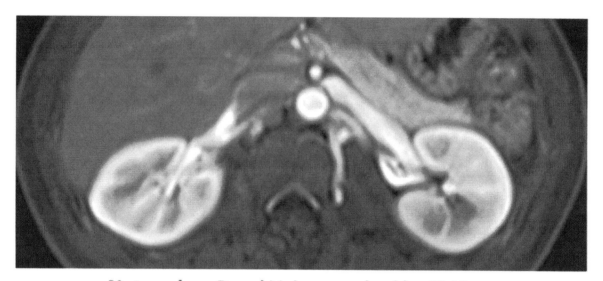

Nutcracker: Renal Vein, smashed by SMA.
Note the prominent venous collateral

Pelvic Congestion Syndrome – This is a controversial entity, sometimes grouped in the fibromyalgia spectrum. Patients often have "chronic abdominal pain." They also often wear a lot of rings and drink orange soda. The classic demographic is a depressed, multiparous, pre-menopausal women with chronic pelvic pain. Venous obstruction at the left renal vein (nutcracker compression) or incompetent ovarian vein valves leads to **multiple dilated parauterine veins**. This very "real" diagnosis can be treated by your local Interventional Radiologist via ovarian vein embolization.

Testicular Varicocele – Abnormal dilation of veins in the pampiniform plexus. Most cases are idiopathic and **most (98%) are found on the left side** *(left vein is longer, and drains into renal vein at right angle)*. They can also occur on the left, secondary to the above mentioned "nutcracker syndrome." They **can cause infertility**. "Non-decompressible" is a buzzword for badness. Some sources state that neoplasm is actually the most likely cause of **non-decompressible varicocele** in men over 40 years of age; (left renal malignancy invading the renal vein). Right sided varicocele can be a sign of malignancy as well. When it's new, and on the right side (in an adult), you should raise concern for a pelvic or abdominal malignancy. New right sided varicocele in an adult should make you think renal cell carcinoma, retroperitoneal fibrosis, or adhesions. **Non-decompressible Bad, Right Bad, Left Ok, Bilateral Ok (probably).**

Gamesmanship - This diagnosis is the classic next step question of all next step questions because you need to recognize when this common diagnosis is associated with something bad.

- Isolated Right Varicocele = Get an ABD CT (or MR, or US)

- Non-decompressible Varicocele = Get an ABD CT (or MR, or US)

- Bilateral Decompressible Varicoceles = Might need treated if infertile etc.. but doesn't need additional cancer hunting imaging.

- Isolated Left Varicocele = Might need treated if infertile etc.. but doesn't need additional cancer hunting imaging.

Uterine AVM – This can present with life threatening massive genital bleeding. Rarely they can present with CHF. They come in two flavors (a) Congenital, and (b) Acquired. **Acquired occurs after D&C**, abortion, or multiple pregnancies. They are most likely to show this on color Doppler with serpiginous structures in the myometrium with low resistance high velocity patterns. This one needs embolization. Could look similar to retained products of conception (clinical history will be different, and *RPOC is usually centered in the endometrium rather than the myometrium*).

May Thurner – A syndrome resulting in DVT of the left common iliac vein. The pathology is **compression of the left common iliac vein by the right common iliac artery**. Treatment is thrombolysis and stenting. *If they show you a swollen left leg, this is probably the answer.*

Popliteal Aneurysm – This is the most common peripheral arterial aneurysm (2nd most common overall, to the aorta). The main issue with these things is distal thromboembolism, which can be limb threatening. There is a strong and frequently tested association with AAA.

- *30-50% of patients with popliteal aneurysms have a AAA*

- *10% of patients with AAA have popliteal aneurysms*

- *50-70% of popliteal aneurysms are bilateral*

The **most dreaded complication of a popliteal artery aneurysm is an acute limb** from thrombosis and distal embolization of thrombus pooling in the aneurysm.

Popliteal Entrapment – Symptomatic compression or occlusion of the popliteal artery due to the developmental relationship with the **medial head of the gastrocnemius** (less commonly the popliteus). Medial deviation of the popliteal artery is supposedly diagnostic. This usually occurs in young men (<30). These patients may have *normal pulses that decrease with plantar flexion or dorsiflexion of the foot.* They will show you either a MRA or conventional angiogram in rest and then stress (dorsi / plantar flexion) to show the artery occlude.

Hypothenar Hammer – Caused by blunt trauma (history of working with a jack-hammer), to the ulnar artery and superficial palmar arch. The impact occurs against the hook of the hamate. Arterial wall damage leads to aneurysm formation with or without thrombosis of the vessel. Emboli may form, causing distal obstruction of digits (this can cause confusion with the main DDx Buergers). Look for **corkscrew configuration of the superficial palmar arch, occlusion of the ulnar artery, or pseudoaneurysm off the ulnar artery.**

Peripheral Vascular Malformations: About 40% of vascular malformations involve the extremities (the other 40% are head and neck, and 20% is thorax). Different than hemangiomas, vascular malformations generally increase proportionally as the child grows. This dude Jackson classified vascular malformation as either low flow or high flow. Low flow would include venous, lymphatic, capillary, and mixes of the like. **High flow has an arterial component.** Treatment is basically determined by high or low flow.

Klippel-Trenaunay Syndrome (KTS) - This is often combined with **Parkes-Weber which is a true high flow AV malformation.** KTS has a triad of port wine nevi, bony or soft tissue hypertrophy (localized gigantism), and a venous malformation. A persistent sciatic vein is often associated. The marginal vein of Servelle (some superficial vein in the lateral calf and thigh) is pathognomonic (it's basically a great saphenous on the wrong side). Additional trivia: 20% have GI involvement and can bleed, if the system is big enough it can eat your platelets (**Kasabach Merritt**). Basically, **if you see a MRA/MRV of the leg with a bunch of superficial vessels (and no deep drainage) you should think about this thing**.

- *KTS* = Low Flow (venous)

- *Parks Weber* = High Flow (arterial)

- *"Klippel Trenaunay Weber"* = Something people say when they (a) don't know what they are talking about, or (b) don't know what kind of malformation it is and want to use a blanket term.

ABIs – So basic familiarity with the so called "Ankle to Brachial Index" can occasionally come in handy, with regard to peripheral arterial disease. This is basically a ratio of systolic pressure in the leg over systolic blood pressure in the arm. Diabetics can sometimes have unreliable numbers, because dense vascular calcifications won't let the vessels compress. 1.0 = normal, 0.5-0.3 = claudication, < 0.3 = rest pain.

Intimal Hyperplasia – "The bane of endovascular intervention." This is not a true disease but a response to blood vessel wall damage. Basically this is an exuberant healing response that leads to intimal thickening which can lead to stenosis. You hear it talked about the most in IR after they have revascularized a limb. Re-Stenosis that occurs 3-12 months after angioplasty is probably from intimal hyperplasia. It's sneaky to treat and often resists balloon dilation, and/or reoccurs. If you put a bare stent in place it may grow through the cracks and happen anyway. If you put a covered stent in, it may still occur at the edges of the stent. The take home point is that it's a pain in the ass, and if they show an angiogram with a stent in place, that now appears to be losing flow, this is probably the answer.

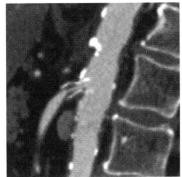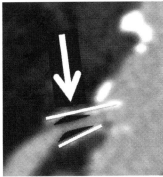

Intimal Hyperplasia
-dark stuff growing along the inside of the stent walls

Vasculitis:

Basically all vasculitis looks the same, with wall thickening, occlusions, dilations, and aneurysm formation. The trick to telling them apart is the age of the patient, the gender / race, and the vessels affected. Classically, they are broken up into large vessel, medium vessel, small vessel ANCA +, and small vessel ANCA negative.

Large:

Takayasu - "The pulse-less disease." This vasculitis loves **young Asian girls** (usually 15-30 years old). If they mention the word "Asian" this is likely to be the answer. Also, if they show you a **vasculitis involving the aorta** this is likely the answer. In the acute phase there will be both **wall thickening and wall enhancement**. There can be occlusion of the major aortic branches, or dilation of the aorta and its branches. The aortic valve is often involved (can cause stenosis or AI). In the late phase there is classically diffuse narrowing distally. The pulmonary arteries are commonly involved, with the typical appearance of peripheral pruning.

If anyone was a big enough jerk to ask, there are 5 types with variable involvement of the aorta and its branches. Which type is which is beyond the scope of the exam, just know type 3 is most common - involves arch and abdominal aorta.

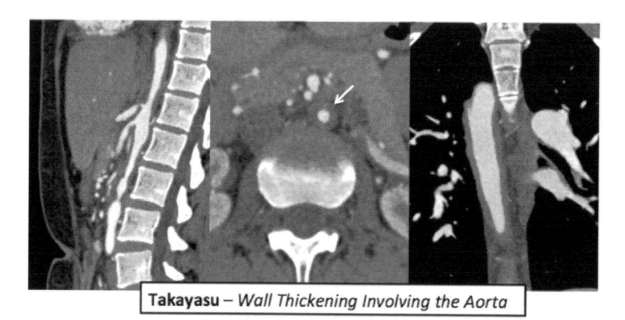

Takayasu – *Wall Thickening Involving the Aorta*

Giant Cell – The most common primary system vasculitis. This vasculitis loves **old men** (usually 70-80). This vasculitis involves the aorta and its major branches particularly those of the external carotid (**temporal artery**). This can be shown in two ways: (1) an ultrasound of the temporal artery, demonstrating wall thickening, or (2) CTA / MRA or even angiogram of the arm pit area (Subclavian/ Axillary/ Brachial), demonstrating wall thickening, occlusions, dilations, and aneurysm. Think about it as the **part of the body that would be compressed by crutches** (old men need crutches). Trivia worth knowing is that ESR and CRP are markedly elevated, and that the disease responds to steroids. "Gold Standard" for diagnosis is temporal artery biopsy (although it's often negative).

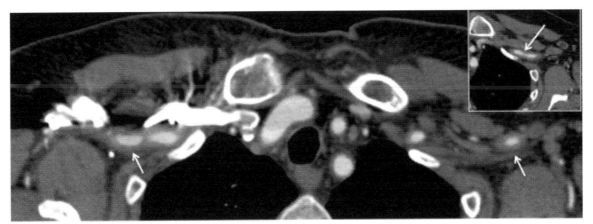

Giant Cell – "Arm Pit" Vessel Thickening

Cogan Syndrome – Total Zebra probably not even worth mentioning. It is a large vessel vasculitis that affects children and young adults. It likes the eyes and ears causing optic neuritis, uveitis, and audiovestibular symptoms resembling Menieres. They can also get aortitis, and those that do have a worse prognosis. Basically, **kid with eye and ear symptoms + or – aortitis.**

Medium

PAN (polyarteritis nodosa) – This is one of two vasculitides (*the other being Buergers*) that is more common in men. **PAN is more common in a MAN.** This can effect a lot of places with the big 3 being Renal (90%), Cardiac (70%), and GI (50-70%). Typically we are talking about **microaneurysm formation**, primarily at branch points, followed by infarction. I would expect this to be shown either as a CTA or angiogram of the **kidneys with microaneurysms**, or a kidney with areas of infarct (multiple wedge shaped areas). Trivia to know is the **association with Hep B.** Also, as a point of trivia the micro-aneurysm formation in the kidney can also be seen in patients who abuse Crystal Meth (sometimes called a "speed kidney").

Kawasaki Disease – Probably the most common vasculitis in children (HSP also common). Think about this as a cause of coronary vessel aneurysm. A **calcified coronary artery aneurysm shown on CXR is a very rare aunt Minnie.** Other trivia includes the buzzwords *"Mucocutaneous lymph node syndrome"* and *"Fever for Five days."*

-Coronary Artery Aneurysms > 8mm are "Giant" and prone to badness including MI
-Coronary Artery Aneurysms < 8mm may regress

Small Vessel Disease (ANCA +)

Wegeners - I think about upper respiratory tract (sinuses), and lower respiratory tract (lungs), and kidneys. cANCA is (+) 90% of the time. Ways this is shown are the **nasal perforation** (like a cocaine addict), and the **cavitary lung lesions**.

> *Vocab Update -*
>
> You aren't supposed to say "Wegener" - apparently he was a Nazi. Instead say "Granulomatosis with polyangiitis."

Churg Strauss – This is a necrotizing pulmonary vasculitis which is in the spectrum of Eosinophilic lung disease. They always have asthma and eosinophilia. **Transient peripheral lung consolidation** or ground glass regions is the most frequent feature. Cavitation is rare (this should make you think Wegeners instead). They are pANCA (+) 75% if the time.

Microscopic Polyangiitis – Affects the kidneys and lungs. Diffuse pulmonary hemorrhage is seen in about 1/3 of the cases. It is pANCA (+) 80% of the time.

Small Vessel Disease (ANCA -)

HSP (Henoch-Schonlein Purpura) – The most common vasculitis in children (usually age 4-11). Although it is a systemic disease, GI symptoms are most common (pain, blood diarrhea). It is a common lead point for intussusception. They could show this two classic ways: (1) ultrasound with a **doughnut sign for intussusception**, or (2) as a ultrasound of the **scrotum showing massive skin edema**. A less likely (but also possible) way to show this case would be multi-focal bowel wall thickening, or a plain film with thumb printing.

Behcets – Classic history is mouth ulcers, and genital ulcers, in someone with Turkish descent. It can cause thickening of the aorta, but for the purpose of multiple choice test I expect the question will be **pulmonary artery aneurysm**.

Buergers – This vasculitis is strongly associated with **smokers**. It affects both small and medium vessels in the arms and legs (more common in legs). Although it is more commonly seen in the legs, it is more commonly tested with a hand angiogram. The characteristic features are extensive arterial occlusive disease with the development of corkscrew collateral vessels. It usually affects more than one limb. **Buzzword = Auto-amputation.**

Gamesmanship Hand Angiograms:

If they are showing you a hand angiogram, it's going to be either Buergers of Hypothenar Hammer Syndrome (HHS).

My strategy centers around the ulnar artery.

(1) Ulnar artery involved = HHS. The most helpful findings is a pseudo-aneurysm off the ulnar artery - this is a slam dunk for HHS.

(2) Ulnar artery looks ok - then look at the fingers - if they are out go with Buergers. It sure would be nice to see some "corkscrew collaterals" - to make it sure thing.

Be careful, because the fingers can be out with HHS as well (distal emboli), but the ulnar artery should be fucked. Look at that ulnar artery first.

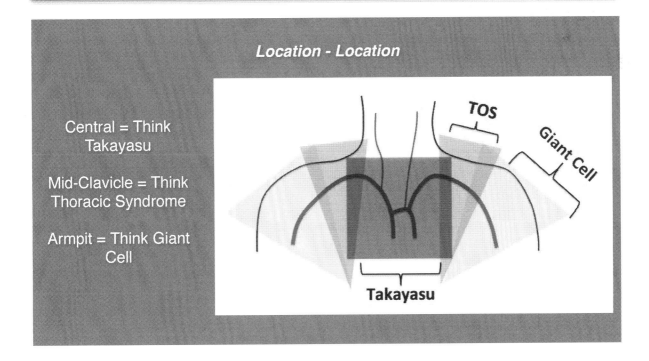

Location - Location

Central = Think Takayasu

Mid-Clavicle = Think Thoracic Syndrome

Armpit = Think Giant Cell

TOS

Giant Cell

Takayasu

Large Vessel	
Takayasu	Young Asian Female – thickened aneurysmal aorta
Giant Cell	Old Person with involvement of the crutches (Subclavian, axillary, brachial).
Cogan Syndrome	Kid with eye and ear symptoms + Aortitis
Medium Vessel	
PAN	More common in man. Renal Micoraneurysm (similar to speed kidney). Associated with Hep B.
Kawasaki	Coronary Artery Aneurysm
Small Vessel (ANCA +)	
Wegeners	Nasal Septum Erosions, Cavitary Lung Lesions
Churg Stauss	Transient peripheral lung consolidations.
Microscopic Polyangitis	Diffuse pulmonary hemorrhage
Small Vessel (ANCA -)	
HSP	Kids. Intussusception. Massive scrotal edema.
Behcets	Pulmonary artery aneurysm
Buergers	Male smoker. Hand angiogram shows finger occlusions.

Misc:

SAM (Segmental Arterial Mediolysis) – Affects the splanchnic arteries in the elderly, and the coronaries in young adults. Not a true vasculitis, with no significant inflammation. It's complicated but essentially the media of the vessel turns to crap, and you get a bunch of aneurysms. The aneurysms are often multiple. The way this is shown is **multiple abdominal splanchnic artery saccular aneurysms** – *this is the disease hallmark.*

Cystic Adventitial Disease – This uncommon disorder classically **affects the popliteal artery, of young men**. Basically you have one or **multiple mucoid filled cysts** developing in the outer media and adventitia. As the cysts grow they compress the artery.

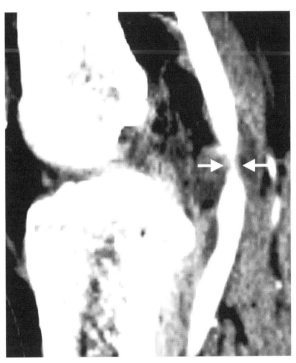

MIP CTA showing Vascular Narrowing

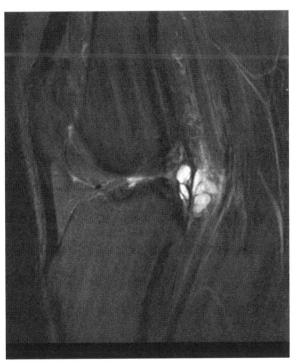

Fluid sensitive MR showing a much of cysts around the vessel, extrinsically narrowing it

Carotid Doppler

There are a couple of high yield topics regarding carotid Doppler.

Stenosis: They will show you an elevated velocity (normal is 125cm/s). They may also show you ICA/CCA ratio (normal is 2), or the ICA end diastolic velocity (< 40 is normal).

Here are the rules:

• Less that 50% stenosis will not alter the peak systolic velocity

• 50-69% Stenosis: ICA PSV 125-230cm/s , ICA/CCA PSV ratio: 2.0-4.0 , ICA EDV 40-100

• >70 % Stenosis: ICA PSV > 230cm/s, ICA/CCA PSV ratio: >4.0 , ICA EDV >100

Proximal Stenosis: OK here is the trick; they will show tardus parvus waveform. **If they show it unilateral, it is stenosis of the innominate. If it's bilateral then it's aortic stenosis.**

Subclavian Steal: This is discussed in greater detail in the cardiac chapter, but this time lets show it on ultrasound. As a refresher, we are talking about stenosis and/or occlusion of the proximal subclavian artery with retrograde flow in the ipsilateral vertebral artery.

How will they show it? They are going to show two things: (1) Retrograde flow in the left vertebral, and (2) a stenosis of the subclavian with a high velocity.

How they can get really sneaky? They can show this thing called "early steal." Steal is apparently a spectrum, which starts with mid-systolic deceleration with antegrade late-systolic velocities. Some people think the "early steal" waveform looks like a rabbit.

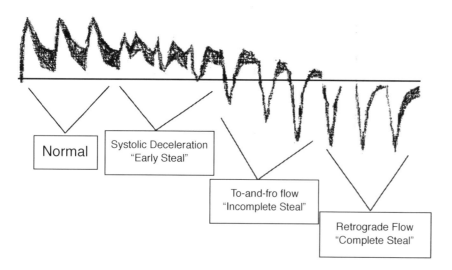

Gamesmanship Internal Carotid vs External Carotid:

This really lends itself well to multiple choice test questions. The big point to understand is that the brain is always on. You need blood flow to the brain all the time, which means diastolic flow needs to be present all the time, and thus continuous color flow throughout the cardiac cycle. The external carotid feeds face muscles… they only need to be on when you eat and talk.

Internal Carotid	External Carotid
Low Resistance	High Resistance
Low Systolic Velocity	High Systolic Velocity
Diastolic velocity does not return to baseline	Diastolic velocity approaches zero baseline
Continuous color flow is seen throughout the cardiac cycle	Color flow is intermittent during the cardiac cycle

Temporal Tap – It is a technique sonographers use to tell the external carotid from the internal carotid. You tap the temporal artery on the forehead and look for ripples in the spectrum. The tech will usually write "TT" on the strip - when they do this.

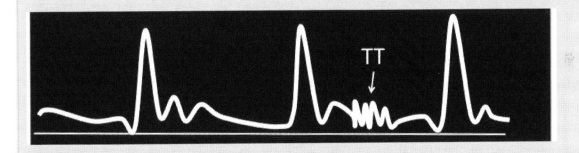

*You can also **look for branches** to tell the external carotid vs the internal.*

Aortic Regurgitation: - Just like aortic stenosis they are going to show you bilateral CCAs. In this case you are going to get **reversal of diastolic flow**.

Brain Death – Apparently in the ever-feuding monarchies of Europe ultrasound can be used for brain death studies. **A loss of diastolic flow suggests cessation of cerebral blood flow.**

Aneurysms: - In case someone asks you, distal formation of an aneurysm (such as one in the skull) cannot be detected by ultrasound, because proximal flow is normal.

Intra-Aortic Balloon Pump - Remember these guys are positioned so that the superior balloon is 2cm distal to the take off of the left subclavian artery, and the inferior balloon is just above the renals (you don't want it occluding importing stuff when it inflates). When the balloon does inflate it will displace the blood in this segment of the aorta - smashing it superior and inferior to the balloon. The balloon will inflate during early diastole (right after the aortic valve closes) because this is when the maximum amount of blood is available for displacement.

What does this do to the internal carotid (ICA) waveform? You are going to see an extra bump or "augmentation" as the balloon inflates and displaces blood superior.

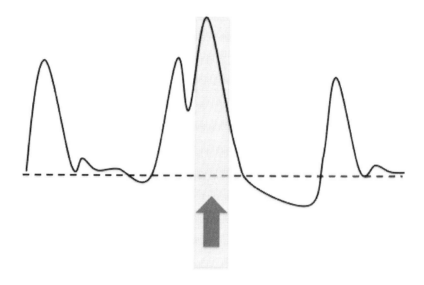

Which wave would you measure to evaluate the velocity? The first one (the one that is not assisted).

Classic Carotid Doppler Cases

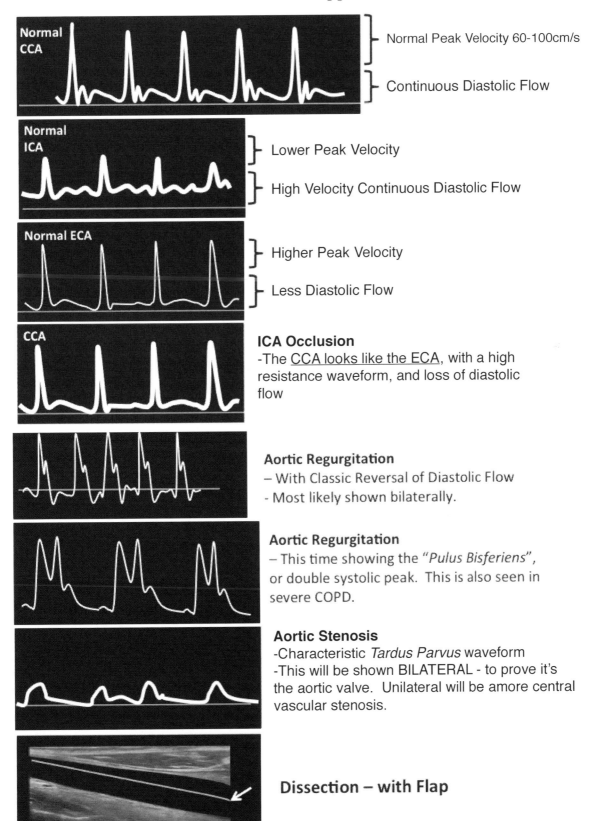

Normal CCA — Normal Peak Velocity 60-100cm/s

Continuous Diastolic Flow

Normal ICA — Lower Peak Velocity

High Velocity Continuous Diastolic Flow

Normal ECA — Higher Peak Velocity

Less Diastolic Flow

CCA

ICA Occlusion
-The CCA looks like the ECA, with a high resistance waveform, and loss of diastolic flow

Aortic Regurgitation
– With Classic Reversal of Diastolic Flow
- Most likely shown bilaterally.

Aortic Regurgitation
– This time showing the *"Pulus Bisferiens"*, or double systolic peak. This is also seen in severe COPD.

Aortic Stenosis
-Characteristic *Tardus Parvus* waveform
-This will be shown BILATERAL - to prove it's the aortic valve. Unilateral will be amore central vascular stenosis.

Dissection – with Flap

Blank for scribbles / Notes

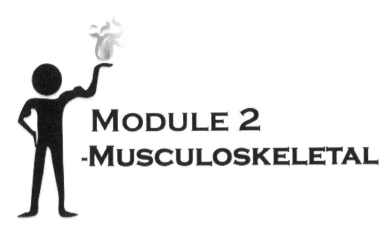

MODULE 2
-MUSCULOSKELETAL

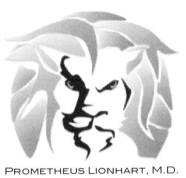

PROMETHEUS LIONHART, M.D.

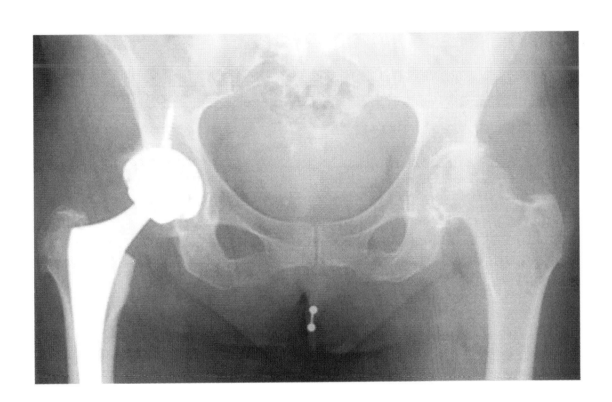

Trauma / Acquired

Basic Fracture Trivia:

- *Stress fracture* is abnormal stress on normal bone.
- An *insufficiency fracture* is normal stress on abnormal bone.
- Bones heal in about 6-8 weeks (months for tibia), and remember that the osteolytic phase precedes new bone formation.

Hand / Wrist:

Scaphoid Fracture:
- Most common carpal bone fracture
- 70% at the waist
- Blood supply is distal to proximal; with the proximal pole most susceptible to AVN.
- The first sign of AVN = Sclerosis (the dead bone can't turn over / recycle)
- Proximal fractures are most susceptible to AVN and non-union
- Avulsion fractures occur at distal pole
- AVN on MRI - This is tricky stuff with lots of papers contradicting each other. Probably the most reliable is sign is DARK ON T1.

SLAC and SNAC Wrists

Both are potential complications of trauma, with similar mechanisms.

SLAC Wrist (Scaphoid-Lunate Advanced Collapse) occurs with injury (or degeneration via CPPD) to the S-L ligament.

SNAC Wrist (Scaphoid Non-Union Advanced Collapse) occurs with a scaphoid fracture.

Just remember that the scaphoid always wants to rotate in flexion - the scaphoid-lunate ligament is the only thing holding it back. If this ligament breaks it will tilt into flexion, messing up the dynamics of the wrist. The radial scaphoid space will narrow, and the capitate will migrate proximally.

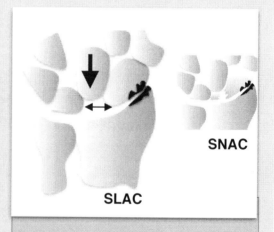

SNAC

SLAC

The things to know are;

- Radioscaphoid joint is first to develop degenerative changes

- Capitate will migrate proximally and there will eventually be a **DISI**

Q: How do you Treat a SLAC Wrist ?

A: Depends on the patient's occupation and needs:

    o   Wrist Fusion = Maximum Strength, Loss of Motion

    o   Proximal Row Carpectomy = Maintain ROM, Lose Strength

Carpal Dislocations - *A spectrum of severity*

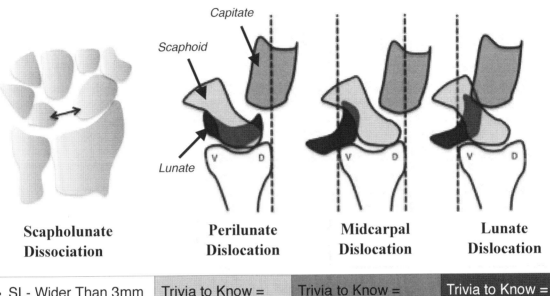

Scapholunate Dissociation	**Perilunate Dislocation**	**Midcarpal Dislocation**	**Lunate Dislocation**
• SL- Wider Than 3mm • Clenched Fist View can worsen it (would make a good next step question) • Chronic SL dissociation can result in a SLAC wrist	Trivia to Know = 60% associated with Scaphoid Fractures	Trivia to Know = (1)Associated with Triquetrolunate interosseous ligament disruption (2) Associated with a Triquetral Fracture	Trivia to Know = It happens with a Dorsal radiolunate ligament injury

DISI vs VISI

This is a very confusing topic - thus high yield. If you have carpal ligament disruption the carpal bones will rotate the way they naturally want to. The reasons for their rotational desires are complex but basically have to do with the shape of the fossa they sit on. Just remember the scaphoid wants to flex (rock volar) and the lunate wants to extend (rock dorsal). The only thing holding them back is their ligamentous attachment to each other.

DISI (dorsal intercalated segmental instability) - I like to call this *dorsiflexion instability* because it helps me remember whats going on. After a "Radial sided injury" (scapholunate side) the lunate becomes free of the stabilizing force of the scaphoid and rocks dorsally. Remember SL ligament injury is common, so this is common.

VISI (volar intercalated segmental instability) - I like to call this *volar-flexion (palmar-flexion) instability* because it helps me remember whats going on. After a "Ulnar sided injury" (lunotriquetral side) the lunate no longer hast the stabilizing force of the lunotriquetral ligament and gets ripped volar with the scaphoid *(remember the scaphoid stays up late every night dreaming of tilting volar)*. Remember LT ligament injury is not common, so this is not common. It's so uncommon in fact that if you see it - it's probably a normal variant due to wrist laxity.

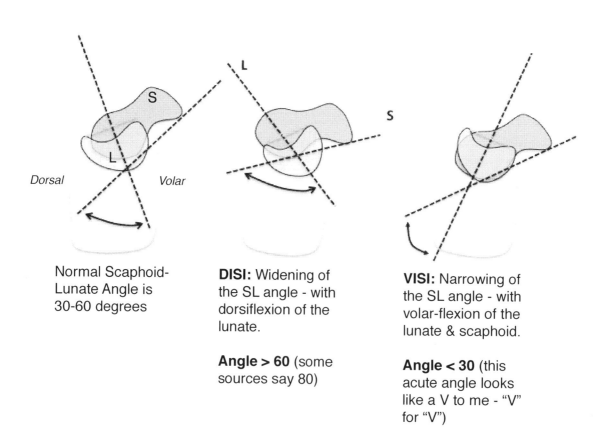

Normal Scaphoid-Lunate Angle is 30-60 degrees

DISI: Widening of the SL angle - with dorsiflexion of the lunate.

Angle > 60 (some sources say 80)

VISI: Narrowing of the SL angle - with volar-flexion of the lunate & scaphoid.

Angle < 30 (this acute angle looks like a V to me - "V" for "V")

Bennett and Rolando Fractures
- They are both fractures at the base of the first metacarpal
- The Rolando fracture is comminuted (Bennett is not)
- *Trivia:* The pull of the **Abductor pollicis longus (APL)** tendon is what causes the dorsolateral dislocation in the Bennett Fracture

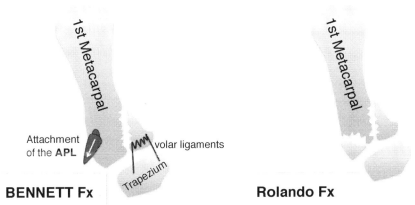

BENNETT Fx   **Rolando Fx**

Gamekeeper's Thumb
- Avulsion fracture at the base of the proximal first phalanx associated with **ulnar collateral ligament** disruption.
- The frequently tested association is that of a "**Stener Lesion**." A Stener Lesion is when the Adductor tendon gets caught in the torn edges of the UCL. The displaced ligament won't heal right, and will need surgery.
- It makes a "yo-yo" appearance on MRI - supposedly...

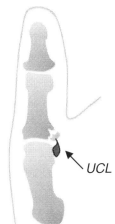

Carpal Tunnel Syndrome (CTS)
- Median Nerve Distribution (thumb-radial aspect of 4th digit), often bilateral, and may have thenar muscle atrophy.
- On Ultrasound, enlargement of the nerve is the main thing to look for
- It's usually from repetitive trauma,
- *Trivia* = **Association with dialysis**

Guyon's Canal Syndrome
- Entrapment of the ulnar nerve as it passes through Guyon's canal (formed by the pisiform and the hamate – and the crap that connects them). Classically caused by handle bars "***handle bar palsy***." Fracture of the hook of the hamate can also eat on that ulnar nerve.

Elbow / Forearm:

- Radial Head Fracture is most common in adults (supracondylar is most common in PEDs)
    - o Sail sign (posterior is positive)
- Capitellum fractures are associated with posterior dislocation

Eponyms:
- *Essex-Lopresti:* Fracture of the radial head + Anterior dislocation of the distal radial ulnar joint
- *Monteggia Fracture (MUGR):* Fracture of the proximal ulna, with anterior dislocation of the radial head.
- *Galeazzi Fracture (MUGR):* Radial shaft fracture, with anterior dislocation of the ulna at the DRUJ.

The Dreaded PEDs elbow *(Covered in the Peds chapter - see volume 2, module 5):*

Cubital Tunnel Syndrome
- The result of repetitive valgus stress
- *Anatomy Trivia:* the site where the ulnar nerve passes beneath the cubital tunnel retinaculum also known as the epicondylo-olecranon ligament or Osborne band
- Can occur from compression by any pathology (tumor, hematoma, etc…) , when it occurs from an **accessory muscle** it's classically the **anconeus epitrochlearis -** *also known as the "accessory anconeus."*

Shoulder (*MRI covered separately*)

Dislocation:
- *Anterior inferior* (subcoracoid) are by far the most common (like 90%).
  - **Hill-Sachs** is on the **H**umerus.
  - Hill-Sachs is on the posterior lateral humerus, and *best seen on internal rotation view.*
  - Bankart – anterior inferior labrum
  - Greater tuberosity avulsion fracture occurs in 10-15% of anterior dislocations in patient's over 40.
- *Posterior Dislocation*: uncommon – probably from seizure or electrocution
  - *Rim Sign* – no overlap glenoid and humeral head
  - *Trough Sign* – reverse Hill Sachs, impaction on anterior humerus
  - Arm may be locked in internal rotation on all views
- *Inferior Dislocation (luxatio erecta humeri)* – this is an uncommon form, where the arm is sticking straight over the head.   The thing to know is 60% get neurologic injury (usually the axillary nerve).

Hill Sacs	Posterolateral humeral head impaction fracture (anterior dislocation)
Bankart	Anterior Glenoid Rim (anterior dislocation)
Trough Sign	Anterior humeral head impaction fracture (posterior dislocation)
Reverse Bankart	Posterior Glenoid Rim (posterior dislocation)

Memory Tool (works for me anyway)

I remember that hip dislocations are posterior - from the straight leg dashboard mechanism. Then I just remember that shoulders are the opposite of that (the other one, is the other one). **Shoulder = Usually Anterior**

Proximal Humerus Fracture: This is usually in an old lady falling on an out stretched arm. Orthopods use the Neer classifications (how many parts the humerus is in ?). Three or four part fractures tend to do worse.

The Post Op Shoulder (Prosthesis)

There are 4 Main Types: Humeral Head Resurfacing, Hemi-Arthroplasty, Total Shoulder Arthroplasty, and the Reverse Total Shoulder Arthroplasty.

Who gets what? - The surgical choice depends on two main factors: (1) is the cuff intact?, and (2) is the Glenoid Trashed ? Here is the breakdown:

	Cuff-Intact	**Cuff- Deficient**
Glenoid Intact	**Resurfacing or Hemi**	**Hemi or Reverse**
Glenoid Deficient	**TSA**	**Reverse**

Complications / Trivia:

—Total Shoulder Most Common Complication = Loosening of the Glenoid Component

—Total Shoulder Complication - *"Anterior Escape"* - This describes anterior migration of the humeral head after subscapularis failure.

—Reverse Total Shoulder Does NOT require an intact rotator cuff - patient rely heavily on the deltoid.

—Reverse Shoulder Complication - *Posterior Acromion Fracture* - from excessive deltoid tugging.

Hip / Femur

Femoral Neck Fractures:
- On the inside (**medial**) is the classic **stress** fracture location
- On the outside (**lateral**) is the classic **bisphosphonate** related fx location

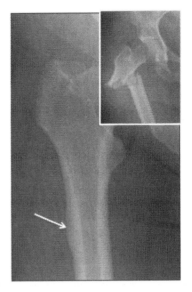

Bisphosphonate Fracture (Lateral Femur)
**Stress would be medial

Hip Fracture / Dislocation: You see these with dash board injuries. The **posterior dislocation** (almost always associated with a fracture as it's driven backwards) is much more common than the anterior dislocation.

> *Anterior Column vs Posterior Column* - the acetabulum is supported by two columns of bone that merge together to form an "inverted Y"
>
> - o Iliopectineal Line = Anterior
> - o Ilioischial Line = Posterior (remember you sit on your ischium)
> - o The both column fracture by definition divides the ilium proximal to the hip joint, so you have no articular surface of the hip attached to the axial skeleton (that's a problem).
>
> *Corona Mortis:* The anastomosis of the inferior epigastric and obturator vessels sometimes rides on the superior pubic ramus. During a lateral dissection - sometimes used to repair a hip fracture this can be injured. I talk about this more in the vascular chapter.

Hip Fracture Leading to AVN: The location of the fracture may predispose to AVN. It's important to remember that since the femoral head gets vascular flow from the circumflex femorals a **displaced intracapsular fracture could disrupt this blood supply – leading to AVN**.

- **Testable Point:** *Degree of fracture displacement corresponds with risk of AVN.*

Avulsion Injury: This is seen more in kids than adults. Adult bones are stronger than their tendons. In kids it's the other way around. One pearl is that if you see an **isolated "avulsion" of the lesser trochanter in a seemingly mild trauma / injury in an adult - query a pathologic fracture.** Now, to discuss what I believe is the highest yield topic in MSK for the exam, "where did the avulsion come from?" The easiest way to show this is a plain film pelvis (or MRI) with a tug/avulsion injury to one of the muscular attachment sites. The question will most likely be *"what attaches there?" or "which muscle got avulsed?"*

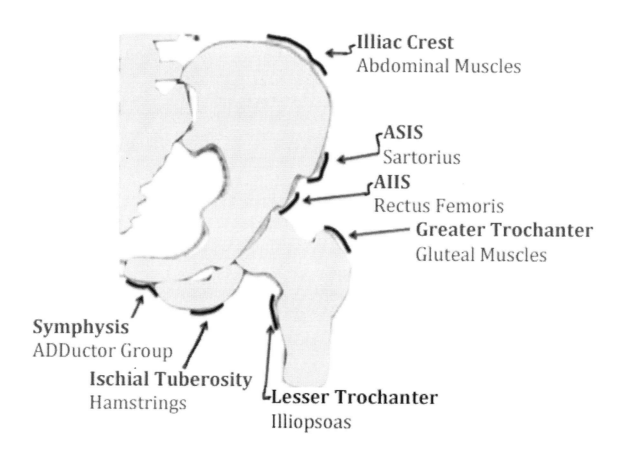

Snapping Hip Syndrome: The clinical sensation of "snapping" or "clicking" with hip flexion and extension. For a multiple choice testing standpoint all you need to know is (1) that it exists, (2) there are three types, and (3) what muscle each type involves.

Snapping Hip Syndrome	
External (most common)	Iliotibial Band over Greater Trochanter
Internal	Iliopsoas over Iliopectineal eminence or femoral head
Intra-Articular	Labral tears / joint bodies

Femoroacetabular Impingement (FAI): This is a syndrome of painful hip movement. It's based on hip / femoral deformities, and honestly might be total BS. Supposedly it can lead to early degenerative changes. There are two described subtypes:

Pincer Impingement	Cam Impingement
Middle Aged Women	Young Man
Over Coverage of the femoral head by the acetabulum	Bony protrusion on the antero-superior femoral head-neck junction
"Cross Over Sign" *anterior acetabular rim "crossing over" the posterior rim.	*"Pistol Grip Deformity"* Describes the appearance of the femur

Femoroacetabular Impingement

Normal   Cam-Type   Pincer-Type

Memory Aid

I remember that the femoral one (cam-type) is more common in men because the femoral head kinda looks like a penis.

Be honest, you were thinking that too.

"Cross Over Sign" – A sign of pincer type FAI. This refers to the anterior and posterior rims of the acetabulum forming a "figure of eight" on AP pelvis. It is extremely unreliable, and heavily based on positioning.

Trivia - Most common location for an acetabular labral tear = Anterior Superior

Sacrum:

You can get fractures of the sacrum in the setting of trauma, but if you get shown or asked anything about the sacrum it's going to be either (a) SI degenerative change - discussed later, (b) unilateral SI infection, (c) a chordoma - discussed later, (d) sacral agenesis, or (e) an insufficiency fracture. Out of these 5 things the insufficiency fracture is probably the most likely.

Sacral Insufficiency Fracture - The most common cause is postmenopausal **osteoporosis.** You can also see this in patients with renal failure, patients with RA, **pelvic radiation, mechanical changes after hip arthroplasty**, or extended steroid use. They are often (usually) occult on plain films. They will have to show this either with a bone scan, or MRI.

The classic "**Honda Sign**" from the "H" shaped appearance is probably the most likely presentation on a multiple choice test.

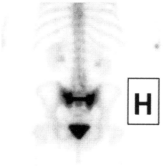

"Honda Sign"
Sacral Insufficiency Fx

Knee / Tibia / Fibula:

Segond Fracture: This is a fracture of the **Lateral** Tibial Plateau (*common distractor is medial tibia*). The thing to know is that it is **associated with ACL tear (75%),** and occurs with **internal rotation.**

Reverse Segond Fracture: This is a fracture of the **Medial** Tibial Plateau. The thing to know is that it is **associated with a PCL tear,** and occurs with **external rotation.** There is also an associated **medial meniscus** injury.

Arcuate Sign This is an avulsion of **proximal fibula** (insertion of arcuate ligament complex). The thing to know is that **90% are associated with cruciate ligament injury (usually PCL)**

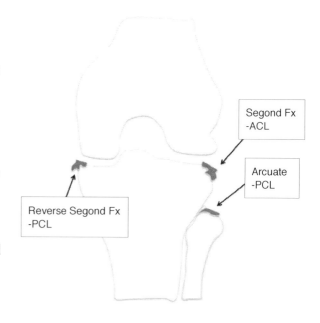

Segond Fx
-ACL

Arcuate
-PCL

Reverse Segond Fx
-PCL

Deep Intercondylar Notch Sign: This is a depression of the lateral femoral condyle (terminal sulcus) that occurs secondary to an impaction injury. This is **associated with ACL tears.**

Patella Dislocation: Basically **always lateral,** and the Medial Patello-Femoral Ligament is injured. There is a characteristic appearance on MRI, which will be shown and discussed later in this chapter.

Patella Alta / Baja: The patella will move up or down in certain traumatic situations. If the quadricep tendon tears you will get unopposed pull from the patellar tendon resulting in a low patella (Baja). If the patella tendon tears you will get unopposed quadriceps tendon pull resulting in a high patella (Alta).

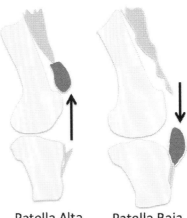

Patella Alta   Patella Baja

The "classic" association with patellar tendon tear (Alta) is **SLE**, (also can see in elderly, trauma, athletics, or RA). "Bilateral patellar rupture" is a buzzword for chronic steroids.

Tibial Plateau Fracture: This injury most commonly occurs from axial loading (falling and landing on a straight leg). The **lateral plateau is way more common than the medial**. If you see medial, it's usually with lateral. Some dude named Schatzker managed to get the classification system named after him, of which type 2 is the most common (split and depressed lateral plateau).

Pilon Fracture (Tibial plafond fracture): This injury also most commonly occurs from axial loading, with the talus being driven into the tibial plafond. The fracture is characterized by comminution and articular impaction. About 75% of the time you are going to have fracture of the distal fibula.

Tibial Shaft Fracture: This is the most common long bone fracture. It was also *listed as the most highly tested subject in american orthopedic OITE exam (with regard to trauma)*, over the last 8 years. Apparently there are a bunch of ways to put a nail or plate in it. It doesn't seem like it could be that high yield for the exam compared to other fractures with French or Latin sounding names.

Tillaux Fractures: This a **salter-harris 3**, through the anterolateral aspect of the distal tibial epiphysis.

Triplane Fracture: This is a **salter-harris 4**, with a vertical component through the epiphysis, horizontal component through the physis, and oblique through the metaphysis.

Maisonneuve Fracture: This is an unstable fracture involving the medial tibial malleolus and/or **disruption of the distal tibiofibular syndesmosis.** The most common way to show this is to first show you the ankle with the widened mortis, and *"next step?"* get you to ask for the proximal fibula - which will show the **fracture of the proximal fibular shaft.** This fracture pattern is unique as the forces begin distally in the tibiotalar joint and ride up the syndesmosis to the proximal fibula. For some reason knowing that the fracture **does not extend into the hindfoot** is a piece of valuable trivia.

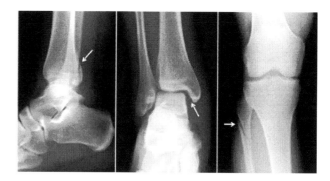

Maisonneuve Fracture:

Foot / Ankle

Casanova Fracture – If you see bilateral calcaneal fractures, you should *"next step?"* look at the spine for a compression or burst fracture. These tend to occur in axial loading patterns (possibly from jumping out a window to avoid an angry husband).

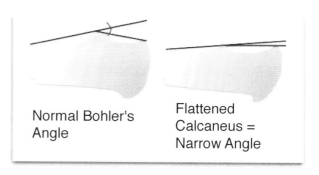

Normal Bohler's Angle

Flattened Calcaneus = Narrow Angle

Trivia: Peroneal tendons can become entrapped with lateral calcaneal fractures.

Bohler's Angle – The line drawn between the anterior and posterior borders of the calcaneus on a lateral view. An angle less than 20, is concerning for a fracture.

Jones Fracture: This is a fracture at the base of the fifth metatarsal, 1.5cm distal to the tuberosity. These are placed in a non-weight bearing cast (may require internal fixation- because of risk of non-union. .

Avulsion Fracture of the 5th Metatarsal: This is more common than a jones fracture. The classic history is a dancer. It may be **secondary to tug from the lateral cord of the plantar aponeurosis or peroneus brevis** (this is controversial).

Stress Fracture of the 5th Metatarsal: This is considered a high risk fracture (hard to heal).

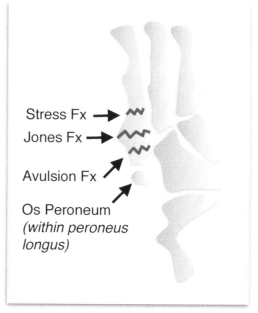

Stress Fx →

Jones Fx →

Avulsion Fx

Os Peroneum *(within peroneus longus)*

LisFranc Injury: This is the **most common dislocation of the foot**. The Lisfranc joint is the articulation of the tarsals and metatarsal heads. This joint would make a good place to amputate if you were a surgeon assisting in the Napoleonic invasion of Russia. The LisFranc ligament connects the medial cuneiform to the 2nd metatarsal base on the plantar aspect. If the ligament goes out you can see two patterns: (1) "Homo-lateral" - everyone moves lateral, (2) "Divergent" - the 1st MT goes medial, the 2nd-5th MT goes lateral.

What you need to know:
- Can't exclude it on a non-weight bearing film
- Associated fractures are most common at the base of the 2nd MT - *"Fleck Sign"*
- Fracture non-union and post traumatic arthritis are gonna occur if you miss it (plus a lawsuit).

"Fleck Sign" - This is a small bony fragment in the LisFranc Space (between 1st MT and 2nd MT) - that is associated with an avulsion of the LF ligament.

Spine: *Fractures and other acquired pathologies of the spine are discussed in detail in the spine section of the neuro chapter (volume 2, module 6).*

Stress / Insufficiency Fractures:

Stress Fracture vs Insufficiency Fracture: A stress fracture is the result of abnormal stress on normal bone. An insufficiency fracture is the result of normal stress on abnormal bone.

Compressive Side vs Tensile Side: This comes up in two main areas - the femoral neck and the tibia. Fractures of the compressive side are constantly getting pushed back together - these do well. Fractures of the tensile side are constantly getting pulled apart - these are a pain in the ass to heal.

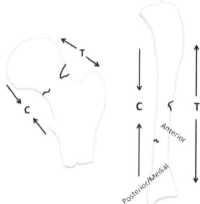

Compressive vs Tensile Forces
-Femoral Neck and Tibia

- **Femoral Stress Fracture:** Fractures along the compressive (medial) side are more common, typically seen in a younger person along the inferior femoral neck. Fractures along the tensile (lateral) side are more common in old people.

- **Tibial Stress Fracture:** This is the *most common site of a stress fracture in young athletes.* These are most common on the compressive side (posterior medial) in either the proximal or distal third. Less common are the tensile side (anterior) fractures, and these favor the mid shaft. They are bad news and don't heal - often called "***dreaded black lines.***"

SONK (Spontaneous Osteonecrosis of the Knee): This is totally named wrong, as it is another type of insufficiency fracture. You see this in old ladies with the classic history of "sudden pain after rising from a seated position." Young people can get it too (much less common), usually seen after a meniscal surgery.

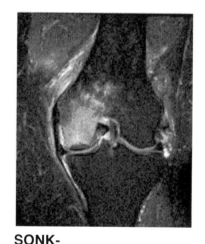

SONK-
-Diffuse Increased Signal (edema)

Things to know about SONK:
- *It's an insufficiency fracture (NOT osteonecrosis)* <u>think SINK not SONK</u>
- *Favors the medial femoral condyle (area of maximum weight bearing) -*
- *Usually unilateral in an old lady without history of trauma*
- *Associated with meniscal injury*

Navicular Stress Fracture – You see these in runners who run on hard surfaces. The thing to know is that just like in the wrist, the navicular is high risk for AVN.

March Fracture: This is a metatarsal stress fracture, which is fairly common. Classically seen in military recruits that are marching all day long.

Calcaneal Stress Fracture – The calcaneus is actually the most fractured tarsal bone. The fractures are usually intra-articular (75%). The stress fracture will be seen, with the fracture line perpendicular to the trabecular lines.

High Risk vs Low Risk Stress Fractures: You can sort these based on the likelihood of uncomplicated healing when treated conservatively.

High Risk	Low Risk
Femoral Neck (tensile side)	Femoral Neck (compressive side)
Transverse Patellar Fracture	Longitudinal Patellar Fracture
Anterior Tibial Fracture (midshaft)	Posterior Medial Tibial Fracture
5th Metatarsal	2nd and 3rd Metatarsal
Talus	Calcaneus
Tarsal Navicular	
Sesamoid Great Toe	

Osteoporosis / Osteopenia & Complications:

Osteopenia: This just means increased lucency of bones. Although this is most commonly caused by osteoporosis that is not always the case.

Osteomalacia: This is a soft bone from excessive uncalcified osteoid. This is typically related to vitamin D issues (either renal causes, liver causes, or other misc causes). It generally looks just like diffuse osteopenia. For the purpose of multiple choice you should think about 4 things; Ill-defined trabeculae, Ill-defined corticomedullary junction, bowing, and "Looser's Zones."

Looser Zones: These things are wide lucent bands that transverse bone at right angles to the cortex. You should think two things: **osteomalacia** and **rickets**. Less common is OI. The other piece of trivia is to understand **they are a type of insufficiency fracture**.

Osteoporosis: The idea is that you have low bone density. Bone density peaks around 30 and then decreases. It decreases faster in women during menopause. The imaging findings are a thin sharp cortex, prominent trabecular bars, lucent metaphyseal bands, and spotty lucencies.

Causes: Age is the big one. Medications (steroids, heparin, dilantin), Endocrine issues (cushings, hyperthryoidism), Anorexia, and Osteogenesis Imperfecta.

Complications: Fractures – Most commonly of the spine (2nd most common is the hip, 3rd most common is the wrist).

DEXA: This is a bone mineral density test and an excellent source of multiple choice trivia.

General Things to know about DEXA
- T score = Density relative to young adult
- T score defines osteopenia vs osteoporosis
- T score > 1.0 = Normal, -1.0 to -2.5 = Osteopenia, < **-2.5 Osteoporosis**
- Z score = Density relative to aged match control "to **Za Zame** Age"
- False negative / positives (see below)

False Positive / Negative on DEXA: DEXA works by measuring the density. Anything that makes that higher or lower than normal can fool the machine.

False Positive:
- Absent Normal Structures: Status post laminectomy

False Negative:
- Including excessive Osteophytes, dermal calcifications, or metal
- Including too much of the femoral shaft when doing a hip - can elevate the number as the shaft normally has denser bone.
- Compression Fx in the area measured

Reflex Sympathetic Dystrophy (RSD):

Can cause severe osteopenia (like disuse osteopenia). Some people say it **looks like unilateral RA, with preserved joint spaces**. Hand and shoulder are most common sites of involvement. May occur after trauma or infection resulting in an overactive sympathetic system. It's one of the many causes of a 3 phase hot bone scan. In fact, *intra-articular uptake* of tracer on bone scan in patients with RSD (secondary to the increased vascularity of the synovial membrane), and this is somewhat characteristic.

Transient Osteoporosis:

There are two types of presentations.:

Transient osteoporosis of the hip: For the purpose of multiple choice tests by far you should expect to see the **female in the 3ʳᵈ trimester of pregnancy** with involvement of the left hip. Having said that, it's actually more common in men in whom it's usually bilateral. The joint space should remain normal. It's self limiting (hence the word transient) and resolves in a few months. *Plain film shows osteopenia, MRI shows Edema, Bone scan shows increased uptake focally.*

Regional migratory osteoporosis - This is an idiopathic disorder which has a very classic history of **pain** in a joint, which gets better then shows up in another joint. It's associated with osteoporosis – which is also self limiting. It's more common in men.

Osteoporotic Compression Fracture: Super Common. On MR you want to see a *"band like"* fracture line - which is typically T1 dark (T2 is more variable). The non-deformed portions of the vertebral body should have normal signal.

Neoplastic Compression Fracture: Most vertebral mets don't result in compression fracture until nearly the entire vertebral body is replaced with tumor. If you see abnormal marrow signal (not band like) with involvement of the posterior margin you should think about cancer. *Next step ?* - look at the rest of the spine - mets are often multiple.

OCDs/ OCLs

Osteochondritis Dissecans (OCD): The new terminology is actually to call these "OCLs" (the "L" is for Lesion). This a spectrum of aseptic separation of an osteochondral fragment which can lead to gradual fragmentation of the articular surface and secondary OA. Most of the time it is secondary to trauma, although it could also be secondary to AVN.

Where it happens: Classic locations include the femoral condyle (most common site in the knee), patella, talus, and capitellum.

Staging: There is a staging system, which you probably need to know exists.

- Stage 1: Stable – Covered by intact cartilage, Intact with Host Bone
- Stage 2: Stable on Probing, Partially not intact with host bone.
- Stage 3: Unstable on Probing, Complete discontinuity of lesion.
- Stage 4: Dislocated fragment

Treatment / Who cares? If the fragment is unstable you can get secondary OA. You want to **look for high T2 signal undercutting the fragment from the bone to call it unstable** (edema can force a false positive). Thus, the absence of high T2 signal at the bone fragment interface is a good indicator of osseous bridging and stability. Granulation tissue at the interface (which will enhance with Gd), does not mean it's stable.

Osteochondroses: These are a group of conditions (usually seen in childhood) that are characterized by involvement of the epiphysis,or apophysis with findings of collapse, sclerosis, and fragmentation – suggesting osteonecrosis.

Kohlers	Tarsal Navicular	Male 4-6. Treatment is not surgical.
Freiberg Infraction	Second Metatarsal Head	Adolescent Girls – can lead to secondary OA
Severs	Calcaneal Apophysis	Some say this is a normal "growing pain"
Panners	Capitellum	Kid 5-10 "Thrower" ; does not have loose bodies.
Perthes	Femoral Head	White kid; 4-8.
Kienbock	Carpal Lunate	Associated with negative ulnar variance. Seen in person 20-40.

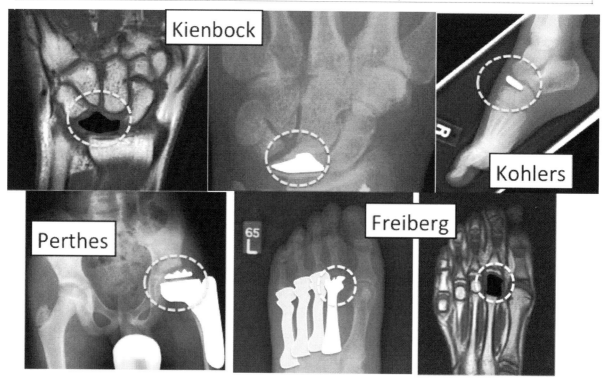

166

Soft Tissue Injury / Acquired *(stuff likely shown with MRI)*

MRI of the Wrist / Hand:

Don't panic if you are shown a MRI of the wrist, there are only a few things that they can show you. First let's briefly review the anatomy. With regard to the extensor tendons there are four things to know:

- There are 6 extensor compartments (5 fingers + 1 for good luck).

- First compartment (APL and EPB) are the ones affected in de Quervain's

- Third compartment has the EPL which courses beside Lister's Tubercle.

- The sixth compartment (Extensor Carpi Ulnaris) – can get an early tenosynovitis in rheumatoid arthritis.

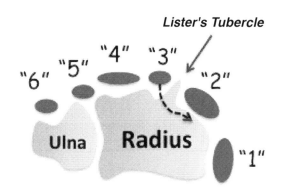

Carpal Tunnel: They could show you the carpal tunnel, but only to ask you about anatomy.

What goes through the carpal tunnel (more easily asked as what does NOT go through)?

Knowing what is in (and not in) the carpal tunnel is high yield for multiple choice testing. The tunnel lies deep to the palmaris longus, and is defined by 4 bony prominences (pisiform, scaphoid tubercle, hook of hamate, trapezium tubercle), with the transverse carpal ligament wrapping the contents in a fibrous sheath.

The tunnel contains 10 things (4 Flexor Profudus, 4 Flexor Superficials, 1 Flexor Pollicis Longus, and 1 Median Nerve). The Flexor Carpi Radialis is not truly in the tunnel. The extensor tendons are on the other side of the hand. Note that flexor pollicis longus goes through the tunnel, but flexor pollicis brevis does not (it's an intrinsic handle muscle). Palmaris longus (if you have one) does NOT go through the tunnel.

Does NOT go through the tunnel
-Flexor Carpi Radialis
-Flexor Carpi Ulnaris
-Palmaris Longus (if you have one)
-Flexor Pollicis BREVIS

Anatomic Trivia Regarding the Spaces of the Wrist:

Which synovial spaces normally communicate ? The answer is **pisiform recess and radiocarpal joint**. I can think of two ways to ask this (1) related to fluid – the bottom line is that excessive fluid in the pisiform recess should not be considered abnormal if there is a radiocarpal effusion, and (2) that either space can be used for wrist arthrography.

Other joint spaces in the body, easily lending to multiple choice testing:

Glenohumeral Joint and Subacromial Bursa	Should NOT communicate. Implies the presence of a full thickness rotator cuff tear.
Ankle Joint and Common (lateral) Peroneal Tendon Sheath	Should NOT communicate. Implies a tear of the calcaneofibular Ligament.
Achilles Tendon and Posterior Subtalar Joint	Should NOT communicate. The Achilles tendon does NOT have a true tendon sheath.
Pisifrom Recess and Radiocarpal Joint	Should normally communicate.

Common Pathology Seen on MRI of the Wrist / Hand:

Triangular Fibrocartilage Tears: These can be acute or chronic. The acute one is going to be a young person with a tear on the ulnar side. The chronic one is more likely to be shown with ulnar abutment syndrome (positive ulnar variance with cystic change in the lunate). Degeneration of this cartilage is common (50% at age 60).

Scapholunate Ligament Tear: The Terry Thomas look (gap between the scaphoid and lunate) on plain film. There are actually 3 parts (volar, dorsal, and middle), with the <u>dorsal band being the most important</u> for carpal stability. Predisposed for DISI deformity and all that crap I talked about earlier.

Kienbocks: AVN of the lunate, seen in people in their 20s-40s. *The most likely testable trivia is the association with negative ulnar variance.* It's going to show signal drop out on T1.

De Quervain's Tenosynovitis: This is the so called "Washer Woman's Sprain" or "Mommy Thumb" from repetitive activity / overuse. The classic history is "new mom - holding a baby." The affected area is the **first dorsal (extensor) compartment** (extensor pollicis brevis and abductor pollicis longus). This is way more common in women. The presence or absence of an intratendinous septum is a prognostic factor.

How it's shown:

- *This can be shown with ultrasound, as increased fluid within the first extensor tendon compartment*
- *This can be shown with MRI, as increased T2 signal in the tendon sheath*

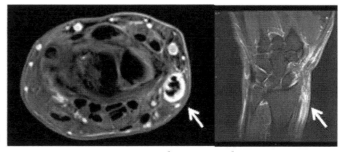

DeQuervain's Syndrome

Intersection Syndrome: A repetitive use issue (classically *seen in rowers*), where the first extensor compartment, cross over those of the second extensor compartment. The result is extensor carpi radialis brevis and longus tenosynovitis .

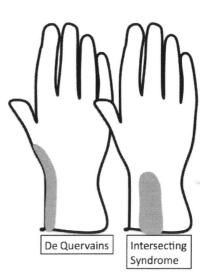

De Quervains | Intersecting Syndrome

Tenosynovitis : This is an inflammation of the tendon, with increased fluid seen around the tendon. This will be shown on MRI.

Diffuse:

- **Nontuberculous Mycobacterial Infection** – The hand and the wrist are the most common areas affected. This is a diffuse exuberant tenosynovitis that spares the muscles. It usually occurs in patients who are immunocompromised.

- **Rheumatoid Arthritis:** A nice trick is to show that multiple flexor tendons , or extensor carpi ulnaris - tenosynovitis can present as an early RA (before bone findings).

Focal:

- **Overuse:** This is going to be classic locations like 1st extensor compartment for De Quervains.

- **Infection:** The hard rule is that tenosynovitis of any flexor tendon is a surgical emergency as it can spread rapidly to the common flexors of the wrist. You can get increased pressures and necrosis of the tendons. Delayed treatment tend to do terrible.

Gamesmanship Wrist Compartments	
Isolated 1st	De Quervains
1st + 2nd	Intersecting
Isolated 6th	Early RA
Multiple Flexors	RA

Dupuytren Contracture: This is the most common of the fibromatoses. The classic scenario is a white person from North Europe with alcoholic liver disease. It's a nodular mass on the palmar aspect of the aponeurosis that progresses to cord–like thickening and eventual contracture (usually involving the 4th finger). It's bilateral about half the time.

Finger Tumor: They can show scalloping on a plain film of the finger, but if they want a single diagnosis they need to show a MRI. There is a long differential, but the only things they are going to show are:

- **Glomus Tumor:** This is a benign vascular tumor seen at the tips of fingers (75% in hand). It will be T1 low, **T2 bright**, and **enhance avidly**.

- **Giant Cell Tumor of the Tendon Sheath:** This is **basically PVNS of the tendon**. Typically found in the hand (palmar tendons). Can cause erosions on the underlying bone. Will be soft tissue density, and be **T1 and T2 dark** (contrasted to a glomus tumor which is T1 dark, T2 bright, and will enhance uniformly). **Will bloom on gradient**.

- **Fibroma:** This is a benign overgrowth of the tendon collagen. It's going to be low on T1 and low on T2. **Will NOT bloom like a GCT will.**

Finger Tip Tumors / Masses		
Glomus	T1 Dark, T2 Bright, Enhances avidly.	T2 Bright, Enhance Avidly.
Giant Cell Tumor Tendon	T1 Dark, T2 Dark, Variable Enhancement, Bloom on Gradient	Bloom on Gradient
Fibroma	T1 Dark, T2 Dark. No Blooming	Does NOT Bloom on Gradient.

Common Pathology Seen on MRI of the Elbow:

If you are shown an MRI of the Elbow don't panic, there are only a few things they can show you.

Cubital Tunnel Syndrome

- The result of repetitive valgus stress
- *Anatomy Trivia:* the site where the ulnar nerve passes beneath the cubital tunnel retinaculum also known as the epicondylo-olecranon ligament or Osborne band
- Can occur from compression by any pathology (tumor, hematoma, etc...) , when it occurs from an **accessory muscle** it's classically the **anconeus epitrochlearis**

Partial Ulnar Collateral Ligament Tear:

For the exam all you really need to know is that <u>throwers</u> (people who <u>valgus over load</u>) hurt their ulnar collateral ligament (which attaches on the medial coronoid - *sublime tubercle*). The ligament has three bundles, and the **anterior bundle is by far the most important**. If you get any images it is most likely going to be of the partial UCL tear, described as the **"T sign,"** with contrast material extending medial to the tubercle.

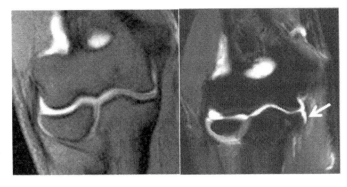

Normal   T-Sign
"UCL Partial Tear"

Panner Disease: This is one of the osteochondroses of the capitellum. It's seen in kids 5-10, and thought to be related to trauma from throwing (baseball playing). It looks a lot like an OCD lesion of the elbow (which also favors the capitellum).

Panner	Osteochondritis Dissecans
Affects the Capitellum	Also favors the Capitellum
Age 5-10	Teenager
Low T1, High T2	Low T1, High T2
No Loose Bodies	Loose Bodies

Lateral Epicondylitis *(more common than medial) – seen in Tennis Players -*
• Extensor Tendon Injury (classically extensor carpi radialis brevis)
• Radial Collateral Ligament Complex – Tears due to varus stress

Medial Epicondylitis *(less common than lateral) – seen in golfers*
• Common flexor tendon and ulnar nerve may enlarge from chronic injury

Epitrochlear Lymphadenopathy – This is a classic look for cat-scratch disease.

Dialysis Elbow: This is the result of olecranon bursitis from constant pressure on the area, related to positioning of the arm during treatment.

—

Common Pathology Seen on MRI of the Shoulder:

Impingement / Rotator Cuff Tears: This is a high yield / confusing subject that is worth talking about in a little more detail. In general, rotator cuff pathology is the result of overuse activity (sports) or impingement mechanisms. There are two types of impingement with two major sub-divisions within those types. Like many things in Radiology if you get the vocabulary down, the pathology is easy to understand.

External: This refers to impingement of the rotator cuff overlying the bursal surfaces (superficial surfaces) that are adjacent to the coracoacromial arch. As a reminder the arch is made up of the coracoid process, acromion, and coracoacromial ligament.

Primary External Causes (Abnormal Coracoacromial Arch) :

- The **hooked acromion** (type III Bigliani) is more associated with external impingement than the curved or flat types.

- **Subacromial osteophyte formation** or thickening of the coracoacromial ligament

- **Subcoracoid impingement**: Impingement of the subscapularis between the coracoid process and lesser tuberosity. This can be secondary to congenital configuration, or a configuration developed post traumatically after fracture of the coracoid or lesser tuberosity.

Secondary External Causes (Normal Coracoacromial Arch):

- "**Multidirectional Glenohumeral Instability**" – resulting in micro-subluxation of the humeral head in the glenoid, resulting in repeated microtrauma. The important thing to know is this is *typically seen in patients with generalized joint laxity*, often involving both shoulders.

Internal: This refers to impingement of the rotator cuff on the undersurface (deep surface) along the glenoid labrum and humeral head.

- **Posterior Superior:** This is a type of impingement that occurs when the posterior superior rotator cuff (junction of the supra and infraspinatus tendons) comes into contact with the posterior superior glenoid. Best seen in the ABER position, where these tendons get pinched between the labrum and greater tuberosity. This is seen in athletes who make overhead movements (throwers, tennis, swimming).

- **Anterior Superior:** This is internal impingement that occurs when the arm is in horizontal adduction and internal rotation. In this position, the undersurface of the biceps and subscapularis tendon may impinge against the anterior superior glenoid rim.

High Yield Trivia Points on Impingement	
Subacromial Impingement – most common form, resulting from attrition of the coracoacromial arch.	Damages **Supraspinatus Tendon**.
Subcoracoid Impingement – Lesser tuberosity and coracoid do the pinching.	Damages **Subscapularis**
Posterior Superior Internal Impingement – Athletes who make overhead movements. Greater tuberosity and posterior inferior labrum do the pinching.	Damage **Infraspinatus** (and posterior fibers of the supraspinatus).

Rotator Cuff Tears: A tear of the articular surface is more common (3x more) than the bursal surface. The underlying mechanism is usually degenerative, although trauma can certainly play a role. The **most common of the four muscles to tear is the Supraspinatus**. The teres minor is the least common to tear. **A partial tear that is > 50% is what the surgeon wants to know**.

"Massive rotator cuff tear" - refers to at least 2 out of the 4 rotator cuff muscles.

A final general piece of trivia is that a tear of the fibrous rotator cuff interval (junction between anterior fibers of the Supraspinatus and superior fibers of the subscapularis), is still considered a rotator cuff tear.

How do you know it's a full thickness tear? You will have high T2 signal in the expected location of the tendon. On T1 you will have **Gad in the bursa.**

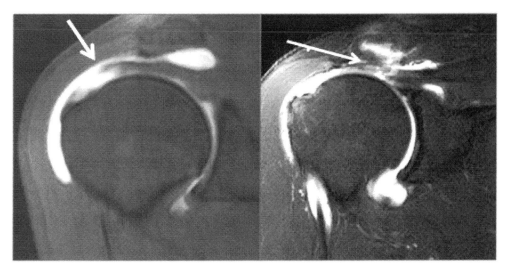

Full Thickness Tear

- With Gad crossing over the cuff into the bursa.

Injury to the Labrum:

SLAP: Labral tears favor the <u>superior</u> margin and track anterior to posterior. As this tear involves the labrum at the insertion of the long head of the biceps ,injury to this tendon is associated and part of the grading system (type 4).

Things to know about SLAP tears:

- When the SLAP extends into the biceps anchor (type 4) the surgical management changes from a debridement to a debridement + biceps tenodesis.

- The mechanism is usually an over-head movement (classic = swimmer)

- People over 40 usually have associated Rotator Cuff Tears injury

- **NOT associated with Instability** *(usually)*

SLAP Mimic - The Sublabral Recess. This is essentially a normal variant where you have incomplete attachment of the labrum at 12 o'clock. The 12 o'clock position on the labrum has the shittiest blood flow - that's why you see injury there and all these development variants.

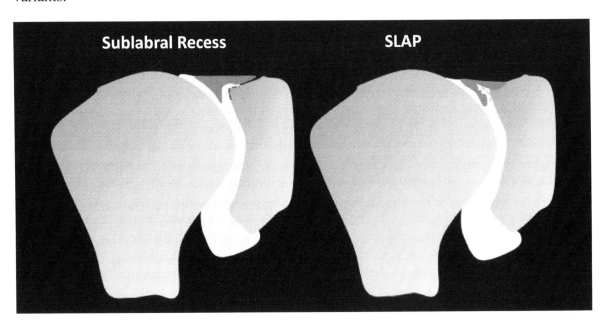

Follows Contour of Glenoid
SMOOTH Margin
Located at Biceps Anchor

Extends Laterally
Ratty Margin
Located at Biceps Anchor & Posteriorly

Labral Tear Mimic - The Sublabral Foramen -
The is an unattached (<u>but present</u>) portion of the
labrum - located at the anterior-superior labrum
(1 o'clock to 3 o'clock).

As a rule it should NOT extend below the equator
(3 o'clock position).

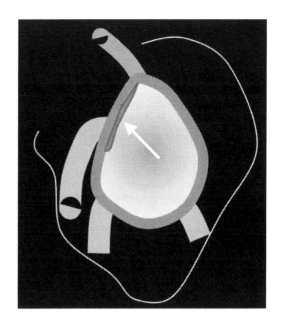

Labral Tear Mimic - The Buford Complex - A commonly tested (and not infrequently
seen) variant is the Buford Complex. It's present in about 1% of the general population. This
consists of an **<u>absent</u> anterior/superior labrum** (1 o'clock to 3 o'clock)**, along with a
thickened middle glenohumeral ligament**.

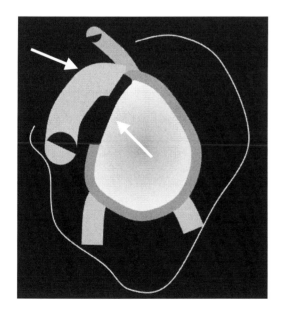

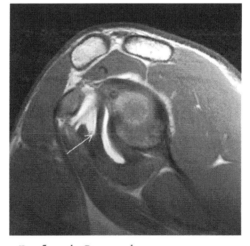

Buford Complex
-Thick Middle GH Ligament

Bankart Lesions: There is an alphabet soup of Bankart (anterior dislocation) related injuries.

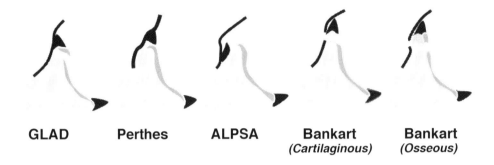

GLAD   **Perthes**   **ALPSA**   **Bankart**   **Bankart**
                                  (Cartilaginous)   *(Osseous)*

GLAD = Glenolabral Articular Disruption. It's the most mild version, and it's basically a superficial anterior inferior labral tear with associated articular cartilage damage ("impaction injury with cartilage defect"). Not typically seen in patient's with underlying laxity. It's common in sports. **No instability** *(aren't you GLAD there is no instability)*

Perthes = Detachment of the anteroinferior labrum (3-6 o'clock) with medially stripped but *intact periosteum*.

ALPSA = Anterior Labral Periosteal Sleeve Avulsion. Medially displaced labroligamentous complex with absence of the labrum on the glenoid rim. *Intact periosteum*. It scars down to glenoid.

True Bankart: Can be cartilaginous or osseous. *The periosteum is disrupted*. There is often an associated Hill Sach's fracture.

GLAD	Perthes	ALPSA	True Bankart
Superficial partial labral injury with cartilage defect	Avulsed anterior labrum (only minimally displaced). Inferior GH complex still attached to periosteum	Similar to perthes but with "bunched up" medially displaced inferior GH complex	Torn labrum
No instability	Intact Periosteum (lifted up)	Intact Periosteum	*Periosteum Disrupted*

Misc - Shoulder

HAGL: A non Bankart lesion that is frequently tested is the **HAGL** (Humeral avulsion glenohumeral ligament). This is an **avulsion of the inferior glenohumeral ligament**, and is most often the result of an anterior shoulder dislocation (just like all the above bankarts). The "J Sign" occurs when the normal U-shaped inferior glenohumeral recess is retracted away from the humerus appearing as a J.

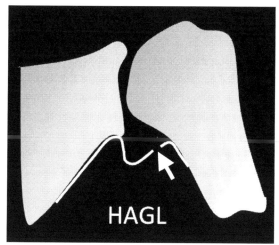
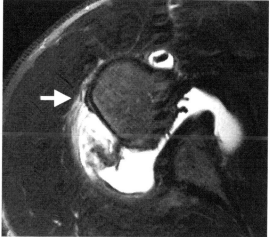

Subluxation of the Biceps Tendon: The subscapularis attaches to the lesser tuberosity. It sends a few fibers across the bicipital groove to the greater tuberosity ,which is called the "transverse ligament". A tear of the subscapularis opens these fibers up and allows the biceps to dislocate (usually medial). **Subscapularis Tear = Medial Dislocation of the Long Head of the Biceps Tendon.**

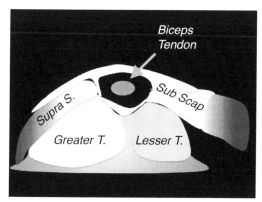

Sub Scap Tendon - Forming portions of the *"Transverse Ligament"* that holds the biceps tendon in the grove

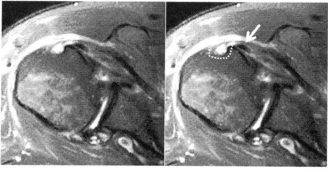

Subluxation of Biceps Tendon
Occurs with Tear of the Subscapularis

179

Nerve Entrapment: *High Yield Trivia:*

Suprascapular Notch vs Spinoglenoid Notch: A cyst at the level of the suprascapular notch will affect the supraspinatus and the infraspinatus. At the level of the spinoglenoid notch it will only affect the infraspinatus.

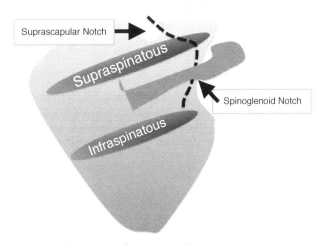

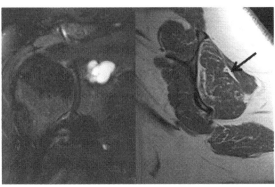

Cyst in the spinoglenoid notch causing fatty atrophy of the Infraspinatus

***Dotted Line = Suprascapular Nerve

Quadrilateral Space Syndrome: Compression of the Axillary Nerve in the Quadrilateral Space (usually from fibrotic bands). They will likely show this with **atrophy of the teres minor**. Another classic question is to name the borders of the quadrilateral space: Teres Minor Above, Teres Major Below, Humeral neck lateral, and Triceps medial.

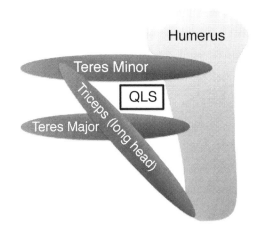

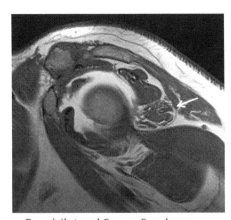

Quadrilateral Space Syndrome
– Atrophy of Teres Minor

Parsonage-Turner Syndrome: Think about this when you see muscles affected by pathology in two or more nerve distributions (suprascapular and axillary etc..). The condition is an idiopathic involvement of the brachial plexus.

MRI of the Knee

I want to focus on how the RCR is likely to ask the questions with two main pathways: (1) Total Trivia (2) Aunt Minnie Images

Anatomy:

Ligaments: The ACL has two bundles. The long one (anteromedial) tightens the knee in flexion. The short one (posterior lateral) tightens the knee in extension. The PCL is the strongest ligament in the knee (you don't want a posterior dislocation of your knee resulting in dissection of your popliteal artery).

Meniscus: The meniscus is "C shaped", thick along the periphery and thin centrally. There are two main things to know about the meniscus:

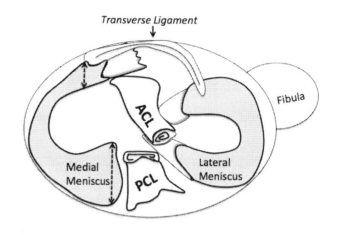

- Medial meniscus is thicker posteriorly. Lateral meniscus has equal thickness between anterior and posterior portion.

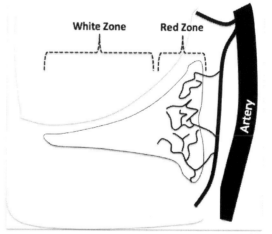

- The Peripheral "Red Zone" is vascular and might heal. The Central "white zone" is avascular and will not heal.

- The blood supply comes from the geniculate arteries (which enter peripherally).

- There are two meniscofemoral ligaments (Wrisberg, Humphry) which can be mimics of meniscal tears. Wrisberg is in the back (*"humping Humphry"*). You could also remember that "H" comes before "W" in the alphabet.

Tendons:

- The conjoint tendon is formed by the biceps femoris tendon and the LCL.

- The PCL and Patellar tendon may have foci of intermediate signal intensity on sagittal images with short echo time (TE) sequences where the tendon forms an angle of 55 degrees with the main magnetic field (***magic angle phenomenon***). This will NOT be seen on T2 sequences (with long TE). This phenomenon is reduced at higher field strengths due to greater shortening of T2 relaxation times.

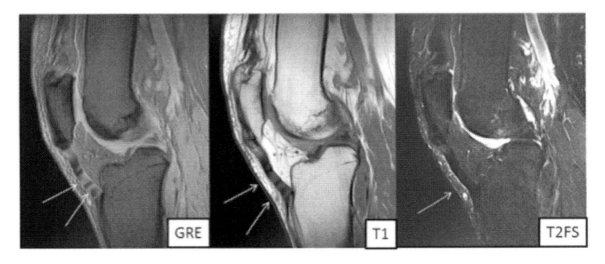

Magic Angle: You see it on short TE sequences (T1, PD, GRE). It goes away on T2.

Pathology:

Meniscal Tears: The peripheral meniscus (red zone) has better vasculature than the inner 2/3s (white zone) and might heal on its own. Broadly you can think about tears as either vertical or horizontal. Vertical tears can be sub divided into radial and longitudinal.

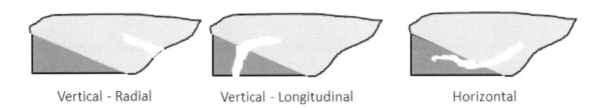

Vertical - Radial   Vertical - Longitudinal   Horizontal

Meniscal cysts are most often seen near the lateral meniscus and are often associated with horizontal cleavage tears.

Meniscocapsular Separation: The deepest layer of the **MCL** complex (capsular ligament) is relatively weak and is the first to tear; therefore there is an association with meniscocapsular separation.

Discoid Meniscus: This is a normal variant of the **lateral meniscus** that is **prone to tear.** It's not C-shaped, but instead shaped like a disc. In other words, it's too big (too many bow-ties!).

There are three types, with the most rare and most prone to injury being the *Wrisberg Variant.*

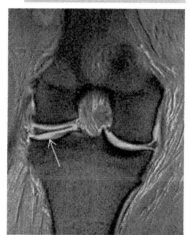

Discoid Meniscus

Bucket Handle Tear: This is a torn meniscus (usually **medial** - 80%), that flips medially to lie anterior to the PCL. The classic Aunt Minnie appearance is that of a "**double PCL.**" Another piece of trivia is that a double PCL can **only occur in the setting of an intact ACL**, otherwise it won't flip that way. Just know it sorta indirectly proves the ACL is intact (I can just see some knucklehead asking that).

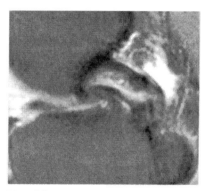

Double PCL
-Bucket Handle Meniscal Tear

Meniscal Ossicle: This is a focal ossification of the posterior horn of the medial meniscus, that can be secondary to trauma or simply developmental. They are often associated with radial root tears.

CL Tear: ACL tears happen all the time, usually in people who are stopping and pivoting.

Things to know about ACL tears:
- Associated with Segond Fracture
- ACL Angle lesser than Blumensaat's Line
- **O'donoghue's Unhappy Triad: ACL Tear, MCL Tear, Medial Meniscal**
- *Classic Kissing Contusion Pattern:* The lateral femoral condyle (sulcus terminals) bangs into the posterior lateral tibial plateau. This is 95% specific in adults.

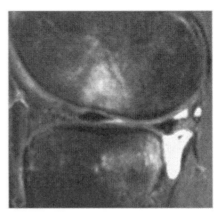

ACL Tear
"Kissing Contusion Pattern"

ACL Mucoid Degeneration: This can mimic acute or chronic partial tear of the ACL. There will be no secondary signs of injury (contusion etc..). It predisposes to ACL **ganglion cysts**, and they are usually seen together. The **T2/STIR buzzword is "celery stalk"** because of the striated look. The **T1 buzzword is "drumstick"** because it looks like a drum stick.

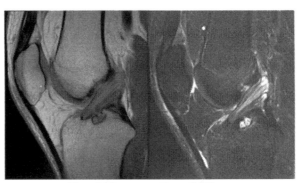

Mucoid Degeneration of ACL
-*"Drumstick / Celery Stick"*

ACL Repair:

- Method 1: Using the middle one-third of the patellar tendon, with the patella bone plug attached to one end and tibial bone plug attached at the other.

- Method 2: Use a four-strand hamstring graft often made of semitendinosus or gracilis tendon, or both. Then fold and braid the segment to form a quadruple-thickness structure. The graft is then attached with interference screws, endobuttons, or staples. There is a lower reported morbidity related to harvest site using this method.

Posterior Lateral Corner (PLC)- The most complicated anatomy in the entire body. My God this posterior lateral corner! Just think about the LCL, the IT band, the biceps femoris, and the popliteus tendon. If you see injury to any of those (or edema in the fibular head), you need to question PLC injury (instability).

Who cares? *Missed PLC injury is a very common cause of ACL reconstruction failure.*

Complications:

"Roof Impingement" – If the tibial tunnel is placed too far anterior (partially or completely anterior to the intersection of the Blumensaat line), the graft may bump up against the anterior inferior margin of the intercondylar roof. The **positioning of the tibial tunnel is the primary factor in preventing impingement.**

"Maintaining Isometry" – "Isometry" is a word Orthopods use to define constant length and tension of the graft during full range of motion. Positioning of the **femoral tunnel** is the primary factor in maintaining isometry.

"Arthrofibrosis" Can be focal or diffuse (focal is more common). The focal form is the so called **"Cyclops" lesion** – so named because of its arthroscopic appearance. It's gonna be a low signal speculated mass-like scar in Hoffa's fat pad. It's bad because it limits extension.

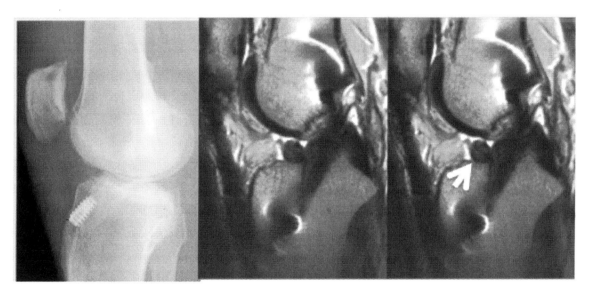

Cyclops Lesion – Scar associated with ventral graft

"Graft Tear" The graft is most susceptible to tear in the remodeling process (4-8 months post op). Signs of graft tear are increased T2 signal, and fiber discontinuity. Uncovering of the posterior horn of the lateral meniscus, and anterior tibial translation are considered good secondary signs.

PCL Tear: The posterior collateral ligament is the strongest ligament in the knee. A tear is actually uncommon, but you should think about it with a posterior dislocation.

Patella Dislocation - Dislocation of the patella is usually lateral because of the shape of the patella and femur. The contusion pattern is classic.

Things to know about Patella Dislocation:
- It's Lateral
- Contusion Pattern - Classic
- Associated tear of the MPFL (medial patellar femoral ligament)

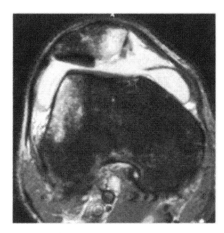

Patella Dislocation
Classic Contusion Pattern

—

The Foot / Ankle:

I'll lead with the most likely anatomic trivia, which is the tendons at the medial and lateral ankle.

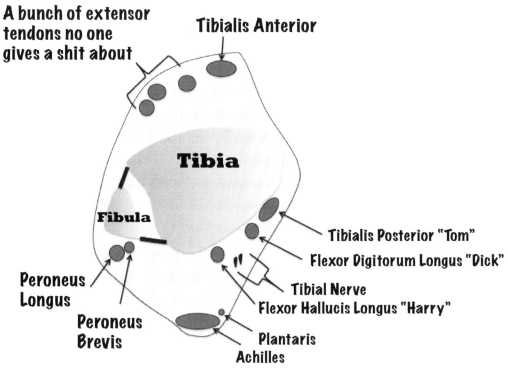

The Mythical **Master Knot of Henry -** This has a funny sounding name, therefore it's high yield. This is where Dick (FDL) crosses over Harry (FHL) at the medial ankle.

Whats the Master Knot of Henry? It's a "Harry Dick"

Common Pathology Seen on MRI of the Ankle / Foot:

Ligamentous Injury: The highest yield fact is that the **anterior talofibular ligament is the weakest ligament and the most frequently injured** (usually from inversion).

Posterior Tibial Tendon Injury / Dysfunction: This results in a progressive flat foot deformity, as the PTT is the primary stabilizer of the longitudinal arch. When chronic, the tear is most common behind the medial malleolus (this is where the most friction is). When acute, the tear is most common at the insertion into the navicular bone. **Acute Flat Arch should make you think of PTT tear.** You will also have a hindfoot valgus deformity (from unopposed peroneal brevis action). The other point of trivia to know is that the spring ligament is a secondary supporter of the arch (it holds up the talar head), and it will thicken and degenerate without the help of the PTT. Don't get it twisted though, the spring ligament is very thick and strong and almost never ruptures in a foot/ankle trauma.

I Say Acute Flat Foot, You Say Posterior Tibial Tendon Injury

Classic Progression - *PTT out then Spring Ligament Out, Then Sinus Tarsi gets jacked, then you heel strike on a painful flat foot and get plantar fasciitis*

Split Peroneus Brevis: You can see longitudinal splits in the peroneus in people with inversion injuries. The history is usually "chronic ankle pain". The tendon will be C shaped or **boomerang shaped** with central thinning and partial envelopment of the peroneus longus. Alternatively, there may be 3 instead of 2 tendons. The tear occurs at the lateral malleolus. There is a strong (80%) association with lateral ligament injury.

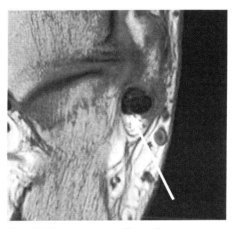

Split Peroneus Brevis
-Boomerang

Anterolateral Impingement Syndrome: Injury to the anterior talofibular ligaments and tibiofibular ligaments (usually from an inversion injury) can cause lateral instability, and chronic synovial inflammation. You can eventually produce a "mass" of hypertrophic synovial tissue in the lateral gutter. The **MRI finding is a "meniscoid mass" in the lateral gutter of the ankle**, which is a balled up scar (**T1 and T2 dark**).

Sinus Tarsi Syndrome: The space between the lateral talus and calcaneus. The syndrome is caused by hemorrhage or inflammation of the synovial recess with or without tears of the associated ligaments (talocalcaneal ligaments, inferior extensor retinaculum). There are associations with rheumatologic disorders and abnormal loading (flat foot in the setting of a posterior tibial tendon tear). The **MRI finding is obliteration of fat in the sinus tarsi space**, and replacement with scar.

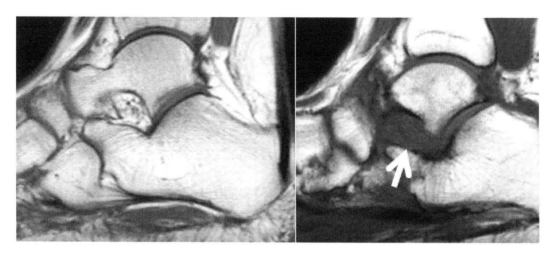

Normal Sinus Tarsi
-Full of Fat

Sinus Tarsi Syndrome
-Full of Scar

Tarsal Tunnel Syndrome: Pain in the distribution of the tibial nerve (first 3 toes), from compression as it passes through the tarsal tunnel (behind the medial malleolus). It's usually unilateral (unlike carpal tunnel which is usually bilateral).

Achilles Tendon Injury: Acute rupture is usually obvious. The ability to plantar flex should be lost on exam (*unless a plantaris muscle is intact - a common trick question*).

Xanthoma: Think about a xanthoma if the Achilles tendon is really enlarged / fusiform thickened. This can be seen in people with familial hypercholesterolemia, and is often bilateral.

Plantar Fasciitis: This is an inflammation of the fascia secondary to repetitive trauma. The pain is localized to the origin of the plantar fascia, and worsened by dorsiflexion of the toes. Buzzword is *"**most severe in the morning.**"* Plain film might show heel spurs, MRI may show a thickened fascia (> 4mm) , with increased T2 signal, most significant near its insertion at the heel. A bone scan may show increased tracer in the region of the calcaneus (from periosteal inflammation).

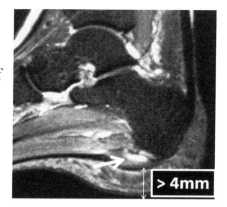

> 4mm

Plantar Fasciitis

Morton's Neuroma: Soft tissue mass shown between the 3rd and 4th metatarsal heads is most likely a Morton's Neuroma (especially on multiple choice tests). They classically show it on short axis, T1 (it will be dark). The proposed pathology results from compression / entrapment of the plantar digital nerve in this location by the intermetatarsal ligament. Over time this results in thickening and development of perineural fibrosis.

It's a big stupid scar, that looks like a dumbbell between the 3rd and 4th metatarsals. It's usually unilateral in a women.

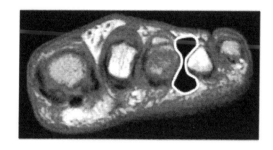

Morton's Neuroma
-Dumbbell Scar Between 3rd and 4th Metatarsals

Infection

Infection

With regard to osteomyelitis, radiographs will be normal for 7-10 days. Essentially, osteomyelitis can have any appearance , occur in any location, and at any age. Children have hematogenous spread usually hitting the long bones (metaphysis). Adults are more likely to have direct spread (in diabetic). However, you can have hematogenous spread in certain situations as well. General rule is that septic joins are more common in adults, osteomyeltitis is more common in kids.

Knee Jerks:
- *Osteomyelitis in Spine = IV Drug User*
- *Osteomyelitis in Spine with Kyphosis = Gibbus Deformity = TB*
- *Unilateral SI joint = IV Drug User*
- *Psoas Muscle Abscess = TB*

Hallmarks are destruction of bone and periosteal new bone formation.

Brodie's Abscess is a chronic infection (bone abscess). It's usually well circumscribed. It may have an osseous sequestrum (piece of necrotic bone surrounded by granulation tissue). As mentioned above, a sequestration has a DDx (Osetomyelitis, EG, Lymphoma, Fibrosarcoma).

Some frequently tested vocabulary:
- *Sequestrum = Piece of necrotic bone surround by granulation tissue*
- *Involucrum = Thick sheath of periosteal bone around sequestrum*
- *Cloaca = The space /tract where there dead bone lives*

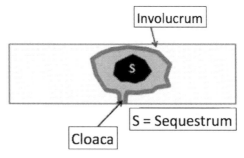

Acute bacterial osteomyelitis can be thought of in three different categories: 1) hematogenous seeding (*most common in child*), 2) contiguous spread, and 3) direct inoculation of the bone either from surgery or trauma.

Acute hematogenous osteomyelitis has a predilection for the long bones of the body, specifically the metaphysis, which has the best blood flow and allows for spreading of the infection via small channels in the bone that lead to the subperiosteal space.

More Trivia that Multiple Choice Writers Love:
- *Age < 1 month = Multicentric involvement,* ***often with joint involvement***
  - *Bone scan often negative (75%) at this age*
- *Age < 18 months = Spread to epiphysis through blood*
- *Age 2-16 years = Trans-physeal vessels are closed (primary focus is metaphysis).*

In the slightly older baby (<18 months) these vessels from the metaphysis to the epiphysis atrophy and the growth plate stops the spread (although spread can still occur). This creates a "septic tank" effect. This same thing happens with certain cancers (leukemia); the garbage gets stuck in the septic tank (metaphysis). Once the growth plates fuse, this obstruction is no longer present.

MRI findings of osteomyelitis: Low signal in the bone marrow on T1 imaging adjacent to an ulcer or cellulitis is diagnostic.

The Ghost Sign: *Neuropathic Bone vs Osteomyelitis in a Neuropathic Bone*
A bone that becomes a ghost (poor definition of margins) on T1 imaging, but then re-appears (more morphologically distinct) on T2, or after giving IV contrast is more likely to have osteomyelitis.

Discitis/ Osteomyelitis:

Infection of the disc and infection of the vertebral body nearly always go together. The reason has to do with the route of seeding; which typically involves seeding of the vertebral endplate (which is vascular), with subsequent eruption and crossing into the disc space, and eventual involvement of the adjacent vertebral body.

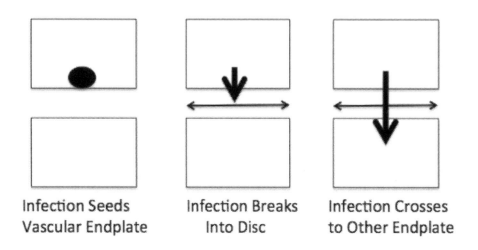

Infection Seeds Vascular Endplate   **Infection Breaks Into Disc**   **Infection Crosses to Other Endplate**

In adults, the source is usually from a recent surgery, procedure, or systemic infection. In children it's usually from hematogenous spread. For the Step 1 trivia: Staph A is the most common bug, and think gram negatives with an IV drug user. Almost always (80% of the time) the ESR and CRP are elevated.

Imaging: Early on it's very hard to see with plain films, you will need MRI. You are looking for paraspinal and epidural inflammation, T2 bright disc signal, and disc enhancement. Remember Gallium is superior to WBC scan in the spine. *This is discussed in the neuro chapter - spine section (volume 2, module 6).*

Pott's Disease: TB of the spine is more common in "developing" countries. It behaves in a few different ways, and that makes it easy to test on.

Things to know about TB in the spine:
- *It tends to **spare the disc space***
- *It tends to have multi-level thoracic "skip" involvement*
- *Buzzword "Large paraspinal abscess*
- *Buzzword "Calcified Psoas Abscess"*
- *Buzzword "Gibbus Deformity" – which is a destructive focal kyphosis*

Mimic - Brucellosis (unpasteurized milk) , can also have some disc space preservation.

Septic Arthritis You see this the most in large joints which have an abundant blood supply to the metaphysis (shoulder, hip, knee). *IV drug users will get it in the SI joint, and sternoclavicular joint.* Conventional risk factors include being old, having AIDS, RA, and prosthetic joints. On plain film you might see a joint effusion, or MRI will show synovial enhancement. If untreated this will jack your joint in less than 48hours.

> ***Pneumoarthrogram Sign***
> - If you can demonstrate air within a joint - you can exclude a joint effusion. No joint effusion = No septic joint.

Necrotizing Fasciitis: This is a very bad actor that kills very quickly. The good news is that it's pretty rare, typically only seen in HIVers, Transplant patients, diabetics, and alcoholics. It's usually polymicrobial (the second form is Group A Strep). **Gas is only seen in a minority of cases, but if you see gas in soft tissue this is what they want.** Diffuse fascial enhancement is what you'd see if the ER is dumb enough to order cross sectional imaging (they often are). Fournier Gangrene is what they call it in the scrotum.

TB: This is a special topic (high yield) with regard to MSK infection. It's not that common, with <5% of patients with TB having MSK involvement. Although on multiple choice tests, I think you'll find it appears with a high frequency.

Key Points to know:
- The vertebral body is involved with sparing of the disc space until late in the disease (very different than more common bacterial infections).
- *"Gibbus Deformity"* is a focal kyphosis seen in "Potts Disease" , among many other things.
- *"Rice Bodies"* – These are sloughed, infarcted synovium seen with end stage RA, and TB infection of joints.
- *Tuberculosis Dactylitis (Spina Ventosa)* – Typically affects kids more than adults with involvement of the short tubular bones of the hands and feet. It is often a smoldering infection without periosteal reaction. Classic look is a **diaphyseal expansile lesion** with soft tissue swelling.

Aggressive Lesions

There are tons of primary osseous malignancies, the most common are myeloma/ plasmacytoma (27%), Osteosarcoma (20%) and Chondrosarcoma (20%). According to Helms, the **wide zone of transition is the best sign that a lesion is aggressive**. This is actually a useful pearl.

Myeloma / Plasmacytoma / Mets - *Discussed in the cystic bone lesion section*

Osteosarcoma: There are a bunch of subtypes, but for the purpose of this discussion there are 4. Conventional Intramedullary (85%), Parosteal (4%), Periosteal (1%), Telangiectatic (rare). All the subtypes produce bone or osteoid from neoplastic cells. Most are idiopathic but you can have secondary causes (*usually seen in elderly*) XRT, Pagets, Infarcts, etc...

Conventional Intramedullary: More common, and higher grade than the surface subtypes (periosteal, and parosteal). Primary subtypes typically occur in young patients (10-20). The most common location is the femur (40%), and proximal tibia (15%).

Buzzwords include various types of aggressive periosteal reactions:

- *"Sunburst"*- periosteal reaction that is aggressive and looks like a sunburst
- *Codman triangle* - With aggressive lesions, the periosteum does not have time to ossify completely with new bone (e.g. as seen in single layer and multi-layered periosteal reaction), so only the edge of the raised periosteum will ossify – creating the appearance of a triangle.
- *Lamellated* (onion skin reaction) – multi layers of parallel periosteum, looks like an onion's skin.

High Yield Trivia:
- *Osteosarcoma met to the lung is a "classic" (frequently tested) cause of occult pneumothorax.*
- **"Reverse Zoning Phenomenon"** – more dense mature matrix in the center, less peripherally (*opposite of myositis ossificans*).

> **Pathologic Fracture - At risk ?**
>
> Reasons to be concerned include:
>
> (1) Lytic lesions,
> (2) Lesions > 3cm in size,
> (3) Lesions involving more than 50% of the cortex.
>
> *These measurements are CT or Plain film... NOT MRI.*

Parosteal Osteosarcoma: Generally low grade, **BULKY** parosteal bone formation. Think Big... just say Big. This guy loves the posterior distal femur (*because of this location it can mimic a cortical desmoid early on*). The lesion is metaphyseal 90% of the time. The buzzword is "***string sign***" – which refers to a radiolucent line separating the bulky tumor from the cortex.

Periosteal Osteosarcoma
Worse prognosis than parosteal but better than conventional osteosarcoma. Tends to occur in the diaphyseal regions, classic medial distal femur.

This vs That: **Parosteal vs Periosteal Osteosarcoma**	
Parosteal	**Periosteal**
Early Adult / Middle Age	Age Group (15-25)
Metaphysis (90%)	Diaphyseal
Likes Posterior Distal Femur	Likes Medial Distal Femur
Marrow extension (50%)	Usually no marrow extension
Low Grade	Intermediate Grade

Telangiectatic Osteosarcoma: About 15% have a narrow zone of transition. Fluid-Fluid levels on MRI is classic. They are High on T1 (from methemoglobin). Can be differentiated from ABC or GCT (maybe) by tumor nodularity and enhancement.

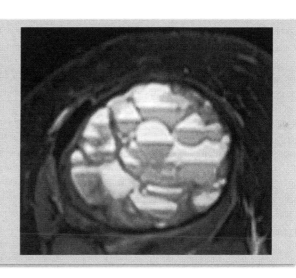

FLUID-FLUID LEVELS DDx:

Telangiectatic Osteosarcoma
Aneurysmal Bone Cyst
Giant Cell Tumor

Chondrosarcoma: Usually seen in older adults (M>F). Likes flat bones, limb girdles, proximal tubular bones. Can be central (intramedullary) or peripheral (at the end of an osteochondroma). Most are low grade.

Risk Factors: Pagets, and anything cartilaginous (osteochondromas, maffucci's etc...)

If you want to say chondroblastoma but it's an adult think clear cell chondrosarcoma

Ewings: *Permeative lesion in the diaphysis of a child = Ewings (could also be infection, or EG)*. Extremely rare in African-Americans. Likes to met bone to bone. Does NOT form osteoid from tumor cells, but can mimic osteosarcoma because of its marked sclerosis (*sclerosis occurs in the bone only, not in the soft tissue – which is NOT the case in osteosarcoma*).

Chordoma Usually seen in adults (30-60) , usually slightly younger in the clivus and slightly older in the sacrum. Most likely questions regarding the chordoma include location (**most common sacrum**, second most common clivus, third most common vertebral body), and the fact that they are **very T2 bright**.

Chordoma Most Commons:
* Most common primary malignancy of the spine.
* Most common primary malignancy of the sacrum.
* When involving the spine, most common at C2.
* Midline, Midline, Midline!

Aggressive Soft Tissue Lesions

Fibrosarcoma / Malignant Fibrous Histiocytoma (MFH)

* **Fibrosarcoma:** Just like osteosarcoma can be primary or secondary (from Pagets, infarct etc..) These are lytic malignant tumors that DO NOT produce osteoid or chondroid matrix. They are almost **"Always Lytic",** and may be permeative or moth eaten. Also **"NOT T2 Bright"** – which most tumors are.

* **MFH: Now called Pleomorphic Undifferentiated Sarcoma "PUS."** This actually used to be lumped in with Fibrosarcoma – but now they are separate. MFHs are way more common than Fibrosarcomas (***most common soft tissue sarcoma in adults***). From a radiology perspective, they look the same. So when you say one you should say the other.

   Trivia: Bone infarcts can turn into MFH - *"sarcomatous transformation of infarct"*

   Pearl: I like the old name "Fibrous" - because it reminds me that parts of the tumor will be dark on MR.

Synovial Sarcoma: Seen most commonly in the lower extremities of patients aged 20-40. They occur close to the joint (but **not in the joint**). To confuse the issue they may have secondary invasion into the joint (10%), however for the purpose of multiple choice tests they "never involve the joint."

They could show this tumor in 3 different ways: (1) as the "**triple sign**", which is high, medium, and low signal all in the same mass (probably in the knee) on T2, (2) as the "**bowl of grapes**" which is a bunch of fluid –fluid levels in a mass (probably in the knee), or (3) as a plain x-ray with a soft tissue component and calcifications – this would be the least likely way to show it.

Synovial Sarcoma Trivia:
- Most sarcomas don't attack bones; Synovial Sarcoma Can
- Most sarcomas present as painless mass; Synovial Sarcomas Hurt
- Soft tissue calcifications + Bone Erosions are highly suggestive
- They are slow growing and small in size often leading to people thinking they are B9.
- 90% have a translocation of X-18.
- Most common malignancy in teens/young adults of the **foot**, ankle, and lower extremity

When I say "Ball like tumor" in the extremity of a young adult, you say Synovial Sarcoma.

Liposarcoma - This is the second most common soft tissue sarcoma. You see it in middle aged people (40-60), with the classic location being the **retroperitoneum** (can also happen in the extremities). The most common type (well-differentiated) is also the least aggressive.

When I say "Fatty Mass in the retroperitoneum," you say Liposarcoma

Things that make you think it is a liposarcoma (and not a lipoma)
- Inhomogenous attenuation - soft tissues masses in the fat
- Infiltration of adjacent structures
- "Deep and Big"

Trivia: Myxoid Liposarcoma is the MC liposarcoma in patients < 20. - They can be T2 Bright (expected), but T1 dark (confusing) - don't call it a cyst. Don't call it a comeback (I've been here for years). They'll need gad+

Treatment High Yields

- *Osteosarcoma:* Chemo first (to kill micro mets) , followed by wide excision
- *Ewings:* Both Chemo and Radiation, followed by wide excision.
- *Chondrosarcoma:* usually just wide excision (they are usually low grade, and main concern is local recurrence).
- *Giant Cell Tumor:* Because it extends to the articular surface usually requires arthroplasty.

"Don't Touch Lesions" – Characteristically Benign Lesions, that look Aggressive but are NOT – and should NOT be biopsied because of possibly misleading pathology.		
Myositis Ossificans	Circumferential calcifications with a lucent center	Can look scary on MRI if imaged early because of edema, and avid enhancement
Avulsion Injury	Typical location near the pelvis	Can have an aggressive periosteal reaction
Cortical Desmoid	Characteristic location on the posterior medial epicondyle of the distal femur	Can be hot on bone scan.
Synovial Herniation Pit "Pitt's Pit"	Characteristic location in the femoral neck	Lytic appearing lesion

Bone Biopsy - The route of biopsy should be discussed with the orthopedic surgeon, to avoid contaminating compartments not involved by the tumor (or not going to be used in the resection process).

Special considerations:
- Pelvis: Avoid crossing gluteal muscles (may be needed for reconstruction).
- Knee: Avoid the joint space via crossing suprapatellar bursa or other communicating bursae. Avoid crossing the quadriceps tendon unless it is involved.
- Shoulder: Avoid the posterior 2/3rd (axillary nerve courses post -> anterior, therefore a posterior resection will denervate the anterior 1/3).

B9 Lesions

FEGNOMASHIC is the mnemonic for cystic bone lesions made popular by Clyde Helms. As it turns out, you can rearrange the letters of FEGNOMASHIC to form a word FOGMACHINES. I find it a lot easier to remember a mnemonic if it actually forms a real word. Having said that the whole idea of memorizing a list of 11 or 12 things is really stupid. You would never give a differential that included all of those, they occur in different places, in different ages, and often look very different. Differentials (for people who know what they are looking at) are usually never deeper than 3 or 4 things. If you are giving a differential of 12 things, just say you don't know what it is.

First a brief discussion of location & Age

> ### Age:
>
> The key to remember is that
> - *< 30 = EG, ABC, NOF, Chondroblastoma, and Solitary Bone Cysts*
> - *Any Age = Infection*
> - *> 40 = Mets and Myeloma (unless it's neuroblastoma mets).*

Epiphysis:

In general, only a few lesions tend to arise in the epiphysis. The "four horseman of the (e)apophysis" is the mnemonic I like to use, and I think about the company AIG that was involved in some scandal a few years ago. **AIG** "the evil" **Company.**

> **Epiphyseal Equivalents:**
>
> Big ones to remember are the carpals, the patella, the greater trochanter, and the calcaneus

ABC, Infection, Giant Cell, and Chondroblastoma.
The caveat is that ABC is usually metaphyseal but after the growth plate closes it can extend into the epiphysis.

For the purpose of multiple choice tests it is important to not forget about the malignant tumor at the end of the bone (epiphysis) – Clear Cell Chondrosarcoma. This guy is slow growing, with a variable appearance (lytic, calcified, lobulated, ill defined, etc…). Just remember **if they say malignant epiphyseal you say Clear Cell Chondrosarcoma.**

Metaphysis

The metaphysis is the fastest growing area of a bone, with the best blood supply. This excellent blood supply results in an increased predilection for Mets and Infection. Most of the cystic bone lesions can occur in the metaphysis.

Diaphysis

Just like the metaphysis, most entities can occur in the diaphysis (they just do it less).

Now a discussion on the pathology:

Fibrous Dysplasia: Fibrous dysplasia is a skeletal developmental anomaly of osteoblasts – failure of normal maturation and differentiation. The disorder can occur at any age . It can be monostotic (20s & 30s) or polyostotic (< 10 year old).

Famously has a very variably appearance, with phases like pagets (lytic, mixed, blastic). The buzzword is "**ground glass**." The catch phrase is "**long lesion in a long bone**." The textbook appearance "lytic lesion with a hazy matrix" The discriminator used by Helms is "**no periosteal reaction or pain**."

Likes the ribs and long bones. If it occurs in the pelvis, it also hits the ipsilateral femur (**Shepherd Crook deformity**). If it's multiple it likes the skull and face (Lion-like faces).

This vs That: McCune Albright vs Mazabraud Syndrome	
McCune Albright	**Mazabraud**
Polyostotic Fibrous Dysplasia	Polyostotic Fibrous Dysplasia
Girl	Woman (*middle aged*)
Café au lait spots	Soft Tissue Myxomas
Precocious Puberty	Increased Risk Osseous Malignant Transformation

Adamantinoma: A total zebra (*probably a unicorn*). A tibial lesion that **resembles fibrous dysplasia** (mixed lytic and sclerotic). It is potentially malignant.

Enchondroma: This guy is a tumor of the medullary cavity composed of hyaline cartilage. It appears as a lytic lesion with irregularly speckled calcification of chondroid matrix, classically described as **ARCS AND RINGS.** Having said that the **chondroid matrix is not found in the fingers or toes** *** *this is a high yield factoid for the purpose of multiple choice tests.* The enchondroma is actually the most common cystic lesion in the hands and feet. Just like fibrous dysplasia this lesion does not have periostitis.

The trick to differentiating enchondroma vs a low grade chondrosarcoma is the history of pain.

This vs That: **Ollier's vs Maffucci's**	
Ollier's	Maffucci's
ONLY Enchondromas	**MO**RE than just Enchondromas (also Hemangiomas) ***Look for those phleboliths!*
	Malignant potential (20% turn into chondrosarcoma, and other cancers GI, Ovary)

Eosinophilic Granuloma (EG): This is typically included in every differential for people less than 30. It can be solitary (usually) or multiple.

There are 3 classic appearances - for the purpose of multiple choice:
(1) Vertebra plana in a kid
(2) Skull with lucent "beveled edge" lesions (also in a kid).
(3) "Floating Tooth" with lytic lesion in alveolar ridge --- this would be a differential case

The appearance is highly variable and can be lytic or blastic, with or without a sclerotic border, and with or without a periosteal response. Can even have an osseous sequestrum.

Classic DDx for Vertebra Plana (MELT)
• Mets / Myeloma
• EG
• Lymphoma
• Trauma / TB

Classic DDx for Osseous Sequestrum:
• Osteomyelitis
• Lymphoma
• Fibrosarcoma
• EG
• *Osteoid Osteoma can mimic a sequestrum

Giant Cell Tumor (GCT): This guy has some key criteria (which lend themselves well to multiple choice tests). They include:
- Physis MUST be closed
- Non Sclerotic Border
- Abuts the articular surface

Another trick is to show you a pulmonary met, and ask if it could be GCT? The answer is yes (although this is rare) GCT is considered "quasi-malignant" because they can be locally invasive and about 5% will have pulmonary mets (which are still curable by resection). As a result of this, they should be resected with wide margins.

Things to know about GCTs:
- Most common in the knee - abutting the articular surface
- Most common at age 20-30 * physis must be closed
- There is an association with ABCs (they can turn into them)
- They are "quasi-malignant" - 5% have lung mets
- Fluid levels on MRI

Nonossifying Fibroma (NOF): These are very common. They are seen in children, and will spontaneously regress (becoming more sclerotic before disappearing). They are *rare in children not yet walking.* Just like GCTs they like to occur around the knee. They are classically described as eccentric with a thin sclerotic border (remember GCTs don't have a sclerotic border). They are called fibrous cortical defects when smaller than 2cm.

Vocab: NOFs are the larger version (>3cm) of a fibrous cortical defect (FCD). A wastebasket term for the both of them is simply "fibroxanthoma."

 Jaffe-Campanacci Syndrome: Syndrome of multiple NOFs, café-au-lait spots, mental retardation, hypogonadism, and cardiac malformations.

Osteoid Osteoma *"Pain at night, relieved by aspirin."* It's classically found in two spots (1) meta/diaphysis of long bones and (2) the posterior elements of the spine. One way to test this is to show a plain film that is probably an osteoid osteoma then follow it with an MRI showing "lots of edema." I'll say that again ***large amount of edema for the size of the lesion.***

Another piece of trivia is that when you have them in the spine (most common in the lumbar spine), you frequently have an associated **painful scoliosis** with the **convexity pointed away from the lesion.** These can be treated with percutaneous radiofrequency ablation (as long as it's not within 1cm of a nerve or other vital structure – *typically avoided in hands, spine, and pregnant patients*).

Association of Osteoid Osteoma
Painful Scoliosis
Growth Deformity: Increased length and girth of long bones
Synovitis: Can be seen if intra-articular, leading to early onset arthritis
Arthritis: Can occur from primary synovitis, or secondarily from altered joint mechanics.

Osteoblastoma: Basically it's an osteoid osteoma that is larger than 2cm. It's seen in patients < 30years old. They are most likely to show this in the posterior elements. It also occurs in the long bones (35%) and when it does it is usually diaphyseal (75%).

Metastatic Disease: Should be on the differential for any patient over 40 with a lytic lesion. As a piece of trivia renal cancer is ALWAYS lytic (usually).

> *Classic Blastic Lesions:* Prostate, Carcinoid, Medulloblastoma
> *Classic Lytic Lesions:* Renal and Thyroid

Multiple Myeloma (MM): Plasma cell proliferation increases surrounding osteolytic activity (in case someone asks you the mechanism). Usually in older patient (40s-80s). Plasmacytomas can precede clinical or hematologic evidence of myeloma by 3 years.

They usually have discrete margins, and can be solitary or multiple. Vertebral body destruction with sparing of the posterior elements is classic. Bone Scan is often negative, *skeletal survey is better* (but horrible pain to read), and MRI is the most sensitive.

Additional classic (testable) scenario: *MM manifesting as Diffuse Osteopenia*

Myeloma Related Conditions:

> ***Plasmacytoma*** *(usually under 40):* This is a discrete, solitary mass of neoplastic monoclonal plasma cells in either bone or soft tissue (*extramedullary sub type*). It is associated with latent systemic disease in the majority of affected patients. It can be considered as a singular counterpart multiple myeloma. The lesions look like a geographic lytic area, sometimes with **expansile** remodeling.
>
> *"Mini Brain Appearance"* – Plasmacytoma in vertebral body
>
> ***POEMS:*** This is basically "*Myeloma with Sclerotic Mets*." It's a rare medical syndrome with plasma cell proliferation (typically myeloma) with neuropathy, and organomegaly.

Aneurysmal Bone Cyst (ABC): Aneurysmal bone cysts are aneurysmal lesions of bone with thin-walled, blood-filled spaces (fluid-fluid level on MRI). Patients are usually < 30. They may develop following trauma.

Location: Tibia > Vert > Femur > Humerus

They can be described as primary ABC, presumably arising denovo or secondary ABC, associated with another tumor (classic GCT). They are commonly associated with other benign lesions.

Classic DDx for Lucent Lesion in Posterior Elements
• Osteoblastoma
• ABC
• TB

Things to know about ABC:
- Up to 40% of secondary ABC's are associated with giant cell tumor of bone.
- It's on the DDx for Fluid - Fluid Level on MRI
- Patient < 30
- Tibia is the most common site

Solitary (Unicameral) Bone Cyst: It would be unusual to see one of these in a patient older than 30. Most common in the tubular bones (90-95)% usually humerus or femur. Unique feature: "Always located centrally."

It's going to be shown one of two ways: (1) With a fracture through it in the humerus (probably with a fallen fragment sign) or (2) As a lucent lesion in the calcaneus (probably with a fallen fragment sign).

The *fallen fragment sign* (bone fragment in the dependent portion of a lucent bone lesion) is pathognomonic of solitary bone cyst.

Brown Tumor (Hyperparathyroidism): The "brown tumor" represents localized accumulations of giant cells and fibrous tissue (in case someone asks). They appear as lytic or sclerotic lesions with other findings of hyperparathyroidism (subperiosteal bone resorption). In other words, they need to tell you he/she has hyperparathyroidism first. They may just straight up tell you, or they will show you some bone resorption first (classically on the side of a finger, edge of a clavicle, or under a rib).

These things have different stages of healing / sclerosis. They resorb and can become totally sclerotic /healed, when the Hyper PTH is treated.

Chondroblastoma: This is seen in kids (90% age 5-25). They classically show it in two ways (1) In the epiphysis of the tibia on a 15 year old, or (2) in an epiphyseal equivalent.

So what are the epiphyseal equivalents???
- *Patella*
- *Calcaneus*
- *Carpal Bones*
- *And all the Apophyses (greater and less trochanter, tuberosities, etc...)*

Features of the tumor include; A thin sclerotic rim, extension across the physeal plate (25-50%), periostitis (30%). Actual location: femur > humerus > tibia . This may show bone marrow edema, and soft tissue edema on MRI (MRI can mislead you into thinking it's a bad thing). This is one of the only bone lesions that is often **NOT T2 bright**. They tend to reoccur after resection (like 30% of the time).

Gamesmanship Hip: When you have a chondroblastoma in the hip, it tends to *favor the greater trochanter (more than the femoral epiphysis).*

Chondromyxoid fibroma*:* This is the least common benign lesion of cartilage. It is usually in patients younger than 30. The typical appearance is osteolytic, elongated in shape, eccentrically located, metaphyseal lesion, with cortical expansion and a "bite" like configuration. Sorta looks like a NOF.

The Hip

Greater Trochanter - Remember this is also an *epiphyseal equivalent* and the chrondroblastomas prefer it to the femoral epiphysis. You can get all the other DDxs (ABC, Infection, GCT here as well). Plus, you can have avulsions of the gluteus medius and minimus.

Lesser Trochanter - An avulsion here - without significant clinical history should make you think pathologic fracture.

The Intertrochanteric Region: Classic DDx here : Lipoma, Solitary Bone Cyst, and Monostotic Fibrous Dysplasia.

The Calcaneus

There are several classic lesions that can be shown in the calcaneus. There are also several non-classic lesions that can be shown (sneaky things).

The classic 3:

Solitary Bone Cyst: This will have sharp edges. A thick sclerotic edge with a multiloculated appearance is helpful. The "fallen fragment" will be more in the bottom if shown – although fractures in the calcaneus are much less common than in the arm.

Pseudo-cyst – This is a variation on the normal trabecular pattern, which creates a central triangular radiolucent area. Supposedly the persistence of thin trabeculae, and visible nutrient foramen, along with the classic location are helpful in telling it from the other benign entities.

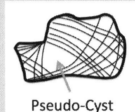

Pseudo-Cyst

Interosseous Lipoma: If they show you this, it will either have to have (a) fat density on CT or MRI, or (b) a **central fragment** – stuck within the middle of the fat. This calcification / fat necrosis occurs about 50% of the time in the real world

Sneaky things:

Just remember that the calcaneus is an *epiphyseal equivalent* so **ABC, Infection, GCT, and Chondroblastoma** can all occur there - think about these when the lesion is more posterior.

In the setting of subtalar degenerative change you can get a **geode** that mimics a cystic lesion (think about this in older patients – 60s with obvious arthritis).

Some Random Benign Lesion Differentials

No Periostitis or Pain
- Fibrous Dysplasia
- Enchondroma
- NF
- Solitary Bone Cyst (unless fractured)

Multiple (FEEMHI)
- Fibrous Dysplasia
- EG
- Enchondroma
- Mets / Myeloma
- Hyperparathyroidism

Misc Conditions:

Liposclerosing Myxofibroma: *Very characteristic location – at the intertrochanteric region of the femur.* Looks like a geographic lytic lesion with a sclerotic margin. Despite non-aggressive appearance, 10% undergo malignant degeneration so they need to be followed.

Osteochondroma: Some people think of this as more of a developmental anomaly (although they still always make the tumor chapter). Actually, it's usually listed as the most common benign tumor. They can be radiation induced, making them the *only benign skeletal tumor associated with radiation.*

They have a very small risk of malignant transformation (which supposedly can be estimated based on size of cartilage cap). Supposedly a cap >1.5cm is concerning.

Key Points:
* They point away from the joint
* The bone marrow flows freely into the lesion

Multiple Hereditary Exostosis: AD condition with multiple osteochondromas. They have an **increased risk of malignant transformation**.

Trevor Disease (Dysplasia Epiphysealis Hemimelica - DEH): Osteochondromas develop in an epiphyses causing significant joint deformity (**most common in ankle** and knee). You see this is young children. The osteochondroma looks more like an irregular mass. They tend to be treated with surgical excision.

Supracondylar Spur (Avian Spur): This is an Aunt Minne, and normal variant. This is an osseous process, that usually does nothing, but can compress the median nerve if the **Ligament of Struthers** smashes it.

This vs That: **Osteochonroma vs Supracondylar Spur**	
Osteochondroma	**Supracondylar Spur**
Points AWAY from joint	Points TOWARD the joint

Periosteal Chondroma (Juxta-Cortical Chondroma): When you see a lesion in the finger of a kid think this. It's a rare entity, or cartilaginous origin. "Saucerization" of the adjacent cortex with sclerotic periosteal reaction can be seen.

Osteofibrous Dysplasia: This is a benign lesion found exclusively in the tibia or fibula in children (10 and under – usually). It looks like an NOF , but centered in the anterior tibia, with associated anterior tibial bowing. It can occur with Adamantinoma, and the two cannot be differentiated with imaging.

When I say looks like NOF in the anterior tibia with anterior bowing, you say Osteofibrous Dysplasia.

Tibial Bowing

Most likely shown as an Aunt Minnie - NF-1 anterior with a fibular pseudoarthrosis, Rickets with wide growth plates, or Blounts tibia vara.

The most likely pure trivia question is that physiology bowing is smooth, lateral, and occurs from 18months - 2 years.

NF-1	**Anterior Lateral** - Unilateral	May be unilateral. May have hypoplastic fibula with pseudarthrosis.
Foot Deformities	Posterior	
Physiologic Bowing	Lateral – Bilateral Symmetric	Self limiting **between 18 months and 2 years**.
Hypophosphatasia	Lateral	"Rickets in a newborn"
Rickets	Lateral	Widening and irregularity of the growth plates.
Blount	Tibial Vara – Often asymmetric	Early walking, Fat, black kid.
Osteogenesis Imperfecta	Involves all long bones	
Dwarfs	Short Limbs	

Arthritis

Arthritis is tricky. Anne Brower wrote a book *called Arthritis in Black and White*, which is probably the best book on the subject. The problem is that book is 415 pages. So, I'm going to try and offer the 10 page version.

Epidemiology

Although there are over 90 different rheumatic diseases recognized by the American College of Rheumatology, only a few tend to show up on multiple choice tests (and at the view box).

You can broadly categorize arthritis into 3 categories:
- Degenerative (OA, Neuropathic)
- Inflammatory (RA, and Variants)
- Metabolic (Gout, CPPD)

Degenerative:

Osteoarthritis is the most common cause. The pathogenesis is that you have mechanical breakdown (hard work) which leads to cartilage degeneration (fissures, micro-fractures) and fragmentation of subchondral bone (sclerosis, and subchondral cysts). You get all the classic stuff, joint space narrowing (NOT symmetric), subchondral cysts, endplate changes, vacuum phenomenon, etc... The poster boy is the osteophyte.

Neuropathic Joint. The way the case is classically shown is a bad joint followed by the reason for a bad joint (syringomyelia, spinal cord injury, etc...). A way to think about this is *"osteoarthritis with a vengeance."* The buzzword is "Surgical Like Margins." Basically nothing else causes this kind of destruction. I like to describe the joints as a **d**eformity, with **d**ebris, and **d**islocation, having **d**ense subchondral bone, and **d**estruction of the articular cortex. The classic scenario is a shoulder that looks like it's been amputated, and then they show you a syrinx.

Inflammatory:

Erosive Osteoarthritis *(Inflammatory Osteoarthritis)*. The buzzword is "gull wing", which describes the central erosions. It is seen in postmenopausal women and favors the DIP joints.

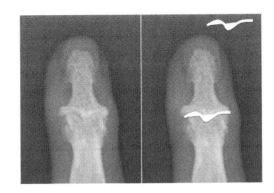

Erosive OA - Gullwing

Rheumatoid Arthritis: There is a ton of trivia related to this disease. It's not a disease of bone production. Instead it is characterized by osteoporosis, soft tissue swelling, marginal erosions and <u>uniform joint space narrowing</u>. It's often bilateral and symmetric. Classically spares the DIP joints (opposite of erosive OA).

Trivia: The 5th Metatarsal head is the first spot in the foot

RA in the Hand Pearls - Expect the IP joints (PIP) to be involved AFTER the MCP joints. The First CMC is classically spared (or is the last carpal to be involved). The first CMC should NOT be first. Obviously OA loves the first CMC so this is helpful in separating them. Psoriasis on the other hand, also tends to make the first CMC go last.

- **Felty Syndrome:** RA > 10 years + Splenomegaly + Neutropenia

- **Caplan Syndrome:** RA + Pneumoconiosis

The distribution of RA vs OA in the hip is a classic teaching point:

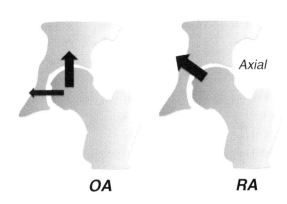

OA   RA

Rheumatoid Variants
- Psoriatic Arthritis
- Reiter's syndrome *(Reactive arthritis)*
- Ankylosing Spondylitis
- Inflammatory Bowel Disease

Psoriatic Arthritis: This is seen in 30% of patients with psoriasis. In almost all cases (90%) the skin findings come first, then you get the arthritis. As a point of trivia, there is a strong correlation between involvement of the nail and involvement of the DIP joint. The classic description is "erosive change with bone proliferation (IP joints > MCP joints). The erosions start in the margins of the joint and progress to involve the central portions (can lead to a "pencil sharpening" effect). The hands are the most commonly affected (second most common is the feet). Up to 40% of cases will have SI joint involvement (asymmetric).

Additional Buzzwords
- "Fuzzy Appearance" to the bone around the joint (bone proliferation)
- Sausage Digit – whole digit has soft tissue swelling
- Ivory Phalanx – sclerosis and/or bone proliferation (most commonly the great toe)
- Pencil in Cup Deformities
- Ankylosis in Finger
- "Mouse Ears"
- Acral osteolysis

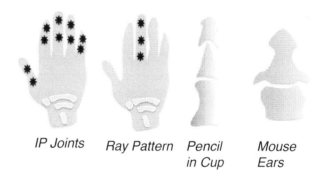

IP Joints   Ray Pattern   Pencil in Cup   Mouse Ears

When I say Ankylosis in the Hand, You Say (1) Erosive OA or (2) Psoriasis

RA	Psoriasis
Symmetric	Asymmetric
Proximal (favors MCP, carpals)	Distal (favors IP joints)
Osteoporosis	No Osteoporosis
No Bone Proliferation	Bone Proliferation - the form of periostitis
Can Cause "Mutilans" When Severe	Can Cause "Mutilans" When Severe

Reiter's (Reactive arthritis): Apparently Reiter was a Nazi (killed a bunch of people with typhus vaccine experiments). So, people try not to give him any credit for things (hence the name change to Reactive arthritis). Regardless of what you call it, it's **a very similar situation to Psoriatic arthritis** – both have bone proliferation and erosions, and asymmetric SI joint involvement. The difference is that **Reiter's is rare in the hands** (tends to affect the feet more). Just remember Reiters below the waist.

Ankylosing Spondylitis: This disease favors the spine and SI joints. The classic buzzword is **"bamboo spine"** from the syndesmophytes flowing from adjacent vertebral bodies. Shiny corners is a buzzword, for early involvement. As you might imagine these spines are susceptible to fracture in trauma. **SI joint involvement is usually the first site (symmetric).** The joint actually widens a little before it narrows. As a point of trivia, these guys can have an upper lobe predominant interstitial lung disease, with small cystic spaces.

Next Step - Any significant Ank Spon / DISH + Even Minor Trauma = Whole Spine CT

Random High Yield Topic: Ankylosing Spondylitis in the Hip
When the peripheral skeleton is involved in patient's with Ank Spond, think about the shoulders and hips (hips more common). Hip involvement can be very disabling.
Heterotopic Ossification tends to occur post hip replacement or revision. It occurs so much that they often get postoperative low dose radiation and NSAIDs to try as prophylactic therapy.
If they show you normal SI joints - then show you anything in the spine it's not AS. It has to hit the SI joints first (especially on multiple choice).

Inflammatory Bowel Disease – This occurs in two distinct flavors.

(A): Axial Arthritis (favors SI joints and spine) – often unrelated to bowel disease
(B): Peripheral Arthritis – this one varies depending on the severity of the bowel disease.

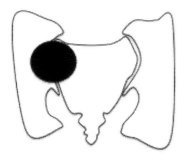
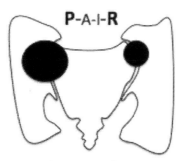
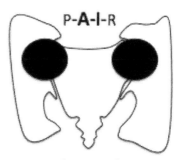

Unilateral = Infection | Asymmetric = Psoriasis, Reiters | Symmetric = Inflammatory Bowel, AS

Psoriatic Arthritis	Reiters (Reactive)	Ankylosing Spondylitis
M = F	M > F	M>F
Asymmetric SI Joint	Asymmetric SI Joint	Symmetric SI Joint
Hands, Feet, Thoracolumbar Spine	Feet, Lumbar Spine, SI joint	SI joint, Spine (whole thing)

——

Metabolic:

Gout: This is a crystal arthropathy from the deposition of uric acid crystals in and around the joints. It's almost always in a man over 40. The big toe is the classic location.

Buzzwords / Things to Know:
- Earliest Sign = Joint Effusion
- Spares the Joint Space (until late in the disease); Juxta-articular Erosions - away from the joint.
- "Punched out lytic lesions"
- "Overhanging Edges"
- Soft tissue tophi

Gout on MR

- Juxta-articular soft tissue masse (LOW ON T2).
- The tophus will typically enhance.

Gout Mimickers: There are 5 entities that can give a similar appearance to a gouty arthritis, although they are much less common. The way I remember them is

"**A**merican **R**oentgen **R**ay **S**ociety **H**ooray"
- *Amyloid*
- *RA (cystic)*
- *Reticular Histocytosis (the most rare)*
- *Sarcoid*
- *Hyperlipidemia*

CPPD: Calcium Pyrophosphate Dihydrate Disease is super common in old people. It often causes chondocalcinosis (although there are other causes). Synovitis + CPPD = "Pseudogout." CPPD loves the triangular fibrocartilage of the wrist, the peri odontoid tissue, and intervertbral disks. Another important phrase is **"degenerative change in an uncommon joint"** – shoulder, elbow, patellofemoral joint, radiocarpal joint. Having said that **pyrophosphate arthropathy is most common at the knee**.

- *If you see isolated disease in the patellofemoral, radiocarpal, or talonavicular joint think CPPD.*
- *Hooked MCP Osteophytes with chondrocalcinosis in the TFCC is a classic look (although hemochromatosis can also look that way).*

Remember - CPPD can (and does commonly) cause SLAC wrist by degenerating the SL Ligament.

"Milwaukee Shoulder" This is a destruction of the shoulder (**almost looks neuropathic**) but is secondary to **hydroxyapatite**. The articular surface changes will be very advanced, and you have a lot of intra-articular loose bodies. It's classically seen in an old women with a history of trauma to that joint.

> ***OA vs CPPD?***
> There are many overlapping features including joint space narrowing, subchondral sclerosis, subchondral cyst, and osteophyte formation. However, CPPD has some unique features such as an "atypical joint distribution" – favoring compartments like the patellofemoral or radiocarpal. Subchondral cyst formation can be bigger than expected.

Hemochromatosis – This iron overload disease also is known for calcium pyrophosphate deposition and resulting chondrocalcinosis. It has a similar distribution to CPPD (MCP joints). Both CPPD and Hemochromatosis will have "hooked osteophytes" at the MCP joint. As a point of trivia, therapy for the systemic disease does NOT affect the arthritis.

Hyperparathyroidism - As you may remember from medical school this can be primary or secondary, and its effects on calcium metabolism typically manifest in the bones. Here are your buzzwords: "Subperiosteal bone resorption" of the radial aspect 2nd and 3rd fingers, rugger-jersey spine, brown tumors, terminal tuft erosions.

The classic ways this is shown:
- *Superior and inferior rib notching – bone resorption*
- *Resorption along the radial aspect of the fingers with brown tumors*
- *Tuft Resorption*
- *Rugger Jersey Spine*
- *Pelvis with Narrowing or "Constricting" of the femoral necks, and wide SI joints.*

Hyperparathyroidism

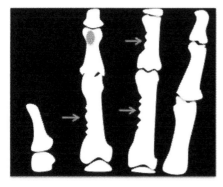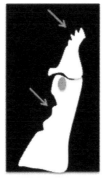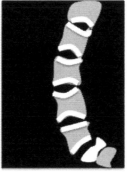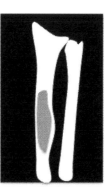

Subperiosteal Resorption, Tuft Resorption *and brown tumors*   Rugger Jersey Spine   Brown Tumor

Problem Solving: If you are given a picture of a hand or foot and asked what the arthritis is, it will probably be obvious (they show a gullwing for erosive OA, or bad carpals for RA, or the pencil in cup for psoriasis, or the 5th metatarsal for RA). If it's not made obvious with an "Aunt Minnie" appearance I like to use this approach to figure it out (I also use this in the real world).

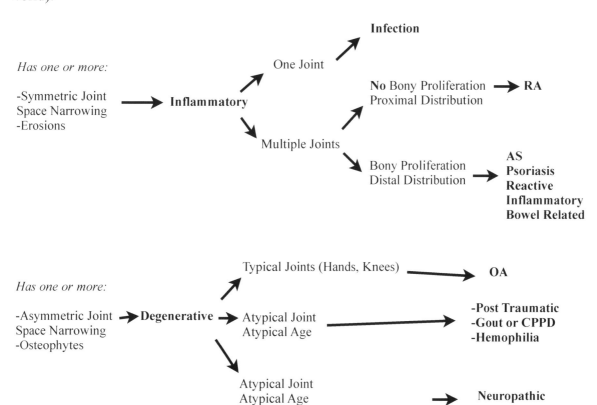

Spine Degenerative Change: In the real world it's usually just multilevel degenerative change. But in multiple choice world you should be thinking about other things. Shiny corners with early AS, or flowing syndesmophytes with later AS. DISH with the bulky osteophytes sparing the disc space. The big bridging lateral osteophyte is classically shown for psoriatic arthritis.

Vertebral Osteophytes	
"Flowing Syndesmophytes"	Ankylosing Spondylitis
Diffuse Paravertebral Ossifications	DISH
Focal Lateral Paravertebral Ossification	Psoriatic Arthritis

Cervical Spine:
Gamesmanship

- **Fusion:** Either congenital (Klippel-Feil) or Juvenile RA.
- **Erosions of the Dens:** CPPD and RA famously do this.
- **Bad Kyphosis** = NF1

Misc Stuff That's Sorta in the Arthritis Category:

Systemic Lupus Erthematous: The Aunt Minnie Look is **reducible deformity of joints without articular erosions**. *Joint space narrowing and erosions are uncommon findings.* They can show you the hands with ulnar subluxations at the MCPs on Norgaard view, then they reduce on AP (because the hands are flat).

This ligamentous laxity also increases risk of **patellar dislocations**.

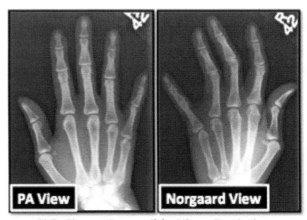

SLE: Shows Reversible Ulnar Deviation

Jaccoud's Arthropathy: This is **very similar to SLE** in the hand (people often say them together). You have non erosive arthropathy with ulnar deviation of the 2nd-5th fingers at the MCP joint. The **history is post rheumatic fever**.

DISH (Diffuse Idiopathic Skeletal Hyperostosis) : You see ossification of the anterior longitudinal ligament involving more than 4 levels with **sparing of the disc spaces**, you say DISH. The **thoracic spine is most commonly used**. These guys often have bony proliferation at pelvis, ischial tuberosities, at the trochanters, and iliac crests. There is **no sacroiliitis** (helps you differentiate from AS).

OPPL (Ossification of the Posterior Longitudinal Ligament): This is an ossification of the posterior longitudinal ligament. It is associated with DISH, ossification of the ligamentum flavum, and Ankylosing Spondylitis. It favors the cervical spine of old Asian men. It **can cause spinal canal stenosis, and lead to cord injury after minor trauma.** A key point is that it's bad news in the cervical spine (where it is most common), in the thoracic spine it is usually asymptomatic.

Destructive Spondyloarthropathy.: This is associated with patients on renal dialysis (for at least 2 years), and it most commonly affects the C-spine. It looks like bad degenerative changes or CPPD. Amyloid deposition is supposedly why it happens.

Mixed Connective Tissue Disease: One unique feature is that it is positive for some antibody – Ribonucleoprotein (RNP), and therefore *serology is essential to the diagnosis.*

Juvenile Idiopathic Arthritis: This occurs before age 16 (by definition). What you see is a washed out hand that has a proximal distribution (**carpals are jacked**), and ankylosed (**premature fusion of growth plates**). Serology is often negative (85%). In the knees, you see enlargement of the epiphyses and widened intercondylar notch – similar to findings in hemophilia.

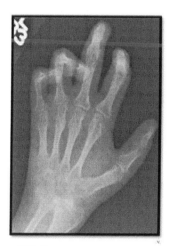

JRA
– Note the effect on the carpals

Amyloid Arthropathy: This is seen with patients on dialysis (less commonly in patients with chronic inflammation such as RA). The pattern of destruction can be severe – similar to septic arthritis or neuropathic spondyloarthropathy. The distribution is key, the **bilateral involvement of the shoulders, hips, carpals, and knees** being typical. **Carpal tunnel syndrome is a common clinical manifestation.** The **joint space is typically preserved** until later in the disease. When associated with dialysis it's rare before 5 years of treatment, but very common after 10 years (80%).

Congenital

Dwarfs, Coalitions, and Feet are discussed in detail in the PEDs chapter (volume 2, module 5)

Total Hip Arthroplasty Complications:

Loosening: This is the most common indication for revision. The criteria on x-ray is **>2mm at the interface** (suggestive). If you see **migration of the component** you can call it *(migration includes varus tilting of the femoral stem).*

Particle Disease: Any component of the device that sheds will cause an inflammatory response. Macrophages will try and eat the particles and spew enzymes all over the place.

Things to know about particle disease (in THA):

* Most commonly seen in non-cemented hips
* Tends to occur 1-5 years after surgery
* X-ray shows "smooth" endosteal scalloping (distinguishes from infection)
* Produces no secondary bone response
* Can be seen around screw holes (particles are transmitted around screws)

Stress Shielding: The stress is transferred through the metallic stem, so the bone around it is not loaded. Orthopods call this "Wolff's Law" – where the unloaded bone just gets resorbed. The trivia to know is that it (1) happens more with uncemented arthroplasty and (2) increases the risk of fracture.

Wear Patterns: It is normal to have a little bit of thinning is the area of weight bearing – this is called "Creep." It is not normal to see wear along the superior lateral aspect.

Polyethylene Wear	Creep
Superior – Lateral	Axial Direction
Pathologic	Normal

Heterotopic Ossifications: This is very common (15-50%). It's usually asymptomatic. The trivia regarding multiple choice tests is that "hip stiffness" is the most common complaint. Also in Ank Spon patients, because they are so prone to heterotopic ossifications, they sometimes give them low dose prophylactic radiation prior to THA.

Marrow

This is a confusing topic and there are entire books on the subject. I'm going to attempt to hit the main points, and simplify the subject.

Bone marrow consists of three components: (1) Trabecular Bone – the support structure, (2) Red Marrow – for making blood, and (3) Yellow Marrow –fat for a purpose unknown at this time.

Marrow Conversion: The basic rules are that yellow marrow increases with age, in a predictable and progressive way. This is usually completed by the mid 20s. You are born with all red marrow, and the conversion of red to yellow occurs from the extremities to the axial skeleton (feet and hands first). Within each long bone the progression occurs epiphyses / apophyses first -> diaphysis -> followed by the distal metaphysis , and finally the proximal metaphysis. **Red marrow can be found in the humeral heads and femoral heads as a normal variant in adults.**

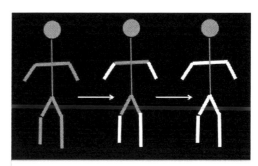

Red Marrow Converts to Yellow Marrow from Distal to Proximal

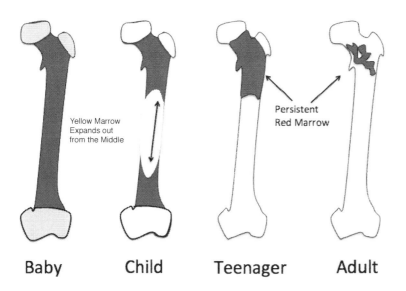

Yellow Marrow Expands out from the Middle

Persistent Red Marrow

Baby   Child   Teenager   Adult

So as a child you have diffuse red marrow except for ossified epiphyses and apophyses. As an adult you have yellow marrow everywhere except in the axial skeleton, and proximal metaphyses of proximal long bones.

Few Pearls on Marrow:

- Yellow marrow increases with age (as trabecular bone decreases with osteoporosis, yellow marrow replaces it).
- T1 is your money sequence: Yellow is bright, Red is darker than yellow (near iso-intense to muscle).
- Red marrow should never be darker than a normal disk or muscle on T1 (think about muscle as your internal control).
- Red marrow increases if there is a need for more hematopoiesis (reconversion – occurs in exact reverse order of normal conversion)
- Marrow turns yellow with stress / degenerative change in the spine

This question can be asked in 3 main ways:

(1) What is the normal pattern of conversion?
(2) What is the normal pattern of reconversion?
(3) What areas are spared / normal variants?

(1) The epiphyses convert to fatty marrow almost immediately after ossification. Distal then proceeds medial (diaphysis first, then metaphysis).

(2) The pattern of reconversion: This occurs in the reverse order of normal marrow conversion, beginning in the axial skeleton and heading peripheral. The last to go are the more distal long bones. Typically the epiphyses are spared unless the hematopoietic demand is very high.

Spine -> Flat Bones -> Long Bone Metaphysis -> Long Bone Diaphysis -> Long Bone Epiphyses

(3) Patchy areas of red marrow may be seen in the proximal femoral metaphysis of teenagers. The **distal femoral sparring is especially true in teenagers and menstruating women.**

Leukemia: Proliferation of leukemic cells results in replacement of red marrow. **Marrow will look darker than muscle (and normal disks) on T1**. On STIR maybe higher than muscle because of the increased water content. T2 is variable often looking like diffuse red marrow.

Gamesmanship: They can show leukemia in two main ways
    (1) *Lucent metaphyseal bands in a kid*
    (2) *T1 weighted MRI showing marrow darker than adjacent disks, and muscle. Remember that Red Marrow is still 40% fat, and should be brighter than muscle on T1.*

Most infiltrative conditions affect the marrow diffusely. The exceptions are *multiple myeloma which has a predilection for focal deposits, and Waldenstrom's macroglobulinemia which causes infarcts.*

Chloroma (Granulocytic Sarcoma) - Just say "destructive mass in a bone of a leukemia patient." It's some kind of colloid tumor.

Metabolic / Misc

Calcium Hydroxyapatite: Most pathologic calcification in the body is calcium hydroxyapatite, which is also the most abundant form of calcium in bone.

Calcium hydroxyapatite deposition disease = **calcific tendinitis.**

The calcium is deposited in tendons around the joint. The most common location for hydroxyapatite deposition is the shoulder. Specifically, the **supraspinatus tendon is the most frequent site of calcification**, usually at the insertion near the greater tuberosity. *The longus coli muscle is also a favorite location for multiple choice test writers.* It may be primary (idiopathic) or secondary. Secondary causes worth knowing are: chronic renal disease, collagen-vascular disease, **tumoral calciniosis** and hypervitaminosis D.

Osteopoikilosis: It's just a bunch of bone islands. Usually in epiphyses (different from blastic mets or osteosarcoma mets). It can be inherited or sporadic but if you are forced to pick a pattern - I'd go with *autosomal dominant.*

Mets vs Osteopoikilosis - Osteopoikilosis tends to joint centered. Sclerotic mets will be all over the place. Sclerotic mets believe in nothing Lebowski.

Osteopathia Striata: Linear, parallel, and longitudinal lines in metaphysis of long bones. Doesn't mean shit (usually - but can in some situations cause pain).

Engelmann's Disease: This is also known as progressive diaphyseal dysplasia or PDD. What you see is *fusiform bony enlargement* with sclerosis of the long bones. This is a total zebra that begins in childhood.

Things to know:

- *It's Bilateral and Symmetric*
- *It likes the long bones - usually shown in the tibia*
- *It's hot on bone scan*
- *It can involve the skull – and can cause optic nerve compression*

Pituitary Gigantism: If they happen to show you x-rays of Andre the Giant, look for **"widening of the joint space in an adult hip"** – can be a classic buzzword. Late in the game the cartilage will actually outgrow its blood supply, and collapse leading to **early onset osteoarthritis.** The formation of endochondral bone at existing chondro-osseous junctions results in widening of osseous structure.

Pigmented Villonodular Synovitis (PVNS) : PVNS is an uncommon benign neoplastic process that may involve the synovium of the joint diffusely or focally It can also affect the tendon sheath.

Intra-Articular Disease : Basically it's **Synovial Proliferation + Hemosiderin Deposition**. The knee is by far the most common joint affected (65-80%). On plain film, features you will probably see are a joint effusion with or without marginal erosions. Osseous erosions with preservation of the joint space, and normal mineralization is typical. It is not possible to distinguish PVNS from *synovial chondromatosis (see below)* on plain film. MRI will be obvious with **blooming on gradient echo**, and this is the most likely way they will show this. Treatment is with complete synovectomy, although recurrence rate is 20-50%.

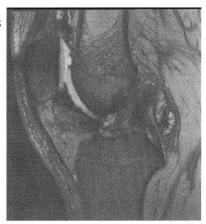
PVNS – Diffuse Blooming

Trivia: Unusual in kids, but when present is typically polyarticular.

Giant Cell Tumor of the Tendon Sheath (PVNS of the tendon): Typically found in the hand (palmar tendons). Can cause erosions on the underlying bone. Will be soft tissue density, and be T1 and T2 dark *(contrasted to a **glomus tumor** which is T1 dark, **T2 bright,** and will enhance uniformly).*

Primary Synovial Chondromatosis: There are both primary and secondary types; secondary being the result of degenerative changes in the joint. The primary type is an extremely high yield topic. It is a metaplastic / true neoplastic process (not inflammatory) that results in the formation of multiple cartilaginous nodules in the synovium of joints, tendon sheaths, and bursea. These nodules will eventually progress to loose bodies. It usually affects one joint, and that one joint is usually the knee (70%). The popular are is usually a person in their 40s or 50s.

Joint bodies (which are usually multiple and uniform in size) may demonstrate the ring and arc calcification characteristic of chondroid calcification. Treatment involves removal of the loose bodies with or without synovectomy.

PVNS	Synovial Chondromatosis
Benign Neoplasia	Benign Neoplasia
Associated with Hemarthrosis	NOT Associated with Hemarthrosis
Never Calcifies	May Calcify

Secondary Synovial Chondromatosis: A lower yield topic than the primary type. This is secondary to degenerative change, and typically seen in an older patient. There will be extensive degenerative changes, and the fragments are usually fewer and larger when compared to the primary subtype.

Diabetic Myonecrosis: This is basically infarction of the muscle seen in poorly controlled type 1 diabetics. It **almost always involves the thigh (80%)**, or calf (20%). MRI will show marked edema with enhancement and irregular regions of muscle necrosis. You **should NOT biopsy this**, it delays recovery time and has a high complication rate.

Soft Tissue Hemangioma: This is a benign vascular tumor, that comes in several varieties (capillary being the most common type). They are more common in women, and *can enlarge during pregnancy*. They can look like a **bunch of phleboliths on plain film** (characteristic of the cavernous subtype). On CT you can see **intralesional fat**. On MR they are going to be T1 and T2 bright, again with intralesional fat. They are typically well defined with a lobulated border, and heterogenous features. They enhance avidly and may have blooming on gradient from the pheboliths.

Next Step - Suspecting hemangioma? think you see intralesional fat ? Plain film can be helpful to look for phleboliths.

Lipoma Arborescens: This is a zebra that affects the synovial lining of the joins and bursa.

The buzzword is "**frond – like**" depositions of fatty tissue.

It's seen in late adulthood (50s-70s), with the most common location being the suprapatellar bursa of the knee. Although it **can develop in a normal knee, it's often associated with OA, Chronic RA, or prior trauma**. It's usually unilateral. On MRI it's going to behave like fat – T1 and T2 bright with response to fat saturation.

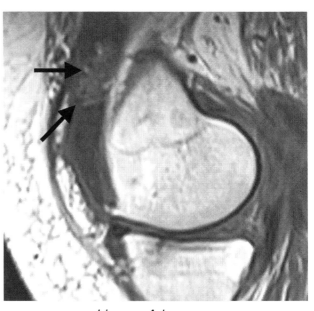

Lipoma Arborescens

A sneaky trick is to show this on gradient – and how you pick up the chemical shift artifact at the fat-fluid interface.

This could also be shown on ultrasound with a "frond-like hyperechoic mass" and associated joint effusions.

AVN of the Hip: Variety of causes including Perthes in kids, sickle cell, gaucher's, steroid use etc…. It can also be traumatic with femoral neck fractures (*degree of risk is related to degree of displacement* / disruption of the retinacular vessels). AVN of the hip typically affects the superior articular surface, beginning more anteriorly.

Double Line Sign: Best seen on T2; inner bright line (granulation tissue), with outer dark line (sclerotic bone) . Seen in 80% of cases

Rim Sign: Best seen on T2; high T2 signal line sandwiched between two low signal lines. This represents *fluid between sclerotic borders of an osteochondral fragment*, and **implies instability**. (Stage III).

Crescent Sign: Seen on X-ray (optimally frog leg); Refers to a subchondral lucency seen most frequently anterolateral aspect of the proximal femoral head. It indicates imminent collapse.

Stages of Osteonecrosis:
- o   Zero = Normal
- o   One = Normal x-ray, edema on MR
- o   Two = Mixed Lytic / Sclerotic
- o   Three = Crescent Sign, Articular Collapse, Joint Space Preserved
- o   Four = Secondary Osteoarthritis

Thalassemia : This is a defect in the hemoglobin chain (can be alpha or beta – major or minor). From the MSK Radiologist prospective we are talking about "hair-on-end" skulls, expansion of the facial bones, "rodent faces" , expanded ribs "jail-bars". It is frequently associated with extramedullary hematopoiesis.

Thalassemia	Sickle Cell
Will Obliterate Sinuses	Will Not Obliterate Sinuses

Pagets
(High Yield Topic)

A relatively common condition that affects 4% of people at 40, and 8% at 80 *(actually 10%, but easier to remember 8%).* M > F. Most people are asymptomatic. The pathophysiology of Pagets is not well understood.

The bones **go through three phases which progress from lytic to mixed to sclerotic** *(the latent inactive phase).* The phrase **"Wide Bones with Thick Trabecula"** make you immediately say Pagets (nothing else really does that).

Lytic	Usually Asymptomatic
Mixed	Elevated Alkaline Phosphate. Fractures
Sclerotic	Elevated Hydroxyproline. More fractures. Sarcomas may develop.

Comes in two flavors: (1) Monostotic and (2) Polyostotic – with the poly subtype being much more common (80-90%).

Paget's Buzzwords / Signs:
* *Blade of Grass Sign:* Lucent leading edge in a long bone
* *Osteoporosis Circumscripta:* Blade of Grass in the Skull
* *Picture Frame Vertebra:* Cortex is thickened on all sides (Rugger Jersey is only superior and inferior endplates)
* *Cotton Wool Bone:* Thick disorganized trabeculae
* *Banana Fracture:* Insufficiency fracture of a bowed soft bone (femur or tibia).
* *Tam O'Shanter Sign:* Thick Skull
* *Saber Shin:* Bowing of the tibia
* *Ivory Vertebra:* This is a differential finding, including mets. Pagets tends to be expansile.

Complications: **Deafness is the most common complication.** Spinal stenosis from cortical thickening is very characteristic. Additional complications, cortical stress fracture, cranial nerves paresis, CHF (high output), secondary hyperparathyroidism (10%), **Secondary development of osteosarcoma (1%) – which is often highly resistant to treatment.** *As a piece of ridiculous trivia - giant cell tumor can arise from pagets.*

Trivia: Of all the tumors to which Paget may devolve to, Osteosarcoma is the Most Common.

Total Trivia: Pagets bone is hypervascular and may be 5 degrees hotter than other bone (get your thermometer ready). Alk Phos will be elevated (up to 20x) in the reparative phase.

Skull	Large Areas of Osteolysis in the Frontal and Occipital Bones "Osteoporosis Circumscripta", in the lytic phase. The skull will look "cotton wool" in the mixed phase. Favors the outer table.
Spine	Cortical Thickening can cause a "picture frame sign" (same as osteopetrosis). Also can give you an ivory vertebral body.
Pelvis	Most common bone affected. "Always" involves the iliopectineal line on the pelvic brim.
Long Bones	Advancing margin of lucency from one end to the other is the so called "blade of grass" or "flame." Will often spare the fibula, even in diffuse disease.

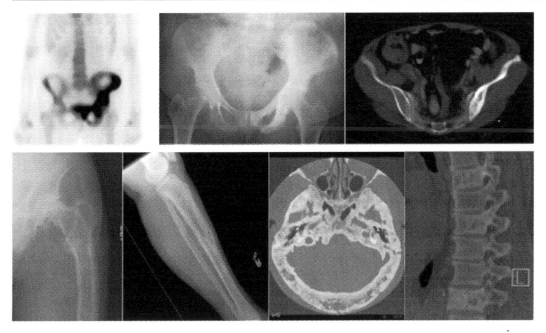

Pagets
-- Femur / Tibia, -- Expanded Bones, -- Coarsened Trabecula, -- Ivory Vertebrae

Other Imaging Modalities:

MRI: There are three marrow patterns that closely (but not exactly) follow the phases on x-ray.

Lytic / Early Mixed	Heterogenous T2, T1 is isointense to muscle, with a "speckled appearance"
Late Mixed	Maintained fatty high T1 and T2 signals
Sclerotic	Low signal on T1 and T2

Nuclear Medicine: The primary utility of a bone scan is in defining the extent of disease and to help assess response to treatment. The characteristic look for Pagets is "Whole Bone Involvement." For example, the **entire vertebral body including the posterior elements**, or the entire pelvis. The classic teaching is that Pagets is hot on all three phases (although often decreased or normal in the sclerotic phase).

Tendon Ultrasound:

It's absolutely incredible that I even need to go over this, but dinosaur radiologist's love this stuff.

Anisotropy: The most common and most problematic issues with ultrasounding tendons is this thing called "anisotropy." The tendon is normally hyperechoic, but if you look at it when it's NOT perpendicular to the sound beam it can look hypoechoic (injured?).

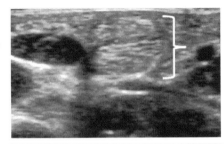

Normal Appearing Hyperechoic Tendon

It's the biggest pain in the ass:

- Supraspinatus tendon – as it curves along the contours of the humeral head
- Long Head of the Biceps – In the bicipital groove

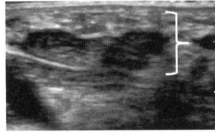

Exact same tendon – now appearing Hypoechoic – when scanned non-parallel

Anisotropy

Tears: The tendon is usually hyperechoic. Focal hypoechoic areas are tears. It can be really tricky to tell if it's partial or complete (that's what MRI is for).

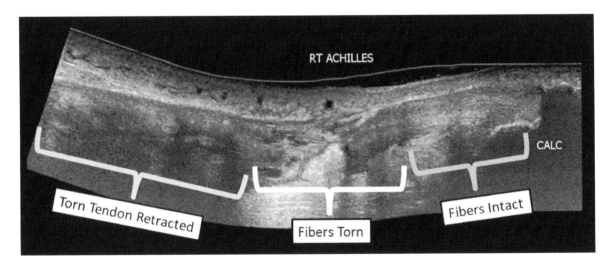

Tenosynovitis: As discussed above there are a variety of causes. If they show it on ultrasound you are looking for increased fluid within the tendon sheath. You could also see associated peritendinous subcutaneous hyperemia on Doppler.

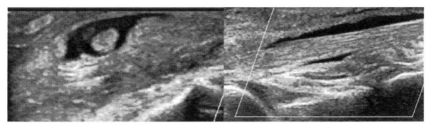

Tenosynovitis – Increased fluid in the tendon sheath

Plantar Fasciitis: This is another pathology that lends itself to a "what is it ?" type of ultrasound question. Hopefully, they at least tell you this is the foot (they could label the calcaneus). The finding will be thickening of the plantar fascia (greater than 4mm), with loss of the normal fibrillar pattern. If you see calipers on the plantar fascia – this is going to be the answer.

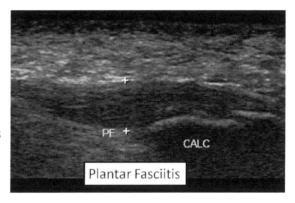

Trivia - <u>Most commonly involves the central band</u> (there are 3 bands - people who don't know anatomy think there are two).

Calcific Tendonitis: As described above, this is very common and related to hydroxyapatite. The most common site is the supraspinatus tendon, near its insertion. It will shadow just like a stone in the GB.

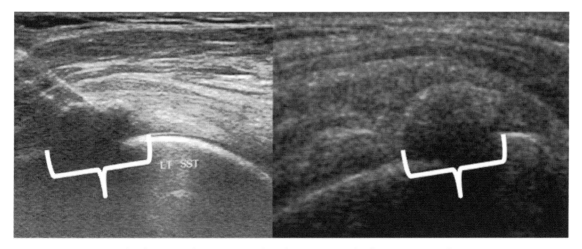

Calcific Tendonitis – Shadowing calcification in the classic location (supraspinatus)

Basic Procedural Trivia - The Arthrogram

An important point to remember is that the target is not actually the joint. The target is the capsule. In other words, you just need the needle to touch a bone within the capsule. The trick is to do this without causing contamination or damaging an adjacent structure (like an artery). *General Tip* - Avoid putting air in the joint, this will cause susceptibility artifact.

Hip: The general steps are as follows: (1) Mark the femoral artery. (2) Internally rotate the hip (slightly) to localize the femoral head-neck junction (your target). (3) Clean and numb the skin. (4) Advance a 20-22 gauge spinal needle into the joint - straight down on the superior head neck junction. (5) Inject a small amount of contrast to confirm position. Contrast should flow away from the tip. If the contrast just stays there it's not in a space. (6) Put the rest of the contrast in.

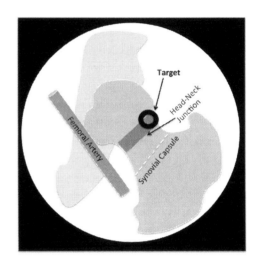

Trivia: The capsule is widest at the head-neck junction.

Trivia: The cocktail injected is around 14cc total (4cc Lidocaine, 10cc Visipaque, and only about 0.1cc Gd).

Shoulder: The general steps are as follows: (1) Supinate the hand (externally rotate the shoulder) (2) Clean and numb the skin. (3) Advance a 20-22 gauge spinal needle into the joint - straight down on the junction between the middle and inferior thirds of the humeral head - 2mm inside the cortex. (4) Once you strike bone, pull back 1mm and turn the bevel towards the humeral head - this should drop into the joint (5) Inject a small amount of contrast to confirm position. Contrast should flow away from the tip. If the contrast just stays there it's not in a space. (6) Put the rest of the contrast in.

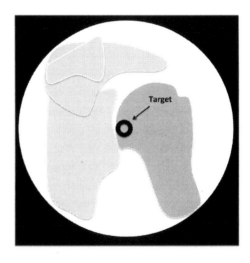

Trivia: The cocktail injected is around 12cc total (4cc Lidocaine, 8cc Visipaque, and only about 0.1cc Gd).

Blank for Notes / Scribbles

Blank for Notes / Scribbles

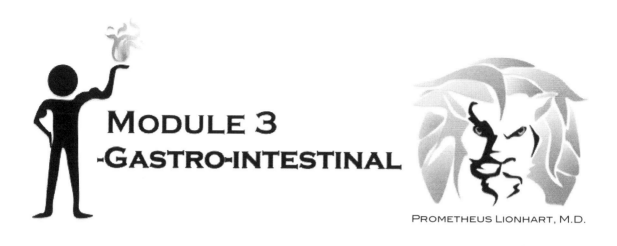

MODULE 3
-GASTRO-INTESTINAL

PROMETHEUS LIONHART, M.D.

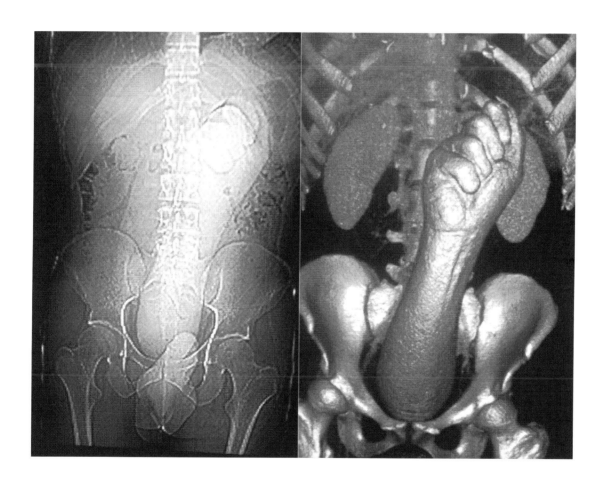

The GI Tract

The reality is that the GI tract is best evaluated with an endoscope, with only few exceptions. The next best option is probably CT Enterography. However, for the purpose of multiple choice tests I expect the majority of GI related questions to be barium related.

Esophagus

Anatomy:

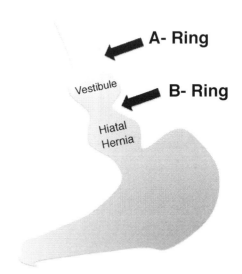

A Ring: The muscular ring above the vestibule.

B Ring: The mucosal ring **B**elow the vestibule. This is a thin constriction at the EG junction. Symptomatic dysphagia can occur if it narrows (historically defined at <13mm in diameter). **If it's narrowed (and symptomatic) you call it a Schatzki.**

Just Say *"Shatz-'B'-Ring"*

Z Line: Represents the squamocolumnar junction (boundary between esophageal and gastric epithelium). This doesn't necessarily correspond with the B-ring. This is an endoscopy finding, and is only rarely seen as a thin serrated line.

Mucosa should have thin, parallel uniform folds.

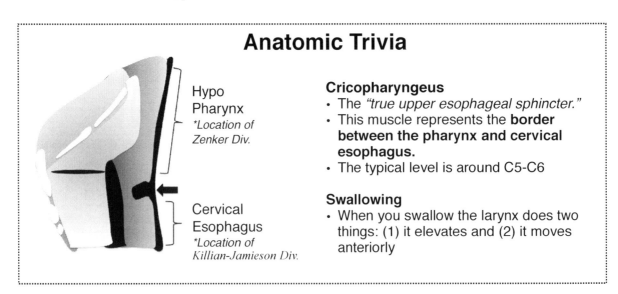

Anatomic Trivia

Hypo Pharynx
Location of Zenker Div.

Cervical Esophagus
Location of Killian-Jamieson Div.

Cricopharyngeus
- The *"true upper esophageal sphincter."*
- This muscle represents the **border between the pharynx and cervical esophagus.**
- The typical level is around C5-C6

Swallowing
- When you swallow the larynx does two things: (1) it elevates and (2) it moves anteriorly

Pathology:

Reflux Esophagitis: A common cause of fold thickening.

Reflux ➡ Thick Folds

More Reflux ➡ Thicker Folds

Still More Reflux ➡ Strictures & Barretts

Still Even More Reflux ➡ Cancer (adeno)

Rx: PPIs, and H2 Blockers, if that fails you can get a fundoplication

Barretts: This is a precursor to adenocarcinoma - that develops secondary to chronic reflux.

The way this will be shown is a **high stricture with an associated hiatal hernia**.

Buzzword = **Reticular Mucosal Pattern**.

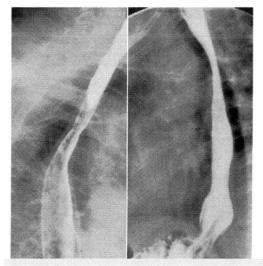

Barrett's - High Stricture + Hiatal Hernia

Eosinophilic Esophagitis: Classically a young man with a long history of dysphagia (and atopia, and peripheral eosinophilia). Barium shows **concentric rings** (distinct look). They fail treatment on PPIs , but get better with steroids.

Buzzword = **"Ringed Esophagus"**

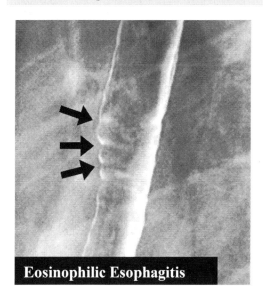

Eosinophilic Esophagitis

Fundoplication Blitz

What is this Fundoplication ? The gastric fundus is wrapped around the lower end of the esophagus and stitched in place, reinforcing the lower esophageal sphincter. The term "nissen" - refers to a 360 degree wrapping. Loser wraps can also be done, and have French sounding names like "toupet," - these are less high yield.

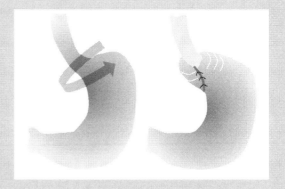

Early Complication: The early problem with these is esophageal obstruction (or narrowing). This occurs from either post op edema, or a wrap made too type. You see this peak around week 2. *Barium will show total or near total obstruction of the esophagus.*

Failure: There are two main indications for the procedure (1) hiatal hernia, and (2) reflux. So failure is defined by recurrence of either of these. The most common reason for recurrent reflux is telescoping of the GE junction through the wrap - or a "slipped nissen."

• *Most common reason for recurrent reflux* ?= slipped nissen

• *Most common reason for slipped nissen ?* = short esophagus

• *WTF is a "short esophagus" ?* The exact definition is allusive (and depends on the phase of the moon). For the purpose of multiple choice test I'd go with *"Hiatal Hernia that is fixed/non-reducible, and greater than 5cm"*

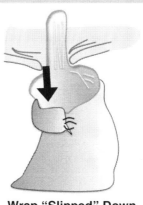
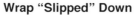

Wrap "Slipped" Down

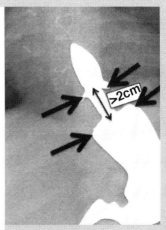

>2cm

• *How can you tell if the wrap has slipped ?* Fundoplication wrap should have length of narrowed esophagus < 2cm (anything greater is slipped wrap)

What is the treatment for a "short esophagus" ? Collis gastroplasty (lengthening + fundoplication).

Trivia: You cannot vomit after a fundoplication

Cancer: On barium you want to see the words *"irregular contour"*, and *"abrupt (shouldered) edges."* I like to use stereotypes to remember the subtypes and associations:

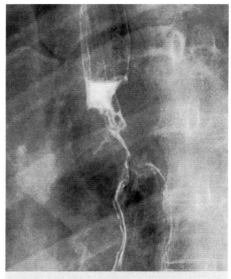

"Apple Core - Abrupt Shoulders"

- *Squamous:* This is a black guy who drinks and smokes, and once tried to kill himself with an alkaloid ingestion (drank lye). The stricture/ulcer/mass is in the mid esophagus.

- *Adeno:* This is a white guy, who is stressed out all the time. He has chronic reflux (history of PPI use). He had a scope years ago that showed Barretts, and he did nothing. The stricture/ulcer/mass is in the lower esophagus.

Esophageal Cancer - Critical Stage: Stage 3 (Adventitia) vs stage 4 (invasion into adjacent structures) - obviously you need CT to do this. The earlier stages are distinguished by endoscopy - so not your problem and unlikely to be tested. 3 vs 4 is in the radiologists world - and therefore the most likely to be tested.

—

Candidiasis: A hint in the question stem might be "HIV Patient" or "Transplant Patient" someone who is immunocompromised. The could also tell you the patient has "achalasia" or "scleroderma" - because motility disorders are also at increased risk. The most common findings is discrete plaque-like lesions. Additional findings include: nodularity, granularity, and fold thickening may occur as a result of mucosal inflammation and edema. When it is most severe, it looks more shaggy with an irregular luminal surface.

Glycogen Acanthosis: This is a mimic of candidiasis, which has multiple elevated nodules in an **asymptomatic elderly patient**.

Ulcers:

- Herpes Ulcer: Small and multiple with a halo of edema (Herpes has a Halo)
- CMV and HIV: Large Flat Ulcer (they look the same)

Varices: Linear often serpentine, filling defects causing a scalloped contour. The differential diagnosis for varices includes varicoid carcinoma (this is why you need them distended on the study).

This vs That: Uphill Varices vs Downhill Varices	
Uphill Varices	**Downhill Varices**
Caused by Portal Hypertension	Caused by SVC obstruction (catheter related, or tumor related)
Confined to Bottom Half of Esophagus	Confined to Top Half of Esophagus

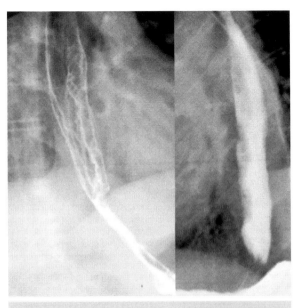

Varices: Varicoid appearance that flattens out with a large barium bolus - this dynamic appearance proves it's not a fixed varicoid looking cancer.

Esophageal (enteric) duplication cysts: If they show one of these it will be on CT (what? GI path not on barium?). Seriously, they would have to show this on CT. It is gonna be in the *posterior mediastinum*, and have an <u>ROI showing water density</u>. This is the only way you can show this.

Most likely questions:

- *What is it ?* - Water density cyst in the posterior mediastinum

- *Most common location ?* - The ileum (esophagus is #2).

- *How can they present ?* Either as an incidental in adult, or if they are big enough - as an infant with dysphagia / breathing problems.

- *Malignant Risk ?* Nope - they are benign

Esophageal Diverticulum

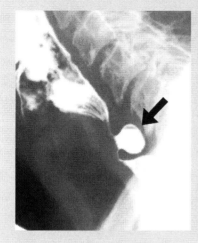 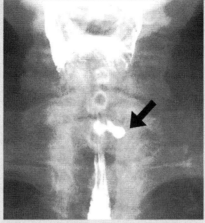 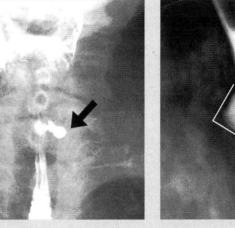

Zenker Diverticulum:
Diverticulum in the back *(Z is in the back of the alphabet)*.

The question they always ask is: site of weakness = **Killian Dehiscence** or triangle.

Another sneaky point of trivia is that the diverticulum **arise from the hypopharynx** (not the cervical esophagus).

Killian-Jamieson Diverticulum:

This one is **anterior and lateral**.

It protrudes through an area of weakness below the attachment of the cricopharyngeus muscle and lateral to the ligaments that help suspend the esophagus on the cricoid cartilage.

This one is **in the cervical esophagus.**

Traction Diverticulum:

Mid esophageal, and often <u>triangular</u> in shape.

These occur from scarring (think granulomatous disease or TB).

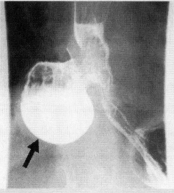

Epiphrenic Diverticula:

Located just above the diaphragm (**usually on the right**). ** The para-esophageal hernia is usually on the left.

They are considered pulsion types (associated with motor abnormality).

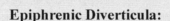

Esophageal Pseudodiverticulosis:

This is an Aunt Minnie. What you have are dilated submucosal glands that cause multiple small out pouchings. **Usually due to chronic reflux esophagitis.**

There is controversy among the whole candida situation. Per the Mayo GI book, candida is often cultured but is not the causative factor.

This vs That: **Traction vs Pulsion Diverticulum**	
Traction	**Pulsion**
Triangular	Round
Will Empty	Will **NOT** Empty (contain no muscle in their walls)

—

Papilloma: The most common benign mucosal lesion of the esophagus. It's basically just hyperplastic squamous epithelium.

Feline Esophagus: Another Aunt Minnie. You have transient, fine transverse folds which course the esophagus. It can be normal. It can be associated with esophagitis..... *correlate clinically.*

Hernias: There are a bunch of ways to classify these, but the most common (and likely tested) is the relationship of the GE junction to the diaphragm.

• *Axial (Sliding)* types have the GE junction above the diaphragm.

• *Paraesophageal (Rolling)* types have the GE junction below the diaphragm, and a piece of the stomach above it. The rolling type has a higher rate of incarceration. There are usually on the left (the epiphrenic diverticulum is usually on the right).

Esophageal Spasm: Basically tertiary contractions with pain. The term *nutcracker esophagus* requires manometric findings (>180mmHg).

Esophageal Web: Most commonly located at the cervical esophagus (near the cricopharyngeus). This thing is basically a ring caused by a thin mucosal membrane. There are 2 things to know about it:

(1) It's a **risk factor for** esophageal and hypopharyngeal **carcinoma**
(2) **Plummer –Vinson Syndrome**: iron def anemia, dysphagia, thyroid issues, "spoon-shaped nails"

Vascular Impressions

This is a very high yield topic for the purpose of multiple choice exams.

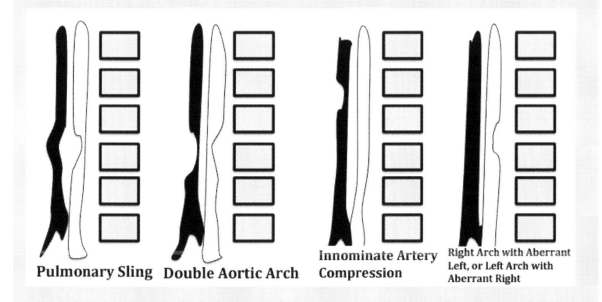

Pulmonary Sling **Double Aortic Arch** **Innominate Artery Compression** **Right Arch with Aberrant Left, or Left Arch with Aberrant Right**

Trivia to Know:

Pulmonary Sling:
- The **only variant that goes between the esophagus and the trachea**.
- Classic question, is that this is **associated with trachea stenosis.**
- High association with other cardiopulmonary and systemic anomalies: hypoplastic right lung, horseshoe lung, TE-fistula, imperforate anus, and complete tracheal rings.

Double Aortic Arch:
- Most Common **SYMPTOMATIC** vascular ring anomaly

Left Arch with Aberrant Right Subclavian Artery
- Most Common Aortic Arch Anomaly — not necessarily symptomatic.
- **"Dysphagia Lusoria"** - fancy Latin speak (therefore high yield) for trouble swallowing in the setting of this variant anatomy
- **"Diverticulum of Kommerell"** pouch like aneurysmal dilatation of the proximal portion of an aberrant right subclavian artery

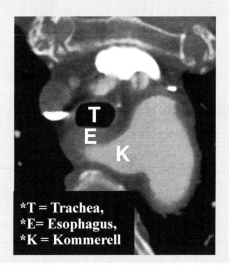

*T = Trachea,
*E= Esophagus,
*K = Kommerell

The Dilated Esophagus

If you get shown a big dilated esophagus (full cheerios, mashed potatoes, and McDonald's french fries… or "freedom fries" as I call them), you will need to think about 3 things.

(1) **Achalasia:** A motor disorder where the distal 2/3 of the esophagus (smooth muscle part) doesn't have normal peristalsis (*"absent primary peristalsis"*), and the lower esophageal sphincter won't relax.

The esophagus will be dilated above a smooth stricture at the GE junction (**Bird's Beak**).

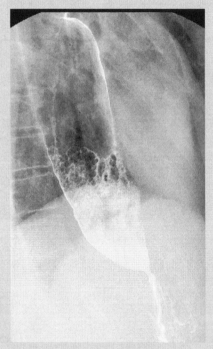

"Vigorous Achalasia" - An early / less severe form which classically has repetitive simultaneous non-propulsive contractions. It's more common in women, but the secondary cancer occurs more in men.

Things to know:

- Failure of the Esophageal sphincter to relax
- Increased Risk of Candida

"Chagas Disease" - More common in the jungle. The esophagus get paralyzed by some parasite transmitted by a fly. The appearance is identical to Achalasia - and some people even lump them together (other's reserve the term "achalasia" for idiopathic types only). You'll simply need to read the mind of the test question writer to know what camp he/she falls into.

(2) **"Pseudoachalasia"** *(secondary achalasia)* has the appearance of achalasia, but is secondary to a cancer at the GE junction. The difference is that real Achalasia will eventually relax, the pseudo won't. They have to show you that the mass - or hint at it, or straight up tell you that the GE junction didn't relax. Alternatively they could be sneaky and just list a bunch of cancer risk factors (smoking, drinking, chronic reflux) in the question stem. Next step would probably be CT (or full on upper GI).

(3) **Scleroderma:** Involves the esophagus 80% of the time. Again the lower 2/3 of the esophagus stops working normally. The LES is incompetent and you end up with chronic reflux, which can cause scarring, Barretts, and even cancer (Adeno). They will show you lung changes (most commonly **NSIP**), and the barium esophagus (or a small bowel series showing closely spaced valvulae conniventes – *hide bound*).

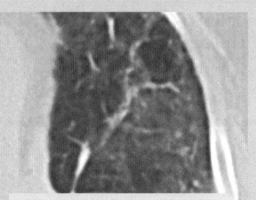

NSIP - Ground Glass - with sub pleural sparring

Esophagus – High Yield Trivia	
Path	**Trivia**
Esophagitis	Fold Thickening. May have smooth stricture at GE junction if severe
Barretts	Buzzword: Reticulated Mucosal Pattern Classically shown as Hiatal Hernia + High Stricture
Medication Induced Esophagitis	Ulcers; Usually at the level of the arch or distal esophagus
Crohns Esophagitis	Ulcers ; can be confluent in severe disease
Candidia	Discrete plaque like lesions that are seen as linear or irregular filling defects that tend to be longitudinally oriented, separated by normal mucosa Buzzword: Shaggy – when severe Not always from AIDS, can also be from motility disorders such as achalasia and scleroderma
Glycogen Acanthosis	Looks like Candidia, but in an asymptomatic old person
Herpes Ulcers	Multiple small, with Edema Halo (herpes has halo)
CMV / AIDS	Large Flat ulcers
Achalasia	Buzzword: Bird Beak, - smooth stricture at GE junction Path is failure of LES to relax (but it will slowly relax) Increased risk of Squamous Cell CA, and Candida
Pseudoachalsia	Cancer at the GE junction. Fixed Obstruction, will not relax
Scleroderma	Involves the Esophagus 80% of the time Looks a little like Achalasia (they will show you lung changes- NSIP) Sequelae of reflux: stricture, barrets, cancer
Long Stricture	DDx: NG tube in too long, Radiation, Caustic Ingestion
Pseudodiverticulosis	Dilated submucosal glands, usually due to chronic reflux esophagitis. Esophageal stricture is seen in 90% of cases
Zenker Diverticula	Zenker in the back (above cricopharyngeus) From the hypopharynx
Killian-Jamieson	Lateral (below cricopharyngeus) From the cervical esophagus.

Stomach

Location Location:

- **H Pylori** Gastritis – Usually in **Antrum**
- **Zollinger-Ellison** – Ulcerations in the stomach (**jeujunal ulcer** is the buzzword). Duodenal bulb is actually the most common location for ulcers in ZE. Remember ZE is from gastrinoma - and might be a way to test MEN syndromes.
- **Crohns** – Uncommon in the stomach, but when it is, it likes the **antrum**
- **Menetrier's** – Usually in the **Fundus** (*classically spares the antrum*)
- **Lymphoma** – "Crosses the Pylorus" – classically described as doing so, although in reality adenocarcinoma does it more.

Selective Polyposis Syndromes	
Path	**Trivia**
Gardner Syndrome	FAP (Hyperplastic Stomach, Adenomatous Bowel Polyps) + Desmoid Tumors, Osteomas, Papillary Thyroid Cancer
Turcots	FAP (Hyperplastic Stomach, Adenomatous Bowel Polyps) + Gliomas and Medulloblastomas
Hereditary nonpolyposis Syndrome (Lynch)	DNA Mismatch Repair They get cancer everywhere in everything
Peutz-Jeghers	Hamartoma Style! Mucocutaneous Pigmentation Small and Large Bowel CA, Pancreatic CA, and GYN CA
Cowden's *THIS IS THE MOST LIKELY TO BE ASKED*	Hamartoma Style! **BREAST CA**, Thyroid CA, Lhermitte-Dulcose (*posterior fossa noncancerous brain tumor*)
Cronkite-Canada	Hamartoma Style! Stomach, Small Bowel, Colon, Ectodermal Stuff (skin, hair, nails, yuck)
Juvenile Polyps	Hamartoma Style!
Zenker Diverticula	Zenker in the back (above cricopharyngeus)

GIST

This is the most common mesenchymal tumor of the GI tract (70% in stomach). Think about this in an old person (it's rare before age 40).

Some tricks to know:

- *Lymph node enlargement is NOT a classic feature*

- *The malignant ones tend to be big angry mother fuckers (>10cm with ulceration - and possible perforation).*

- *The association with Carney's triad - Extra-Adrenal Pheochromocytoma, GIST, Pulmonary Chordoma (hamartoma)*

- *The association with NF-1*

Carneys Triad
"Carney's **E**at **G**arbage"
Chordoma **E**xtra Adrenal Pheo **G**IST

Stomach Ulcers - Benign vs Malignant
— 1960s style medicine --

Malignant	Benign
Width > Depth	Depth > Width
Located within Lumen	Project behind the expected lumen
Nodular, Irregular Edges	Sharp Contour
Folds adjacent to ulcer	Folds radiate to ulcer
Aunt Minnie: Carmen Meniscus Sign	Aunt Minnie: Hampton's Line
Can be anywhere	Mostly on Lesser Curvature

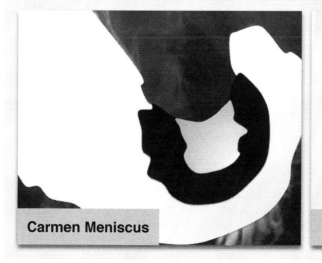

Carmen Meniscus

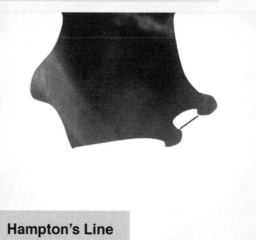

Hampton's Line

Gastric Cancer

It's Either Lymphoma (<5%) or Carcinoma (95%).

Gastric carcinoma is usually a disease of an old person (median age 70). H. Pylori is the most tested risk factor.

Trivia to know:

- Ulcerated carcinoma (or the "penetrating cancer") has the look of an advanced cancer

- Metastatic spread to the ovary is referred to as a **Krukenberg Tumor.**

- Gastroenterostomy performed for gastric ulcer disease (old school – prior to PPIs) have a 2x – 6x- increased risk for development of carcinoma within the gastric remnant.

- Step 1 trivia question: swollen left supraclavicular node = **Virchow Node.**

Gastric Lymphoma, can be primary (MALT), or secondary to systemic lymphoma. The stomach is the most common extranodal site for non-Hodgkin lymphoma. Even when extensive, it **rarely causes gastric outlet obstruction.** It was classically described as *"crossing the pylorus"* , although since gastric carcinoma is like 10x more common it is actually more likely to do that. Has multiple looks and can be big, little, ulcerative, polypoid, or look like target lesions. It can also look like Linitis Plastica.

Trivia: It can rupture with treatment (chemo).

Linitis Plastica: The leather bottle stomach. It's the result of a scirrhous adenocarcinoma, with diffuse infiltration. Can be from **breast** or lung mets.

Ulcerative Trivia:
Gastric Ulcers - They have 5% chance of being cancer.
Duodenal Ulcers - Are never cancer (on multiple choice)
Gastric Ulcers occurs from "altered mucosal resistance"
Duodenal Ulcers occur from "increased peptic acid"
Duodenal Ulcers are usually solitary, when not think ZE.

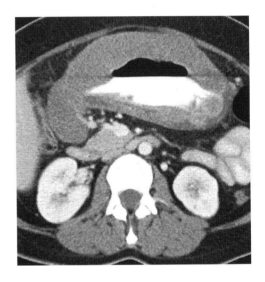

Gastric Cancer is "More Likely" Than Lymphoma to…

- *More Likely to Cause Gastric Outlet Obstruction*

- *More Likely to be in the distal stomach*

- *More Likely to extend beyond the serosa and obliterate adjacent fat plains*

- *More Likely to be a focal mass (95% of primary gastric tumors are adenocarcinoma)*

Misc. Gastric Conditions

Menetrier's Disease: Rare and has a French sounding name, so it's almost guaranteed to be on the test. It's an idiopathic gastropathy, with rugal thickening that classically involves the fundus and spares the antrum. Bimodal age distribution (childhood form thought to be CMV related). They end up with low albumin, from loss into gastric lumen.

Essential Trivia: Involves the fundus, and spares the antrum.

Ram's Horn Deformity *(Pseudo Billroth 1)* Tapering of the antrum causes the stomach to look like a Ram's Horn. This is a differential case, and can be seen with Scarring via peptic ulcers, Granulomatous Disease (Crohns, Sarcoid, TB, Syphillis), or Scirrhous Carcinoma.

Essential Trivia: **The stomach is the most common location for sarcoid (in the GI tract).**

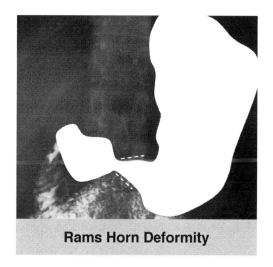
Rams Horn Deformity

Gastric Volvulus

Two Flavors:

- *Organoaxial* – the greater curvature flips over the lesser curvature. This is seen in old ladies with paraesophageal hernias. It's way more common.

- *Mesenteroaxial* – twisting over the messentary. Can cause ischemia and needs to be fixed. Additionally this type causes obstruction. This type is more common in kids.

Gastric Diverticulum: The way they always ask this is by trying to get you to call it an adrenal mass (it's most commonly in the posterior fundus). Find the normal adrenal.

Gastric Varices: This gets mentioned in the pancreas section, but I just want to hammer home that test writers love to ask **splenic vein thrombus casing isolated gastric varices**. Some sneaky ways they can ask this is by saying "pancreatic cancer" or "Pancreatitis" causes gastric varices. Which is true…. because they are associated with splenic vein thrombus. So, just watch out for that.

Areae Gastricae: This is a **normal** fine reticular pattern seen on double contrast. Multiple choice writers have been known to ask when does this "enlarge"? The answer is that it enlarges in elderly and patient's with H. Pylori. Also it can focally enlarge next to an ulcer. It becomes obliterated by cancer or atrophic gastritis.

Chronic Aspirin Therapy: "Multiple gastric ulcers" is the buzzword. Obviously this is non-specific, but some sources say it occurs in 80% of patient's with chronic aspirin use. As a point of trivia, <u>aspirin does NOT cause duodenal ulcers</u>. If you see multiple duodenal ulcers (most duodenal ulcers are solitary) you should think Zollinger-Ellison.

Upper GI Surgical Complications:

Afferent Loop Syndrome: An uncommon complication post billroth 2. The most common cause is obstruction (adhesions tumor, intestinal hernia) of the afferent. The acute form may have a closed loop obstruction. The result of this afferent obstruction is the build up of biliary, pancreatic, and intestinal secretions resulting in afferent limb dilation. The back pressure from all this back up dilates the gallbladder, and causes pancreatitis. A much less common cause is if the stomach preferentially drains into the afferent loop.

Billroth 2

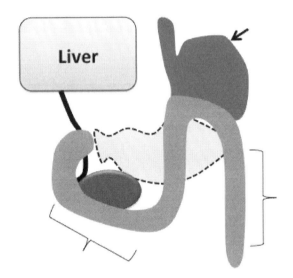

Afferent Limb Syndrome

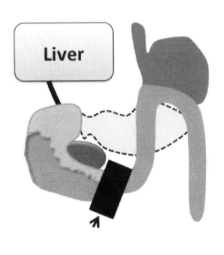

Jejunogastric Intussusception: This is a rare complication of gastroenterostomy. The Jejunum herniates back into the stomach (usually the efferent limb) and can cause gastric obstruction. High mortality is present with the acute form.

Bile Reflex Gastritis: Fold thickening and filling defects seen in the stomach after Billroth I or II are likely the result of bile acid reflux.

Gastro-Gastric Fistula: This is seen in Roux-en-Y patients who gain weight years later. The anastomotic breakdown is a chronic process, and often is not painful.

Cancer: With regard to these old peptic ulcer surgeries (billroths), there is a 3-6 times increased risk of getting adenocarcinoma in the gastric remnant (like 15 years after the surgery).

Small Bowel

Bowel Folds:

Let's be honest Fluoro is pretty useless compared to endoscopy and CT. But just for fun let's pretend it's 1950.

One search pattern to organize your thinking on the subject:

(1) Folds
(2) Filling Defects
(3) Loop Separation

With regard to fold thickening, the best way to think about this is categorically:

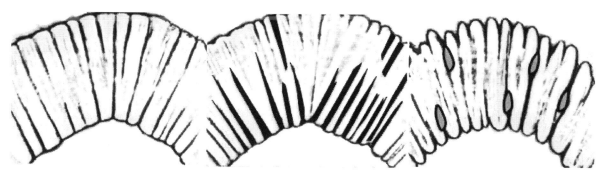

Thin Straight Folds with a dilated lumen

Thick (>3mm) Straight folds — *of which they can be diffuse or segmental*

Thick Nodular folds — of which they can be diffuse or segmental.

Each subtype will carry a different differential.

Fold Pattern				
Thin Folds, with Dilation	Thick Folds > 3mm		Thick Folds with Nodularity	
	Segmental	Diffuse	Segmental	Diffuse
Mechanical Obstruction	Ischemia	Low Protein	Crohns	Whipples
Paralytic Ileus	Radiation	Venous Congestion	Infection	Lymphoid Hyperplasia
Scleroderma	Hemorrhage	Cirrhosis	Lymphoma	Lymphoma
Sprue	Adjacent Inflammation		Mets	Mets
				Intestinal Lymphangiectasia

With regard to filling defects, the way to think about this is:

- Uniform 2-4mm nodules = Lymphoid Hyperplasia
- Nodules of larger or varying sizes = Cancer (probably mets and therefore probably melanoma).

Loop Separation can be thought about as with or without tethering

- Without Tethering = Ascites, Wall Thickening (Crohns, Lymphoma), Adenopathy, or Mesenteric Tumors
- With Tethering = Just say carcinoid
- A pearl is that extrinsic processes will spare the mucosa, intrinsic process with alter the mucosa.

Selected Small Bowel Path:

The Target Sign:

•Single Target: GIST, Primary Adenocarcinoma, Lymphoma, Ectopic Pancreatic Rest, Met (Melanoma).

•Multiple Target: Lymphoma, Met (Melanoma)

Clover Leaf Sign: This is an Aunt Minnie for Healed Peptic Ulcer of the Duodenal Bulb.

Whipples: Rare infection (Tropheryma Wipplei)

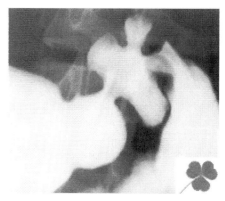

Clover Leaf Sign
- Healed Duodenal Ulcer

Just like a stripper - it prefers white men in their 50s. The bug infiltrates the lamina propria with large macrophages infected by intracellular whipple bacilli leading to marked swelling of intestinal villi and thickened irregular mucosal folds primarily in duodenum and proximal jejunum. The buzzword is "sand like nodules" referring to diffuse micronodules in jejunum. Jejunal mucosal folds are thickened. This is another cause of low density (near fat) enlarged lymph nodes.

Pseudo Whipples: MAI infection. Seen in AIDS patients with CD4<100. Nodules in the jejunum, just like regular Whipples is the finding (plus a big spleen, and retroperitoneal lymph nodes).

Celiac Sprue: Small bowel malabsorption of gluten.

- High yield points:
    o Can cause malabsorption of iron, and lead to iron deficiency anemia.
    o Associated with Idiopathic Pulmonary Hemosiderosis (Lane Hamilton Syndrome
    o Increased Risk of bowel wall **lymphoma**
    o Gold standard is biopsy (*surprisingly not barium*)
    o Dermatitis Herpetiformis – some skin thing (remember that from step 1)

- Findings (CT / Barium)
    o **Fold Reversal** is the Buzzword (Jejunum like Ileum, Ileum like Jejunum)
    o Moulage Sign – dilated bowel with effaced folds (tube with wax poured in it)
    o **Cavitary Lymph Nodes (low density)**
    o Splenic Atrophy

Intestinal Lymphangiectasia: Lymphangiectasia results from obstruction to the flow of lymph from the small intestine into the mesentery. This results in dilation of the intestinal and serosal lymphatic channels. This can be primary from lymphatic hypoplasia, or secondary from obstruction of the thoracic duct (or any place in between).

SMA Syndrome: This is an obstruction of the 3rd portion of the duodenum by the SMA (it pinches the duodenum in the midline). It is seen in **patients who have recently lost a lot of weight.**

Graft vs Host: Buzzword = **Ribbon bowel.** It occurs in patients after bone marrow transplant. It's less common with modern anti-rejection drugs. Skin, Liver, and GI tract get hit. Small bowel is usually the most severely affected. Bowel is featureless, atrophic, and has fold thickening (ribbon like).

Meckel's Diverticulum / Diverticulitis: This is a congenital true diverticulum of the distal ileum. A piece of total trivia is that it is a persistent piece of the omphalomesenteric duct. Step 1 style, "rule of 2s" occurs in 2% of the population, has 2 types of heterotopic mucosa (gastric and pancreatic), located 2 feet from the IC valve, it's usually 2 inches long (and 2cm in diameter), and usually has symptoms before the child is 2. If it has gastric mucosa (the ones that bleed typically do) it will take up Tc-Pertechnetate just like the stomach (hence the Meckel's scan).

High Yield Meckel's Trivia (Regarding Complications)

- *Can get diverticulitis in the Meckels (mimic appendix)*
- *GI Bleed from Gastric Mucosa (causes 30% of symptomatic cases)*
- *Can be a lead point for intussusception (seen with inverted diverticulum)*
- *Can cause Obstruction*

Duodenal Inflammatory Disease: You can have fold thickening of the duodenum from adjacent inflammatory processes of the pancreas or gallbladder. You can also have thickening and fistula formation with Crohn's (usually when the colon is the primary site). Primary duodenal Crohns can happen, but is super rare. **Chronic dialysis patients may get severely thickened duodenal folds** which can mimic the appearance of pancreatitis on barium.

Jejunal Diverticulosis: Less common than colonic diverticulosis, but does occur. They occur along the mesenteric border. Important **association is bacterial overgrowth and malabsorption**. They could show this with CT, but more likely will show it with barium (if they show it at all).

Small Bowel Cancer

Adenocarinoma: Most common in the proximal small bowel (<u>usually duodenum</u>). Increased incidence with celiac disease and regional enteritis. Focal circumferential bowel wall thickening in proximal small bowel is characteristic on CT. The duodenal web does NOT increase the risk.

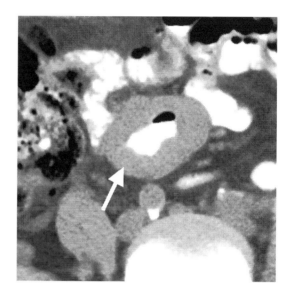

Lymphoma: It's usually the non-Hodgkin flavor. Patient's with celiac, Crohns, AIDS, and SLE are higher risk. It can look like anything (infiltrative, polypoid, multiple nodules etc….). **Key piece of trivia is they usually do NOT obstruct, even with massive circumferential involvement.** The Hodgkin subtype is more likely to cause a desmoplastic reaction.

Carcinoid: This has an **Aunt Minnie look with a mass + desmoplastic stranding.** "Starburst" appearance of the mesenteric mass with calcifications. This tumor most commonly occurs in young adults. The <u>primary tumor is often not seen</u>. That calcified crap you are seeing in the desmoplastic reaction. Liver mets are often hyper vascular. Step 1 style, you don't get carcinoid syndrome (flushing, diarrhea) until you met to the liver. The **most common primary location is the distal appendix** (50%). The appendix + terminal ileum makes it 90%. The appendix, has the best prognosis of all GI primary sites. Systemic serotonin degrades the heart valves (right sided), and classically causes tricuspid regurgitation - *more on this in the cardiac chapter.* MIBG or Octreotide scans can assist with diagnosis and staging - *more on this in the nuclear medicine chapter.*

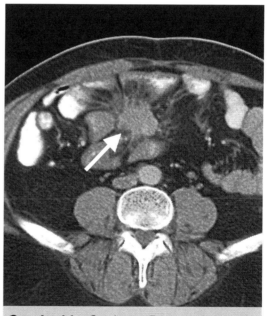

Carcinoid - *Sunburst Desmoplastic Rx*

Mets: This is usually **melanoma** (which hits the small bowel 50% in fatal cases). You can also get hematogenous seeding of the small bowel with breast, lung, and Kaposi sarcoma. Melanoma will classically have multiple targets.

Hernias:

Inguinal Hernias: - the most common type of abdominal wall hernia. M>F (7:1)

Direct	Indirect
Less common	More Common
Medial to inferior epigastric artery	Lateral to inferior epigastric artery
Defect in Hesselback Triangle	Failure of processus vaginalis to close
NOT covered by internal spermatic fascia	Covered by internal spermatic fascia

Femoral: Likely to obstruct, and seen in old ladies. They are medial to the femoral vein, and posterior to the inguinal ligament (usually on the right).

Obturator Hernia: Another old lady hernia. Often seen in patients with increased intraabdominal pressure (Ascites, COPD – chronic cougher). Usually asymptomatic – but can strangulate.

Lumbar Hernia: Can be superior (Grynfeltt-Lesshaft) through the superior lumbar triangle, or inferior (Petit) through the inferior lumbar triangle. Superior is more common than inferior. Otherwise, they are very similar and usually discussed together. Causes are congenital or acquired (post-surgery or acquired).

Spigelian Hernia: The question is probably the location along the **S**emilunar line *("S" for "S")* through the transversus abdominus aponeurosis close to the level of the arcuate line.

Littre Hernia : Hernia with a Meckel Diverticulum in it.

Amyand Hernia: Hernia with the appendix in it.

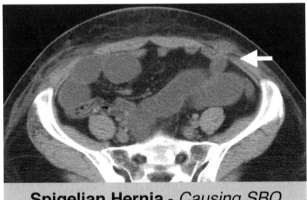

Spigelian Hernia - *Causing SBO*

Richter Hernia: Contains only one wall of bowel and therefore **does not obstruct**. This are actually at higher risk for strangulation.

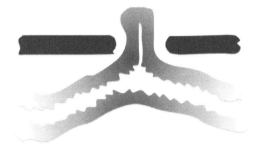

Richter - *Only one wall herniates*

Hernias Post Laparoscopic Roux-en-Y Gastric By Pass:

Factors that promote internal hernia by bypass: (1) Laproscopic over Open – supposedly creates less adhesion, so you have more mobility (2) Degree of weight loss ; more weight loss = less protective, space occupying mesenteric fat.

There are 3 potential sites.

(1) At the defect in the transverse mesocolon, through which the Roux-Loop Passes (if it's done in the retrocolic position).
(2) At the mesenteric defect at the enteroenterostomy
(3) Behind the Roux limb mesentery placed in a retrocolic or antecolic position (**retrocolic Petersen** and **antecolic Petersen** type). ** This is the one they will likely ask because it has an eponym with it.

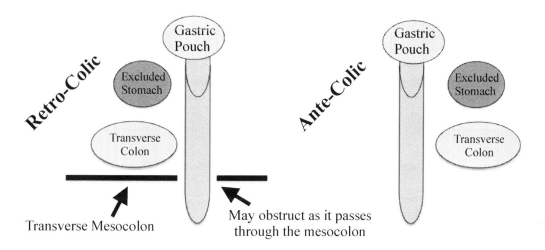

Internal Hernia: These can be sneaky. The most common manifestation is closed loop obstruction (often with strangulation). There are 9 different subtypes, of which I refuse to cover. I will touch on the most common, and the general concept.

General Concept: This is a herniation of viscera, through the peritoneum or mesentery. The herniation takes place through a known anatomic foramina or recess, or one that has been created post operatively.

Paraduodenal (right or left): This is by far the most common type of internal hernia. They can occur in 5 different areas, but it's much simpler to think of them as left or right. Actually, **75% of the time they are on the left**. The exact location is the duodenojejunal junction ("fossa of Landzert"). Here is the trick, the herniated small bowel can become trapped in a "**sac of bowel**," between the pancreas and stomach to the left of the ligament of Treitz.   The sac characteristically contains the IMV and the left colic artery.

The right sided PDHs are located just behind the SMA and just below the transverse segment of the duodenum, at the "Fossa of Waldeyer." The classic setting for right sided PDHs is non-rotated small bowel, with normally rotated large bowel.

Large Bowel

Crohns Disease vs Ulcerative Colitis:

Crohns Disease: Typically seen in a young adult (15-30), but has a second smaller peak 60-70. Discontinuous involvement of the entire GI tract (mouth -> asshole). Stomach, usually involves antrum (Ram's Horn Deformity). Duodenal involvement is rare, and NEVER occurs without antrum involvement. Small bowel is involved 80% of the time, with the terminal ileum almost always involved (Marked Narrowing = String Sign). After surgery the "neo-terminal ileum" will frequently be involved. The colon involvement is usually right sided, and often spares the rectum / sigmoid. Complications include fistulae, abscess, gallstones, fatty liver, and sacroiliitis.

Crohns Buzzwords	
Squaring of the folds	An early manifestation from obstructive lymphedema
Skip lesions	Discontinuous involvement of the bowel
Proud loops	Separation of the loops caused by infiltration of the mesentery, increase in mesenteric fat and enlarged lymph nodes
Cobblestoning	Irregular, appearance to bowel wall caused by longitudinal and transverse ulcers separated by areas of edema
Pseudopolyps	Islands of hyperplastic mucosa
Filiform	Post-inflammatory polyps – long and worm like
Pseudodiverticula	Found on anti-mesenteric side. From bulging area of normal wall opposite side of scarring from disease,
String-sign	Marked narrowing of terminal ileum from a combination of edema, spasm and fibrosis;

Ulcerative Colitis: Just like Crohns, it typically occurs in a "young adult" (age 15-40), with a second peak at 60-70. Favors the male gender. It **involves the rectum 95% of the time, and has retrograde progression**. Terminal ileum is involved 5-10% of the time via backwash ileitis (wide open appearance). It is continuous and does not "skip" like Crohns. It is associated with Colon Cancer, Primary Sclerosing Cholangitis, and Arthritis (similar to Ankylosing Spondylitis). On Barium, it is said that the colon is ahaustral, with a diffuse granular appearing mucosa. "Lead Pipe" is the buzzword (shortened from fibrosis). Here is a key clinical point; UC has an increased risk of cancer (probably higher than Crohns), and it doesn't classically have enlarged lymph nodes (like Crohns does), so if you see a big lymph node in a UC patient (especially one with long standing disease) you have to think that might be cancer.

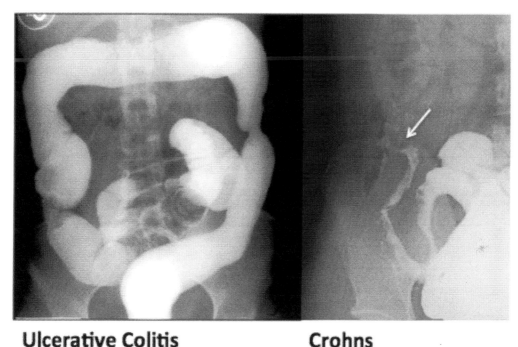

Ulcerative Colitis
- Haustral Loss, Lead Pipe Appearance

Crohns
- String Sign at IC Valve

More Common In : Crohns vs UC	
Path	**More Common IN**
Gallstones	Crohns
Primary Sclerosing Cholangitis	Ulcerative Coliits
Hepatic Abscess	Crohns
Pancreatitis	Crohns

Crohns vs Ulcerative Colitis	
Crohns	**UC**
Slightly less common in the USA	Slightly more common in the USA
Discontinuous "Skips"	Continuous
Terminal Ileum – *String Sign*	Rectum
Ileocecal Valve "Stenosed"	Ileocecal Valve "Open"
Mesenteric Fat Increased *"creeping fat"*	Perirectal fat Increased
Lymph nodes are usually enlarged	Lymph nodes are NOT usually enlarged
Makes Fistula	Doesn't Usually Make Fistula

—

Diverticulosis / Diverticulitis: Some trivia worth knowing is that diverticulosis actually bleeds more than diverticulitis. Right sided is less common (but is seen in young Asians). Fistula formation is actually most common with diverticulitis, and can occur to anything around it (another piece of bowel, the bladder, etc..).

Epiploic Appendagitis / Omental Infarct: Epiploic apppendages along the serosal surface of the colon can torse, **most commonly on the left**. There is not typically concentric bowel wall thickening (unlike diverticulitis). *Omental infarction* is typically a larger mass with a more oval shape, and central low density. It is **more commonly on the right** (*ROI – right omental infarct*). Both entities are self limiting.

—

Appendicitis – The classic pathways are: obstruction (fecalith or reactive lymphoid tissue) -> mucinous fluid builds up increasing pressure -> venous supply is compressed -> necrosis starts -> wall breaks down -> bacteria get into wall -> inflammation causes vague pain (umbilicus) -> inflamed appendix gets larger and touches parietal peritoneum (pain shifts to RLQ). It occurs in an adolescent or young adult (or any age). The measurement of 6mm, was originally described with data from ultrasound compression, but people still generally use it for CT as well. Secondary signs of inflammation are probably more reliable for CT.

Appendix Mucocele – Mucinous cystadenomas are the most common mucinous tumor of the appendix. They produce mucin and can really dilate up and get big. They look similar to cystadenocarcinomas and can perforate leading to pseudomyxoma peritonei. On ultrasound the presence of an "**onion sign**" – layering within cystic mass is a suggestive feature of a mucocele.

Colonic Volvulus: Comes in several flavors:

- *Sigmoid:* Most common adult form. Seen in the nursing home patient (chronic constipation is a predisposing factor). Buzzword is coffee bean sign (or inverted 3 sign). Another less common buzzword is Frimann Dahl's sign – which refers to 3 dense lines converging towards the site of obstruction. Points to the RUQ. Recurrence rate after decompression = 50%.

This vs That: Sigmoid Volvulus vs Cecal Volvulus	
Sigmoid	**Cecal**
Old Person	Younger Person
Points to the RUQ	Points to the LUQ

- *Cecal:* Seen in a younger person (20-40). Associated with people with a "long mesentery." More often points to the LUQ. Much less common than sigmoid.

- *Cecal Bascule:* Anterior folding of the cecum, **without twisting**. A lot of surgical text books dispute this thing even being real (they think it's a focal ileus). The finding is supposedly dilation of the cecum in an ectopic position in the middle abdomen, without a mesenteric twist.

—

Toxic Megacolon: Ulcerative colitis, and to a lesser degree Crohns is the primary cause. C-Diff can also cause it. Gaseous dilation distends the transverse colon (on upright films), and the right and left colon on supine films. **Lack of haustra** and pseudopolyps are also seen. Some people say the presence of normal hausta excludes the diagnosis. **Don't do a barium enema** because of the risk of perforation. Another piece of trivia is that peritonitis can occur without perforation.

Behcets: Ulcers of the penis and mouth. Can also affect GI tract (and **looks like Crohns**) – *most commonly affects the ileocecal region.* It is also cause of **pulmonary artery aneurysms** (test writers like to ask that).

Colonic Pseudo-Obstruction *(Colonic Ileus, Ogilvie Syndrome):* Usually seen after serious medical conditions, and nursing home patients. It can persist for years, or progress to bowel necrosis and perforation. The classic look is marked diffuse dilation of the large bowel, without a discrete transition point.

Diversion Colitis: Bacterial overgrowth in a blind loop through which stool does not pass (any surgery that does this).

Colitis Cystica: This cystic dilation of the mucous glands comes in two flavors: Superficial or Profunda (Deep).

Superficial: The superficial kind consists of cysts that are small in the entire colon. It's associated with vitamin deficiencies, and tropical sprue. Can also be seen in terminal leukemia, uremia, thyroid toxicosis, and mercury poisoning.

Profunda: These cysts may be large and are seen in the pelvic colon and rectum.

 Rectal Cavernous Hemangioma: Obviously very rare. Just know it's associated with a few syndromes; Klippel-Trenaunay-Weber, and Blue Rubber Bleb. They might show you a ton of phleboliths down there.

Gossypiboma: This isn't really a GI pathology but it's an abscess mimic. It's a retained cotton product or surgical sponge, and can elicit an inflammatory response.

—

Infections:

Entamoeba Histolytica: Parasite that causes bloody diarrhea. Can cause liver abscess, spleen abscess, or even brain abscess. Within the colon it is one of the causes of toxic megacolon. They are typically "flask shaped ulcers" on endoscopy. With regard to barium, the buzzword is *"coned cecum"* referring to a change in the normal bulbous appearance of the cecum, to that of a cone. It affects the cecum and ascending colon most commonly, and unlike many other GI injections **spares the terminal ileum.**

Colonic TB: Typically involves the terminal ileum, and is another cause of the "**coned cecum**" appearance. Causes both ulcers and areas of narrowing. Two other signs: (1) *Fleischner sign* – enlarged gaping IC valve, and (2) *Stierlin sign* – narrowing of the TI.

Colonic CMV: Seen in patients who are immunosuppressed. Causes deep ulcerations – which can lead to perforation. Pathology Trivia = Cowdry Type A intranuclear inclusion bodies

C-Diff: Classically seen after antibiotic therapy, the toxin leads to a super high WBC count. CT findings of the *"accordion sign"* with contrast trapped inside mucosal folds is always described in review books and is fair game for multiple choice. The barium findings include thumbprinting, ulceration, and irregularity. Of course it can cause toxic megacolon as mentioned on the prior page.

Neutropenic Colitis (Typhlitis): Infection **limited to the cecum** occurring in severe neurotropenia.

Infections that like the Duodenum *(and proximal small bowel)*	Infections that like the Terminal Ileum
Giardia	TB
Strongyloides	Yersinia

Colon Cancer:

Adenocarcinoma: Common cause of cancer death (#2 overall). The cancer on the right tends to bleed (present with blood stools, anemia), the cancer on the left tends to obstruct. **Apple core** is a buzzword.

Squamous Carcinoma – Occasionally arises in the anus *(think HPV)*.

Lipomas: The second most common tumor in the colon

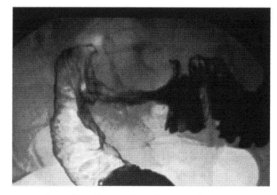

Apple Core Lesion - Cancer

Adenoma – The most common benign tumor of the colon and rectum. The *villous adenoma has the largest risk for malignancy.*

McKittrick-Wheelock Syndrome:

This is a <u>villous adenoma</u> that causes a mucous diarrhea leading to severe fluid and electrolyte depletion.

The clinical scenario would be something like "80 year old lady with diarrhea, hyponatremia, hypokalemia, hypochloremia… and this" and they show you a mass in the rectum / bowel.

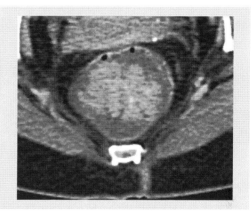

Rectal Cancer:

Things to know:
- Nearly always (98%) adenocarcinoma
- If the path says Squamous - the cause was HPV *(use your imagination on how it got there)*.
- Total mesorectal excision is standard surgical method
- Lower rectal cancer (0-5 cm from the anorectal angle), have the highest recurrence rate.
- MRI is used to stage - and you really only need T2 weight imaging - contrast doesn't matter
- Stage T3 - called when tumor breaks out of the rectum and into the perirectal fat. This is the critical stage that changes management (they will get chemo/rads prior to surgery).

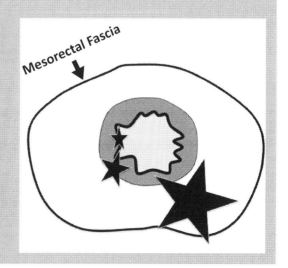

Mesorectal Fascia

Peritoneal Cavity

Pseudomyxoma Peritonei: This is a gelatinous ascites that results from either (a) ruptured mucocele (usually appendix), or interperitoneal spread of a mucinous neoplasm (ovary, colon, appendix, and pancreas). It's usually the appendix (least common is the pancreas). The buzzword is "**scalloped appearance of the liver.**" Recurrent bowel obstructions are common.

Peritoneal Carcinomatosis: The main thing to know regarding peritoneal implants is that the natural flow of ascites dictates the location of implants. This is why the **retrovesical space is the most common spot** , since it's the most dependent part of the peritoneal cavity.

Omental Seeding/Caking: The omental surface can get implanted by cancer, and become thick (like a mass). The catch-phrase is "posterior displacement of the bowel - from the anterior abdominal wall."

Primary Peritoneal Mesothelioma: This is super rare. People think about mesothelioma involving the pleura (and it does 75% of the time), but the other 25% of the time it involves the peritoneal surface. The thing to know is that it <u>occurs 30-40 years after the initial asbestosis exposure.</u>

 Cystic Peritoneal Mesothelioma: This is the even more rare benign mesothelioma, that is <u>NOT associated with prior asbestos exposure</u>. It usually involves a women of child bearing age (30s).

Mesenteric Lymphoma: This is usually non-Hodgkin lymphoma, which supposedly involves the mesentery 50% of the time. The **buzzword is "sandwich sign."** The typical appearance is a lobulated confluent soft tissue mass encasing the mesenteric vessels "sandwiching them."

Barium Gone Bad

Complications of barium use are rare, but can be very serious. They come in two main flavors: (1) Peritonitis, and (2) Intravasation.

Barium Peritonitis: This is why you use a water soluble contrast any time you are worried about leak. The pathology is an attack of the peritoneal barium by the leukocytes which creates a monster inflammatory reaction (often with massive ascites and sometimes hypovolemia and resulting shock). If no "real doctor" is available, you should give IV fluids to reduce the risk of hypovolemic shock. The long term sequela of barium peritonitis is the development of granulomas and adhesions (causing obstructions and an eventual lawsuit).

Barium Intravasation: This is super rare, but can happen. If barium ends up in the systemic circulation it kills via pulmonary embolism about 50% of the time. Risk is increased in patient's with inflammatory bowel or diverticulitis (altered mucosa).

The Liver and Biliary System

Anatomy Trivia

The liver is covered by visceral peritoneum except at the porta hepatis, bare area, and the gallbladder fossa. An injury to the "bare area" can result in a retroperitoneal bleed. Functional division of the liver into multiple segments is done by the Couinaud system. The caudate lobe (segment 1) has a direct connection to the IVC through it's own hepatic veins, which do not communicate with the primary hepatic veins. Additionally, the caudate is supplied by branches of both the right and left portal veins – which matters because the caudate may be spared or hypertrophy as the result of various pathologies, Budd Chiari, etc… (as discussed below). Along the same lines of anatomy explaining pathology, the intra-hepatic course of the right portal vein is longer than the left, which is why it is more susceptible to fibrosis *(this is why the right liver shrinks, and the left liver grows in cirrhotic morphology).*

Trivia: Most common vascular variant = Replaced right hepatic (origin from the SMA)

Trivia: Most common biliary variant = Right posterior segmental branch emptying into the left hepatic duct.

Normal MRI Signal Characteristics: I like to think of the spleen as a bag of water/blood (T2 bright, T1 dark). The pancreas is the "brightest T1 structure in the body" because it has enzymes. The liver also has enzymes and is similar to the pancreas (T1 Brighter, T2 darker), just not as bright as the pancreas

Fetal Circulation: The fetal circulation anatomy is high yield anatomic trivia.

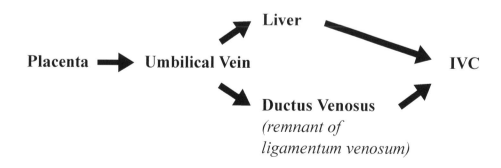

Classic Ultrasound Anatomy: There are 5 high yield looks, that are classically tested with regard to ultrasound anatomy.

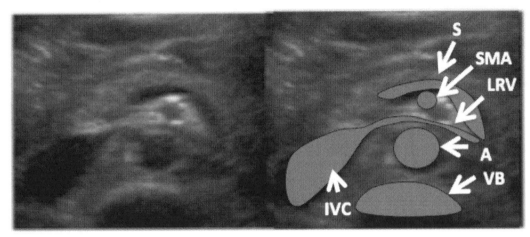

S = Splenic Vein, SMA = SMA, LRV = Left Renal Vein,
A= Aorta, VB = Vertebra Body, IVC = IVC

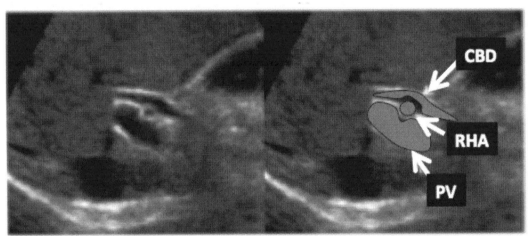

RHA - Right Hepatic Artery, CBD = Common Bile Duct,
PV = Portal Vein

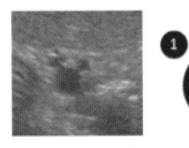
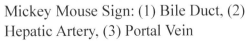

Mickey Mouse Sign: (1) Bile Duct, (2) Hepatic Artery, (3) Portal Vein

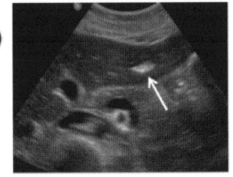

Fat in the Falciform Ligament / Ligamentum Teres

Promethean Dialogue on the Liver -

"A discourse on the liver, cirrhosis, portal HTN, and the development of HCC"

My idea is that by leading with a discussion of normal physiology, and the changes that occur with diffuse liver injury, that a lot of the processes and changes that occur with cirrhosis will make more sense (and be easier to remember). If you are in a rush to cram for the test just skip this discussion and move on to the charts. If you have more time, I think understanding the physiology is worthwhile.

Hepatocyte injury can occur from a variety of causes including viruses, alcohol, toxins (*alfatoxins i.e. peanut fungus*), and nonalcoholic fatty liver disease. These injuries result in increased liver cell turnover, to which the body reacts by forming regenerative nodules. The formation of regenerative nodules is an attempt by the liver not just to replace the damaged hepatocytes but also to compensate for lost liver function. In addition to activation of hepatocytes, stellate cells living in the space of Disse become active and proliferate changing into a *myofibroblast –like cell* that produces collagen. This collagen deposition causes fibrosis.

The development of fibrosis first puts the squeeze on the right portal vein (which <u>*usually*</u> has a longer intrahepatic course). This causes atrophy of segments 6 and 7, and compensatory hypertrophy of the caudate, segments 2, and 3. Because these changes, some people will try and use a caudate / right lobe ratio (*C/RL >0.75 is 99% specific*), to call cirrhosis.

All this squeezing can lead to portal hypertension. Portal hypertension is usually the result of increased hepatic resistance from pre-hepatic (*portal vein thrombosis, tumor compression*), hepatic (*cirrhosis, schistosomiasis*) and post hepatic (*Budd-Chiari*) causes. Obviously, most cases are hepatic with schistosomiasis being the most common cause world-wide, and EtOH cirrhosis being the most common cause in the US. Once portal venous pressure exceeds hepatic venous pressure by 8 mmHg – portal hypertension has occurred. In reaction to this increased resistance offered by the liver, collaterals will form to decompress the liver by carrying blood away from it. These tend to be esophageal and gastric varices. As a point of trivia, in pre-hepatic portal hypertension, collaterals will form above the diaphragm and in the hepatogastric ligaments to bypass the obstruction.

The liver has a dual blood supply (70% portal, 30% hepatic artery) with compensatory relationships between the two inflows; arterial flow increases as portal flow decreases. This helps explain the relationship between these two vessels with regard to Doppler US. As fibrosis leads to portal hypertension, velocity in the hepatic artery increases.

You will sometimes see perfusion related changes in the setting of cirrhosis. Since the fibrosis blockade takes place at the level of the central lobular vein (into sinusoids), flow remains adequate for the central zones of the liver, but not for the peripheral zones. The arterial response produces enhancement of the peripheral subcapsular hepatic parenchyma with relative hypodensity of the central perihilar area. The consequent CT pattern is referred to as the "central–peripheral" phenomenon.

Sometimes you will see reversal of flow (hepatofugal – *directed away from the liver*). As an aside, apparently "fugal" is latin for "flee." So the blood is fleeing the liver, or running away from it. Reversed flow in the portal system is seen in cirrhosis between 5-25%. Why you might ask, does the portal vein reverse flow instead of just clotting off in the setting of high resistance to inflow? The answer has to do with the unique dual hepatic blood supply (70 P / 30 A). As mentioned above, in cirrhosis, the principal area of obstruction to blood flow is believed to be in the outflow vessels (the hepatic venules and distal sinusoids). The outflow obstruction also affects the hepatic artery, causing increased resistance as well. So why doesn't the artery clot or reverse ? The difference is that the portal system can decompress through the creation of collaterals, and the artery cannot. So the artery does something else, it opens up tiny little connections to the portal system. The enlargement of these tiny communications has been referred to as "parasitizing the portosystemic decompressive apparatus." If the resistance is high enough, hepatic artery inflow will be shunted into - and can precipitate hepatofugal flow in the portal vein. So, in patients with hepatofugal flow in the main portal vein or intrahepatic portal vein branches, the shunted blood comes from the hepatic artery.

With increased resistance in the liver to the portal circulation, you also start to have colonic venous stasis (worse on the right). This can lead to *"Portal Hypertensive Colopathy"* ,which is basically an edematous bowel that mimics colitis. Why is it worse on the right? The short answer is that collateral pathways develop more on the left (splenorenal shunt, short gastrics, esophageal varices), and decompress that side. The trivia question is that it does resolve after transplant. The same process can affect the stomach *"Portal Hypertensive Gastropathy"* *causing a thickened gastric wall on CT, and well as cause upper GI bleeding in the absence of varices.*

Earlier I mentioned that hepatocytes react to injury by turning into regenerative nodules. This is how multi-focal HCC starts. Regenerative nodules -> Dysplastic nodules (increased size and cellularity) -> HCC. As this process takes place, the nodule changes from preferring to drink portal blood to only wanting to drink arterial blood. This helps explain why HCC has arterial enhancement and rapid washout. The transformation also follows a progression from T2 dark (regenerative) -> T2 bright (HCC). A buzzword is *"nodule within nodule"* where a central bright T2 nodule, has a T2 dark border. This is concerning for transformation to HCC.

Regenerative	Dysplastic	HCC
Contains Iron	Contains Fat, Glycoprotein	
T1 Dark, T2 Dark	T1 Bright, T2 Dark	T2 Bright
Does NOT Enhance	Usually Does NOT Enhance	Does Enhance

Another thing that happens with hepatocarcinogenesis is the decrease in a thing called the OATP bile uptake transporter. This is the transporter that moves biliary contrast agents (example = Eovist) into the cells. It's the reason normal liver cells look bright on the delayed phase when using a hepatocyte specific agent. It's also the reason FNHs look super bright on delayed images as they are basically hypertrophied hepatocytes. As hepatocytes become cancer they lose function in this transporter and become dark on the delayed phase. The exception (highly testable) is the well differentiated HCC which retains OATP function and is therefore bright on the 20 min delayed Eovist sequence.

There is one last concept, that I wanted to "squeeze" in. The squeezing that causes portal hypertension, also squeezes out most benign liver lesions (cysts, hemangiomas). So, lesions in a cirrhotic liver should be treated with more suspicion.

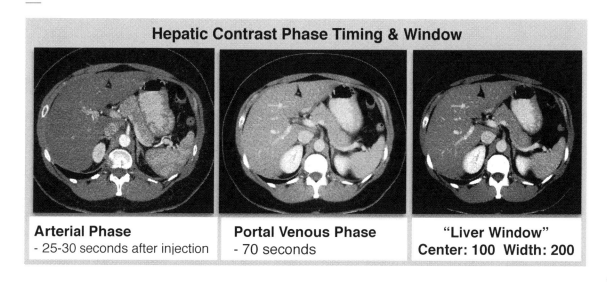

Hepatic Contrast Phase Timing & Window

Arterial Phase
- 25-30 seconds after injection

Portal Venous Phase
- 70 seconds

"Liver Window"
Center: 100 Width: 200

Congenital

Cystic Kidney Disease (both AD and AR): Patient's with AD polycystic kidney disease will also have cysts in the liver. This is in contrast to the AR form in which the liver tends to have fibrosis.

 Hereditary Hemorrhagic Telangectasia (Osler-Weber-Rendu) Autosomal dominant disorder characterized by multiple AVMs in the liver and lungs. It leads to cirrhosis, and a *massively dilated hepatic artery*.

Trivia: The lung AVMs set you up for brain abscess.

Infection

Infection of the liver can be thought of as either viral, abscess (pyogenic or amoebic), fungal, parasitic, or granulomatous.

Viral: Hepatitis which is chronic in B and C, and acute with the rest. A point of trivia is the **HCC in the setting of hepatitis can occur in the acute form of Hep B** (as well as chronic). Obviously, chronic hep C increases risk for HCC. On ultrasound the "starry sky" appearance can be seen. Although, this is non-specific and basically just the result of liver edema making the fat surrounding the portal triads look brighter than normal.

Pyogenic: These can mimic cysts. For the purpose of multiple choice, *a single abscess is Klebsiella, and multiple are E. Coli*. The presence of gas is highly suggestive of pyogenic abscess. "Double Target" sign with central low density, with rim enhancement, surrounded by more low density can be seen with CT. If the amebic abscess is in the left lobe, it needs to be emergently drained (can rupture into the pericardium).

Infection Buzzwords	
Viral Hepatitis	Starry Sky
Pyogenic Abscess	Double Target
Candida	Bull's Eye
Amoebic Abscess	"Extra Hepatic Extension"
Hydatid Disease	Water Lilly, Sand Storm
Schistosomiasis	Tortoise Shell

Liver Masses:

Hemangioma: This is the most common benign liver neoplasm. Favors women 5:1. They may enlarge with pregnancy. On US will be bright (unless it's in a fatty liver, than can be relatively dark). On US, flow can be seen in vessels adjacent to the lesion but NOT in the lesion. On CT and MRI tends to match the aorta in signal and have "peripheral nodular discontinuous enhancement". Should totally fill in by 15 mins. Atypical hemangioma can have the "reverse target sign."

Trivia: A hemangioma can change its sonographic appearance during the course of a single examination. No other hepatic lesion is known to do this.

Hemangioma US Pearls:
- Need to core for biopsy, FNA does not get enough tissue (only blood)
- Hyperechoic (65%)
- Enhanced thru transmission is common
- NO Doppler flow inside the lesion itself
- Atypical appearance – hyperechoic periphery, with hypoechoic center (inverse target)
- Calcifications are extremely rare

Focal Nodular Hyperplasia (FNH): This is the second most common benign liver neoplasm. Believed to start in utero as an AVM. It is NOT related to OCP use. It is composed of normal hepatocytes, abnormally arranged ducts, and Kupffer cells (reticuloendothelial cells). May show spoke wheel on US Doppler. On CT, should be "homogenous" on arterial phase. Can be a **"Stealth" lesion** on MRI – T1 and T2 isointense. Can have a central scar. Scar will demonstrate delayed enhancement (like scars do). *Biopsy Trivia: You have to hit the scar, otherwise path results will say normal hepatocytes.* Sulfur Colloid is always the multiple choice test question (reality is that its only hot 30-40%). Unlike hepatic adenomas, they are not related to the use of birth control pills, although as a point of confusing trivia and possibly poor multiple choice test question writing, birth control pills may promote their growth.

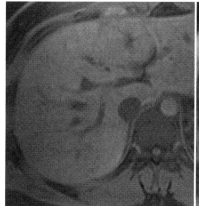 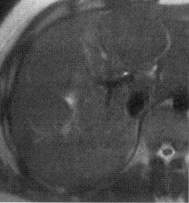 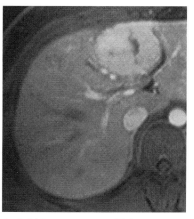

T1 - Stealth   T2 - Stealth   Arterial Homogenous Enhancement
                                -Also has a Central Scar

Hepatic Adenoma: Usually a solitary lesion seen in a female on OCPs. Alternatively could be seen in a man on anabolic steroids. When it's multiple you should think about glycogen storage disease (von Gierke) or liver adenomatosis. No imaging methods can reliably differentiate hepatic adenoma from hepatocellular carcinoma. Rarely, they *may degenerate into HCC* after a long period of stability. They *often regress after OCPs are stopped.* Their propensity to bleed sometimes makes them a surgical lesion if they won't regress.

Gamesmanship: To prove there is fat - they may show signal drop out on in & out of phase

Trivia:
    Q: Most common location for hepatic adenoma (75%)
    A: Right Lobe liver

Management: You stop the OCPs and re-image, they should get smaller. Smaller than 5cm, watch them. Larger than 5cm they often resect because (1) they can bleed and (2) they can rarely turn into cancer.

———

HCC Occurs typically in the setting of cirrhosis and chronic liver disease; Hep B, Hep C, hemochromatosis, glycogen storage disease, Alpha 1 antitrypsin. AFP elevated in 80-95% Will often invade the portal vein, although invasion of the hepatic vein is considered a more "specific finding."

"Doubling Time" – the classic Multiple Choice Question. This is actually incredibly stupid to ask because there are 3 described patterns of growth (slow, fast, and medium). To make it an even worse question, different papers say different stuff. Some say: Short is 150 days, Medium to 150-300, and Long is >300. I guess the answer is 300 – because it's in the middle. Others define medium at around 100 days. A paper in Radiology (*May 2008 Radiology, 247, 311-330*) says 18-605 days. The real answer would be to say follow up in 3-4.5 months.

Other Random Trivia: HCCs like to explode and cause spontaneous hepatic bleeds.

Fibrolamellar Subtype of HCC: This is typically seen in a younger patients (<35) without cirrhosis and a normal AFP. The buzzword is central scar. The scar is similar to the one seen in FNH with a few differences. This scar does NOT enhance, and is T2 dark (usually). As a point of trivia, this tumor is Gallium avid. This tumor calcifies more often than conventional HCC.

This vs That: HCC vs Fibrolamellar Subtype HCC	
HCC	**FL HCC**
Cirrhosis	No Cirrhosis
Older (50s-60s)	Young (30s)
Rarely Calcifies	Calcifies Sometimes
Elevated AFP	Normal AFP

This vs That: Central Scars of FNH and Fibrolamellar HCC	
FNH	**FL HCC**
T2 Bright	T2 Dark (usually)
Enhances on Delays	Does NOT enhance
Mass is Sulfur Colloid Avid (sometimes)	Mass is Gallium Avid

MR Contrast - Hepatobiliary Considerations

I want to clarify a few issues that can be confusing (and may also be testable) regarding MRI contrast.

How they work: Gadolinium (which is super toxic) is bound to some type of chelation agent to keep it from killing the patient. The shape and function of the chelation agent determine the class and brand name. The paramagnetic qualities of gadolinium cause a local shortening of the T1 relaxation time on neighboring molecules (remember short T1 time = bright image).

Types of Agents: I want you to think about MRI contrast in two main flavors: (1) Extracellular, and (2) Hepatocyte Specific.

Extracellular: These are nonspecific agents that are best thought of as Iodine contrast for CT. They stay outside the cell and are blood flow dependent (just like CT contrast). The imaging features in lesions will be the same as CT - although the reason they look bright is obviously different - CT contrast increases the density (attenuation), MR contrast shortens the T1 time locally – which makes T1 brighter. The classic imaging set up is a late hepatic arterial phase (15-30 seconds), and portal venous phase (70 seconds), and a hepatic venous or interstitial phase (90 seconds – 5 mins) - just like CT.

Classic Example of a Non-Specific Extracellular Agent = Gd-DTPA (Magnevist)

Hepatocyte Specific: Certain chelates are excreted via the bile salt pathway. In other words, they are taken up by a normal hepatocytes and excreted into the bile. This gives you great contrast between normal hepatocytes and things that aren't normal hepatocytes (cancer). The 20 min delay is the imaging sequence that should give you a homogenous bright liver (dark holes are things that don't contain normal liver cells / couldn't drink the contrast). The problem is that it's pretty non-specific with a handful of benign things still taking it up (classical example is FNH), and at least one bad thing taking it up (well-differentiated HCC). Plus, a handful of benign things won't take it up (cysts...etc..). There are at least three good reasons to use this kind of agent: (1) it's great for proving an FNH is an FNH - as most lesions won't hold onto the Gd at 20 mins, (2) it's great for looking for bile leaks, and (3) once you've established a baseline MRI (characterized all those benign lesions) it's excellent for picking up new mets (findings black holes on a white background is easy).

Classic Example of a Hepatocyte Specific Agent = Gd-EOB-DTPA (Eovist).

Is Eovist a pure Hepatocyte Specific Agent ? Nope – It also acts like a non-specific extracellular agent early on (although less intense). About 55% is excreted in the bile – and gives a nice intense look at 20 mins.

What about Gd-BOPTA (Multihance) ? This is mostly an extra-cellular agent, but has a small amount (5%) of biliary excretion. The implication is that you can use Multihance to look for a bile leak you just have to wait longer (45mins-3 hours) for the Gd to accumulate.

What about Manganese instead of Gd ? This is the old school way to do biliary imaging. It works the same as Gd – by causing T1 shortening.

Cholangiocarcinoma: Where HCC is a cancer of the hepatocyte, cholangiocarcinoma is a cancer of the bile duct. It is usually seen in an elderly (70s) man. There are multiple risk factors (**Primary sclerosing cholangitis**, recurrent pyogenic cholangitis, clonorchis senesis (the liver fluke), HIV, Hep B&C, EtOH, and of course thorotrast). Primary sclerosing cholangitis is the major risk factor in western countries. Just like a pancreatic head cancer the buzzword is "painless jaundice."

These tumors have an infiltrative growth pattern, and will not have a capsule. On imaging it will show dilation of the biliary system, and possible persistent enhancing soft tissue on delayed phase (the scar enhances). **Capsular retraction is a buzzword,** mainly for the mass forming subtype. Encasement of a portal or hepatic vein without formation of a visible tumor thrombus is one of the distinguishing features of cholangiocarcinoma versus HCC.

Key Findings:
- *Delayed Enhancement*
- *Peripheral biliary dilation*
- *Capsular Retraction*

Klatskin Tumor: A Klastskin tumor is a type of cholangiocarcinoma that occurs at the bifurcation of the right and left hepatic ducts. The tumor has dense fibrosis (which enhances on delayed imaging).

—

Hepatic Angiosarcoma: This used to be the go to for thorotrast questions. Even though everyone who got thorotrast died 30 years ago, a few dinosaurs writing multiple choice test questions still might ask it. Hepatic Angiosarcoma is very rare, although technically the most common primary sarcoma of the liver. It is associated with toxic exposure - arsenic use (latent period is about 25years), Polyvinyl chloride exposure, Radiation, and yes... thorotrast. Additional trivia, is that you can see it in Hemochromatosis and NF patients.

It's usually multifocal, and has a propensity to bleed.

Biliary Cystadenoma Uncommon benign cystic neoplasm of the liver. Usually seen in middle aged women. Can sometimes present with pain, or even jaundice. They can be unilocular or multilocular and there are no reliable methods for distinguishing from biliary cystadenocarcinoma (which is unfortunate).

Mets to the Liver: If you see mets in the liver first think colon. Calcified mets are usually the result of a mucinous neoplasm (colon, ovary, pancreas).

With regard to ultrasound: Hyperechoic mets are often hypervascular (renal, melanoma, carcinoid, choriocarcinoma, thyroid, islet cell). Hypoechoic mets are often hypovascular (colon, lung, pancreas).

"Too Small Too Characterize" - even in the setting of breast cancer (with no definite hepatic mets) tiny hypodensities have famously been shown to be benign 90-95% of the time.

Lymphoma: Hodgkins lymphoma involves the liver 60% of the times (Non Hodgkins is around 50%), and may be hypoechoic.

Kaposi Sarcoma: Seen in patient's with AIDS. Causes diffuse periportal hypoechoic infiltration. Looks similar to biliary duct dilation.

—

Sulfur Colloid HOT or COLD		
Hepatic Adenoma	COLD	
FNH	40% HOT, 30% COLD, 30% Warm	
Cavernous Hemangioma	COLD	RBC Scan HOT
HCC	COLD	Gallium HOT
Cholangiocarcinoma	COLD	
Mets	COLD	
Abscess	COLD	Gallium HOT
Focal Fat	COLD	Xenon HOT

Benign Liver Masses

	Ultrasound	CT	MR	Trivia	
Hemangioma	Hyperechoic with increased though transmission	Peripheral Nodular Discontinuous Enhancement	T2 Bright	Rare in Cirrhotics	Kasabach-Merritt; the sequestration of platelets from giant cavernous hemangioma
FNH	Spoke Wheel	Homogenous Arterial Enhancement	"Stealth Lesion - Iso on T1 and T2"	Central Scar	Bright on Delayed Eovist (Gd-EOB-DTPA)
Hepatic Adenoma	Variable	Variable	Fat Containing on In/Out Phase	OCP use, Glycogen Storage Disease	Can explode and bleed
Hepatic Angiomyolipoma	Hyperechoic	Gross Fat	T1/T2 Bright	Unlike renal AML, 50% don't have fat	Tuberous Sclerosis

Diffuse Liver Processes:

Fatty Liver: Very common in America. Can be focal (next to gallbladder or liagmentum teres), can be diffuse, or can be diffuse with sparing. You can call it a few different ways.

For CT: If it's a non-contrast study 40 H.U. is a slam dunk. If it's contrasted some people say you can NEVER call it. Others say it's ok if (a) it's a good portal venous phase (b) the H.U. is less than 100, and (c) it's 25 H.U. less than the spleen.

On US: If the liver is brighter than the right kidney you can call it. Hepatosteatosis is a fat liver. NASH (hepatitis from a fat liver) has abnormal LFTs.

On MRI: Two standard deviation difference between in and out of phase imaging. Remember the drop out is on the out of phase images (india ink ones - done at T.E 2.3ms - assuming 1.5T).

What causes it? McDonalds, Burger King, and Taco Bell. Additional causes include chemotherapy (breast cancer), steroids, cystic fibrosis.

Hemochromatosis: Iron overload. They can show this two main ways.

(1) The first is just liver and spleen being T1 and T2 dark.
(2) The second (and more likely) way this will be shown is *in and out of phase changes the opposite of those seen in hepatic steatosis.* **Low signal on in phase, and high signal on out of phase. ("Iron on In-phase")**

> **Watch out now — this is the opposite of the fat drop out**
> ****FAT - Drop out on OUT of phase (india ink one - T.E. 2.3ms)**
> ****IRON - Drop out on IN phase (non india ink one - T.E. 4.6ms)**

The second main piece of trivia is to tell *primary vs secondary.*

Primary is the inherited type, caused by more GI uptake, with resulting iron overload. The key point is the pancreas is involved and the spleen is spared.

Secondary is the result of either chronic inflammation or multiple transfusions. The body reacts by trying the "Eat the Iron" , with the reticuloendothelial system. The key point is the pancreas is spared and the spleen is not. **"Primary = Pancreas" , "Secondary = Spleen"**

Hemochromatosis	
Primary	Secondary
Genetic - increased absorption	Acquired - chronic illness, and multiple transfusions
Liver, **Pancreas**	Liver, **Spleen**
Heart, Thyroid, Pituitary	

Budd Chiari Syndrome Classic multiple choice scenario is a pregnant woman, but can occur in any situation where you are hypercoagulable (*most common cause is idiopathic*). The result of hepatic vein thrombosis.

The characteristic findings of Budd-Chiari syndrome include hepatic venous outflow obstruction, intrahepatic and systemic collateral veins, and large regenerative (hyperplastic) nodules in a dysmorphic liver. The caudate lobe is often massively enlarged (spared from separate drainage into the IVC). In the acute phase, the liver will show the *classic "flip-flop pattern"* on portal phase with low attenuation central, and high peripherally. The liver has been described as "nutmeg" with an inhomogeneous mottled appearance, and delayed enhancement of the periphery of the liver.

Who gets a "nutmeg liver" ???
- *Budd Chiari*
- *Hepatic Veno-occlusive disease*
- *Right Heart Failure (Hepatic Congestion)*
- *Constrictive Pericarditis*

Regenerative (hyperplastic) nodules are very difficult to distinguish from multifocal hepatocellular carcinoma. They are bright on both T1 and T2. Multiple big (>10cm) and small (<4cm) nodules in the setting of Budd-Chiari suggest a benign process.

Presentation can be acute or chronic. Acute from thrombus into the hepatic vein or IVC. These guys will present with **rapid onset ascites**. Chronic from fibrosis of the intrahepatic veins, presumably from inflammation.

Who gets massive caudate lobe hypertrophy???
- *Budd Chiari*
- *Primary Sclerosing Cholangitis*
- *Primary Biliary Cirrhosis*

Hepatic Veno-occlusive Disease: This is a form of Budd Chiari that occurs from occlusion of the small hepatic venules. It is endemic in Jamaica (from Alkaloid bush tea). In the US it's typically the result of XRT and chemotherapy. The main hepatic veins and IVC will be patent, but portal waveforms will be abnormal (slow, reversed, or to-and fro).

———

Passive Congestion: Passive hepatic congestion is caused by stasis of blood within the liver due to compromise of hepatic drainage. It is a common complication of congestive heart failure and constrictive pericarditis. It is essentially the result of elevated CVP transmitted from the right atrium to the hepatic veins.

Findings include:
- *Refluxed contrast into the hepatic veins*
- *Increased portal venous pulsatility*
- *Nutmeg liver*

Misc Liver Conditions:

Portal Vein Thrombosis: Occurs in hypercoaguable states (cancer, dehydration, etc…). Can lead to _cavernous transformation_, with the development of a bunch of serpiginous vessels in the porta hepatis which may reconstitute the right and left portal veins. This takes like 12 months to happen (_it proves portal vein is chronically occluded_).

Pseudo Cirrhosis: Treated breast cancer mets to the liver can cause contour changes that mimic cirrhosis. Specifically multifocal liver retraction and enlargement of the caudate has been described. Why this is specific for breast cancer is not currently known, as other mets to the liver don't produce this reaction.

Cryptogenic Cirrhosis: Essentially cirrhosis of unknown cause. Most of these cases are probably the result of nonalcoholic fatty liver disease.

Liver Transplant: The liver has great ability to regenerate and may double in size in as little as 3 weeks making it ideal for partial donation. Hepatitis C is the most common disease requiring transplantation (followed by EtOH liver disease, and cryptogenic cirrhosis). In adults, right lobes (segments 5-8) are most commonly implants. This is the opposite of pediatric transplants, which usually donates segments 2-3. The modern surgery has four connections (IVC, artery, portal vein, CBD).

Contraindications include, extrahepatic malignancy, advanced cardiac disease, advanced pulmonary disease, or active substance abuse. Portal HTN is NOT a true contraindication although it does increase the difficulty of the surgery and increase mortality.

Normal Transplant US
- _Normal Doppler should have a RAPID systolic upstroke_
  - _Diastolic -> Systolic in less than 80msec (0.08 seconds)_
- _Resistive Index is Normally between 0.5 – 0.7_
- _Hepatic Artery Peak Velocity should be < 200 cm/sec_

Syndrome of Impending Thrombosis
3-10 days post transplant
(1st) Initial Normal Waveform
(2nd) No diastolic flow
(3rd) Dampening Systolic flow
Tardus Parvus
RI < 0.5
(4th) Loss of Hepatic Waveform

As mentioned before, the normal liver gets 70% blood flow from the portal vein, making it the key player. In the transplanted liver, the _hepatic artery is the king_ and is the primary source of blood flow for the bile ducts (which undergo necrosis with hepatic artery failure). Hepatic artery thrombosis comes in two flavors: early (<15 days), and later (years). The late form is associated with chronic rejection and sepsis.

Trivia: Tardus Parvus is more likely secondary to stenosis than thrombosis

277

Biliary

Jaundice: You always think about common duct stone, but the most common etiology is actually from a benign stricture (post traumatic from surgery or biliary intervention).

Bacterial Cholangitis: Hepatic abscess can develop secondary to cholangitis, usually as the result of stasis (so think stones). The triad of jaundice, fever, and right upper quadrant pain is the step 1 question.

Primary Sclerosing Cholangitis (PSC) Chronic cholestatic liver disease of unknown etiology characterized by progressive inflammation which leads to multifocal strictures of the intra and or extrahepatic bile ducts. The disease often results in cirrhosis, and is **strongly associated with cholangiocarcinoma**. The buzzword for the **cirrhotic pattern is "central regenerative hypertrophy"**. It is associated with inflammatory bowel disease (Ulcerative Colitis 80%, Crohns 20%). It is an indication for transplant, with a post transplant recurrence of about 20%.

AIDS Cholangiopathy: Infection of the biliary epithelium (*classically Cryptosporidium*) can cause ductal disease in patients with AIDS. The appearance mimics PSC with intrahepatic and/ or extrahepatic multifocal strictures. The classic multiple choice test question is the association with papillary stenosis (which occurs 60% of the time).

This vs That: AIDS Cholangiopathy vs Primary Sclerosing Cholangitis	
AIDS	**PSC**
Focal Strictures of the extrahepatic duct > 2cm	Extrahepatic strictures rarely > 5mm
Absent saccular deformities of the ducts	Has saccular deformities of the ducts
Associated Papillary Stenosis	

Oriental Cholangitis *(Recurrent pyogenic cholangitis):* Common in Southeast Asia (hence the name). They always show it as **dilated ducts, that are full of pigmented stones**. A buzzword is "straight rigid intrahepatic ducts." The cause of the disease is not known, but it may be associated with clonorchiasis, ascariasis, and nutritional deficiency . These guys don't do as well with endoscopic decompression, and often need surgical decompression.

Primary Biliary Cirrhosis: An autoimmune disease that results in the destruction of small & medium bile ducts *(intra not extra)*. It primarily affects **middle aged women**, who are often asymptomatic. In the early disease, normal bile ducts help distinguish it from PSC. In later stages, there is irregular dilation of the intrahepatic ducts, with **normal extrahepatic ducts**. There is increased risk of HCC. If caught early it has an excellent prognosis and responds to medical therapy with ursodexycholic acid. The step 1 trivia is "**antimitochondrial antibodies (AMA)**" which are present 95% of the time.

Choledochal Cysts / Caroli's: Choledochal cysts are congenital dilation of the bile ducts – classified into 5 types by some dude named Todani. *The high yield trivia is type 1 is focal dilation of the CBD and is by far the most common.* Type 2 and 3 are super rare. Type 2 is basically a diverticulum of the bile duct. Type 3 is a "choledochocele." Type 4 is both intra and extra. Type 5 is Caroli's, and is intrahepatic only.

Caroli's is an AR disease *associated with polycystic kidney disease and medullary sponge kidney*. The hallmark is intrahepatic duct dilation, that is large and sacular. **Buzzword is "central dot sign"** which corresponds to the portal vein surrounded by dilated bile ducts.

Complications
- **Cholangiocarcinoma**
- *Cirrhosis*
- *Cholangitis*
- *Intraductal Stones*

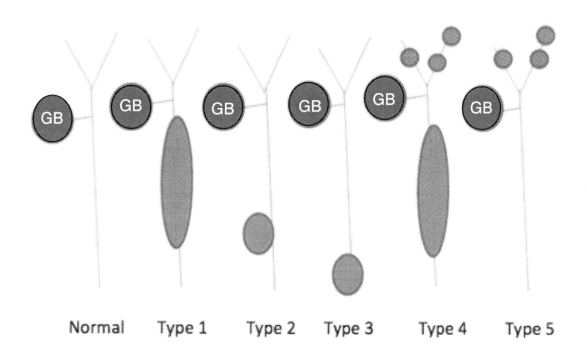

Gamesmanship: If they give you imaging of dilated biliary ducts and a history of repeated cholangitis, think choledocal cyst. These things get stones in them and can be recurrently infected.

Gall Bladder

Normal Gallbladder

The normal gallbladder is found inferior to the interlobar fissure between the right and left lobe. The size varies depending on the last meal, but is supposed to be <4 x <10cm. The wall thickness should be <3mm. The lumen should be anechoic.

Variants / Congenital

Phyringian Cap: A phyringian cap is seen when the GB folds on itself. It means nothing.

Intrahepatic Gallbladder: Variations in gallbladder location are rare, but the intrahepatic gallbladder is probably the most frequently recognized variant. Most are found right above the interlobar fissure.

Duplicated Gallbladder: It can happen.

Duct of Luschka: An accessory cystic duct. This can cause a big problem (persistent bile leak) after cholecystectomy. There are several subtypes which is not likely to be tested.

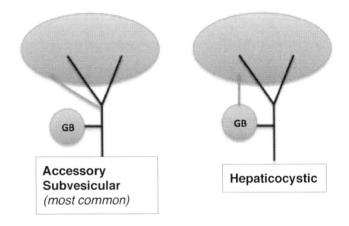

Wall Thickening: Very non-specific. Can occur from biliary (Cholecystitis, AIDS, PSC…) or non-biliary causes (hepatitis, heart failure, cirrhosis, etc….).

Gallstones: Gallstones are found in 10% of asymptomatic patients/ Most (75%) are cholesterol, the other 25% are pigmented. They cast shadows.

Reasons a stone might not cast a shadow
* *It's not a stone*
* *It's a stone, but < 3mm in size*
* *The sonographer sucks*

(WES) - Wall Echo Shadow GB

Can occur for three reasons.
(1) Gallbladder full of stones
   Clean shadowing.

(2) Porcelain Gallbladder
   Variable shadowing

(3) Emphysematous Cholecystitis
   Dirty shadowing.

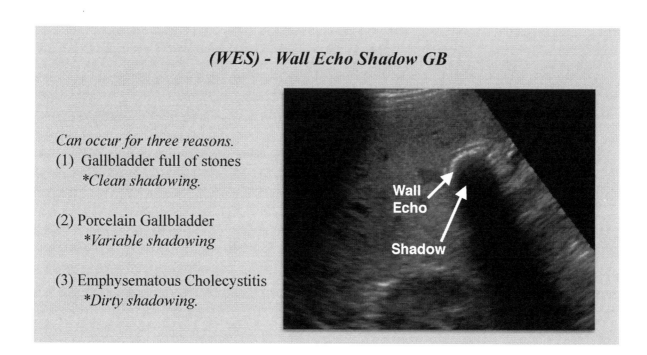

Porcelain Gallbladder: Extensive wall calcification. The key point is increased risk of GB Cancer. These are surgically removed.

Gallbladder Polyps: These can be cholesterol (by far the most common), or not cholesterol (adenomas, papillomas). Cholesterol polpys aren't real polyps, but instead are essentially enlarged papillary fronds full of lipid filled machrophages, that are attached to the wall by a stalk.

The non-cholesterol subtypes are almost always solitary and are typically larger. The larger polyps may have Doppler flow. They are NOT mobile, and do NOT shadow. *Once they get to be 1cm , people start taking them out.*

Adenomyomatosis: Results from hyperplasia of the wall with formation of intramural mucosal diverticula (Rokitansy-Aschoff sinuses) which penetrate into the wall of the gallbladder. These diverticula become filled with cholesterol crystals – which manifest from the unique acoustic signature as comet-tail artifact (highly specific for adenomyomatosis).

Comes in 3 flavors: Generalized (diffuse), Segmental (annular), and Fundal (localized or adenomyoma). The Localized form can't be differentiated from GB cancer.

Clinically Meaningless *This vs That*
Gallbladder Adenomyomatosis vs Cholesterolosis

Radiologists love to spend time distinguishing between two very similar appearing benign processes. They believe this "adds value" and will save them from the eventual avalanche of reimbursement cuts.

The classic one in the gallbladder is adenomyomatosis vs gallbladder cholesterolosis. These things are actually different - and even though it makes zero difference clinically, this is just the kind of thing people who write questions love to write questions about.

Gallbladder Adenomyomatosis: You have hypertrophied mucosal and muscularis propria, with the **cholesterol crystals deposited an intraluminal** location (within Rokitansky-Aschoff sinuses).

Cholesterolosis: Cholesterol and triglyceride deposition is **within the substance of the lamina propria**, and associated with formation of cholesterol polyps.

Gallbladder Cancer: Key points are that most GB cancers are associated with gallstones. The outcomes are terrible with 80% having direct tumor invasion of the liver or portal nodes at the time of diagnosis.

Mirizzi Syndrome: This occurs when the common hepatic duct is obstructed secondary to an impacted cystic duct stone. The stone can eventually erode into the CHD or GI tract. Key point is the increased co-incidence of *gallbladder CA (5x more risk)* with Mirizzi. Another key piece of trivia is that Mirizzi **occurs more in people with a low cystic duct insertion (normal variant),** allowing for a more parallel course and closer proximity to the CHD.

Doppler of the Liver

Brief introduction to terminology.

- *"Duplex" means color.*
- *"Spectral" means color with a waveform.*

Concept of Arterial Resistance:

Some organs require continuous flow (brain), whereas others do not (muscles). The body is smart enough to understand this, and will make alterations in resistance / flow to preserve energy. When an organ needs to be "on," its arteriolar bed dilates, and the waveform becomes low resistance. This allows the organ to be appropriately perfused. When an organ goes to "power save" mode, its arterioles constrict, the waveform switches to high resistance, and blood flow is diverted to other more vital organs.

To help quantify this low resistance high resistance thing. We use this **"Resistive Index (RI)"** - which is defined **as V1-V2 / V1.**

Just remember that things that need blood all the time, will have continuous diastolic flow – and thus a low resistance wave form.

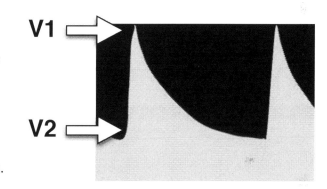

What is this "Tardus Parvus" ?

Tardus: Refers to a slowed systolic upstroke. This can be measured by acceleration time, the time from end diastole to the first systolic peak. An acceleration time >0.07 sec correlates with >50% stenosis of the renal artery

Parvus: Refers to decreased systolic velocity. This can be measured by calculating the acceleration index, the change in velocity from end diastole to the first systolic peak.

An acceleration index <3.0 m/sec- correlates with >50% stenosis of the renal artery

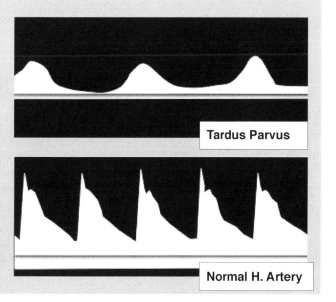

What does RI mean in the Liver:

- The "normal" RI in the liver is between 0.5 and 0.7.

What if it's > 0.7 (too high) ?

- Basically, a high RI (> 0.7) doesn't mean shit as an isolated finding. A high RI is not specific for liver disease. An RI that is too high may be the result of the postprandial state, advanced patient age, or diffuse distal microvascular disease, which has a wide variety of causes including chronic liver disease from cirrhosis or chronic hepatitis.

What if it's <0.5 (too low) ?

- A low RI is either the result of proximal stenosis or distal vascular shunting. The most common cause of this shunting is the arteriovenous or arterioportal fistulas seen in severe cirrhosis. Other more rare causes would be trauma (including iatrogenic injury – liver biopsy) or total zebras like Osler-Weber-Rendu syndrome.

Causes of Low RI (< 0.5)		Causes of High RI (> 0.7)
Proximal Arterial Narrowing	Peripheral Vascular Shunts	Postprandial
Atherosclerotic Disease (Celiac, or Hepatic)	Shunting seen with Cirrhosis	Advanced Age
Stenosis at an anastomosis (transplant)	Post Traumatic (liver biopsy)	Cirrhosis
Median Arcuate Ligament Compression (severe)	Osler-Weber-Rendu	Hepatic Congestion (Acute or Chronic)
		Transplant Rejection

How can Cirrhosis cause low RI and high RI?

- Essentially, the shunts that develop decrease RI, BUT the fibrosis that develops increases RI. So, it's a balance between these two things. As a result, they may be high, normal, or low – and RI is NOT useful for diagnosing cirrhosis or predicting how severe it is.

Understanding Stenosis:

The vocabulary of "Upstream vs Downstream" is somewhat confusing. Try and remember, that the flow of blood defines the direction.

- Upstream = Blood that has NOT yet passed through the stenosis
- Downstream = Blood that has passed area of stenosis

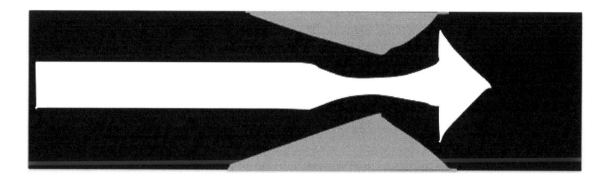

So there are direct signs, and indirect signs of stenosis.

<u>Direct Signs:</u> The direct signs, are those found at the stenosis itself and they include elevated peak systolic velocity, and spectral broadening (immediate post stenotic).

<u>Indirect Signs:</u> The indirect signs are going to be tardus parvus (downstream) – with time to peak < 70msec. The RI downstream will be low (< 0.5) , because the liver is starved for blood. The RI upstream will be elevated (> 0.7) because that blood needs to overcome the area of stenosis.

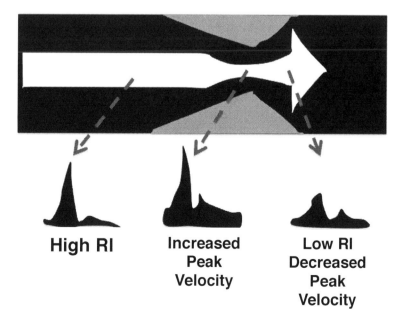

High RI   **Increased Peak Velocity**   **Low RI Decreased Peak Velocity**

Hepatic Veins

Flow in the hepatic veins is complex, with alternating forward and backward flow. The bulk of the flow should be forward "antegrade" (liver -> heart). Things that mess with the waveform are going to be pressure changes in the right heart are transmitted to the hepatic veins (CHF, Tricuspid Regurg) or compression of the veins directly (cirrhosis).

Anything that increases right atrial pressure (atrial contraction) will cause the wave to slope upward. "A" represents atrial contraction.

Anything that decreases right atrial pressure will cause the wave to slope downward.

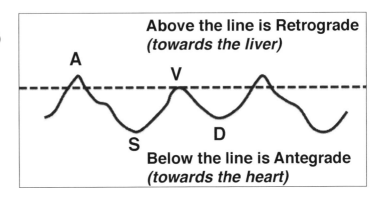

Abnormal Hepatic Vein Waveforms can manifest in one of three main categories: (1) More pulsatile, (2) Less Pulsatile, (3) Absent – Budd Chiari.

Increased HV Pulsatility	Decreased HV Pulsatility
Tricuspid Regurg	Cirrhosis
Right Sided CHF	Hepatic Venous Outflow Obstruction (any cause)

LOW YIELD - TRIVIA - *Study only on second time through*
This vs That: Tricuspid Regurg vs Right Sided CHF

Although certain dinosaur radiologists still love this stuff, it's unlikely to show up on the test, and if it does probably won't be more than one question. If they ask it at all - I would bet the question is something regarding the "D Wave to S Wave" relationship.

- Tricuspid Regurg - D deeper than S
- Right Heart Failure - S deeper than D

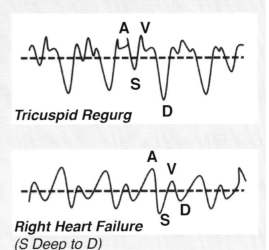

Tricuspid Regurg

Right Heart Failure
(S Deep to D)

Portal Vein

Flow in the portal vein should always be towards the liver (antegrade). You can see some normal cardiac variability from hepatic venous pulsatility transmitted through the hepatic sinusoids. Velocity in the normal portal vein is between 20-40 cm/s. The waveform should be a gentle undulation , always remaining above the baseline.

You have three main patterns:

(1) Normal

(2) Pulsatile

(3) Reversed

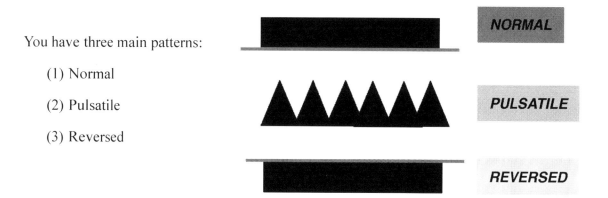

Cause of Portal Vein Pulsatility: **Right sided CHF, Triscupid Regurg, Cirrhosis** with Vascular AP shunting.

Causes of Portal Vein Reversed Flow: The big one is **Portal HTN** (any cause).

Absent Flow: This could be considered a fourth pattern. It's seen in thrombosis, tumor invasion, and stagnant flow from terrible portal HTN.

Slow Flow: Velocities less than 15 cm/s. Portal HTN is the most common cause. Additional causes are grouped by location:

- Pre – Portal Vein Thrombosis
- Intra – Cirrhosis (any cause)
- Post – Right sided Heart Failure, Tricuspid Regurg, Budd-Chiari

Final Doppler Trivia:

An ultra common quiz question is to ask **"what should the Doppler angle be?"** Now even though ultrasound physics is covered in more detail in the dedicated section this is a high yield enough point to warrant repetition. **The answer is "less than 60. "**

Why? If you look at the; Cos 90 = 0, Cos 60 = 0.5, Cos 0 = 1.0 - the doppler strength follows the Cos.

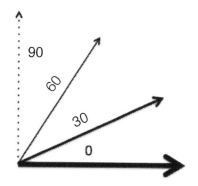

The Pancreas

Trivia regarding the pancreas can be broadly clustered into: Solid Lesions, Cystic Lesions, Pancreatitis, and Misc Trivia (mostly developmental stuff).

Misc Pancreas Trivia:

Anatomy: The pancreas is a retroperitoneal structure (the tail may be intraperitoneal).

Cystic Fibrosis: The pancreas is involved in 85-90% of CF patients. Inspissated secretions cause proximal duct obstruction leading to the two main changes in CF:
(1) Fibrosis (decreased T1 and T2 signal) and the more common one
(2) fatty replacement (increased T1).

Patient's with CF, who are diagnosed as adults, tend to have more pancreas problems than those diagnosed as children. Just remember that those with residual pancreatic exocrine function tend to have bouts of recurrent acute pancreatitis (they keep getting clogged up with thick secretions). Small (1-3mm) pancreatic cysts are common.

High Yield Trivia:
• ***Complete fatty replacement*** is the most common imaging finding in adult CF

• Markedly enlarged with fatty replacement has been termed lipomatous **pseudohypertrophy of the pancreas**. *This is a buzzword.

• ***Fibrosing Colonopathy:*** Wall thickening of the proximal colon as a complication of enzyme replacement therapy.

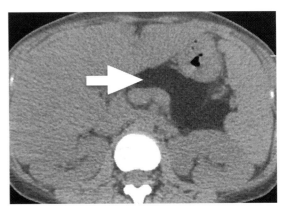

CF - Fatty Replacement of the Pancreas

Shwachman-Diamond Syndrome: The 2nd most common cause of pancreatic insufficiency in kids (CF #1). Basically, it's a kid with diarrhea, short stature (metaphyseal chondroplasia), and eczema. *Will also cause lipomatous pseudohypertrophy of the pancreas.*

Pancreatic Lipomatosis: Most common pathologic condition involving the pancreas. The most common cause in childhood is CF (in adults it's burger king). Additional causes worth knowing are Cushing Syndrome, Chronic Steroid Use, Hyperlipidemia, and Shwachman-Diamond Syndrome.

This vs That: Pancreatic Agenesis vs Pancreatic-Lipomatosis	
Agenesis	Lipomatosis
Does NOT have a duct	Does have a duct

Dorsal Pancreatic Agenesis - All you need to know is that (1) this sets you up for diabetes *(most of your beta cells are in the tail)*, and (2) it's associated with polysplenia.

Annular Pancreas: Essentially an embryologic screw up *(failure of ventral bud to rotate with the duodenum)*, that results in encasement of the duodenum. Results in a rare cause of duodenal obstruction (10%), that typically presents as duodenal obstruction in children and pancreatitis in adults. Can also be associated with other vague symptoms (post-prandial fullness, "symptoms of peptic ulcer disease", etc...).

- Remember in adults this can present with pancreatitis (the ones that present earlier - in kids - are the ones that obstruct).
- On imaging, look for an annular duct encircling the descending duodenum.

Pancreatic Trauma: The pancreas sits in front of the vertebral body, so it's susceptible to getting smashed in blunt trauma. Basically, **the only thing that matters is integrity of the duct.** If the duct is damaged they need to go to the OR. The most common delayed complication is pancreatic fistula (10-20%), followed by abscess formation. Signs of injury can be subtle, and may include focal pancreatic enlargement, or adjacent stranding/fluid.

Imaging Pearls:
- Remember it can be subtle with just focal enlargement of the pancreas
- If you see low attenuation fluid separating two portions of the enhancing pancreatic parenchyma this is a laceration, NOT contusion.
- The presence of fluid surrounding the pancreas is not specific, it could be from injury or just aggressive hydration — on the test they will have to show you the liver and IVC to prove it's aggressive fluid resuscitation.

Suspected Pancreatic Duct Injury? - Next Step - MRCP or ERCP

Pancreatitis:

Acute Pancreatitis:

Etiology: By far the most common causes are gallstones and EtOH which combined make up 80% of the cases in the real world. However, for the purpose of multiple choice tests a bite from the native scorpion of the island of Trinidad and Tobago is more likely to be the etiology. Additional causes include, ERCP (*which usually results in a mild course*), medications (*classically valproic acid*), trauma (*the most common cause in a child*), pancreatic cancer, infectious (*post viral in children*), hypercalcemia, hyperlipidemia, autoimmune pancreatitis, pancreatic divisum, groove pancreatitis, tropic pancreatitis, and parasite induced.

Clinical Outcomes: Prognosis can be estimated with the "Balthazar Score." Essentially, you can think about pancreatitis as "mild" *(no necrosis)* or "severe" *(having necrosis)*. Patient's with necrosis don't start doing terrible until they get infected, then the mortality is like 50-70%.

Key Point: Outcomes are directly correlated with the degree of pancreatic necrosis.

Severe Pancreatitis: Severe acute pancreatitis has a biphasic course. With the first two weeks being a pro-inflammatory phase. This is a sterile response in which infection rarely occurs. The third and fourth weeks transition to an anti-inflammatory period in which the risk of translocated intestinal flora and the subsequent development of infection increases.

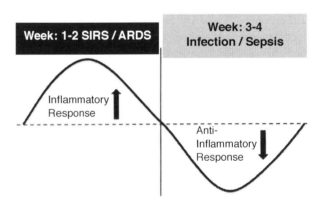

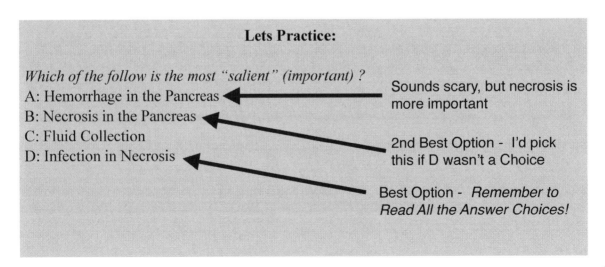

NO Necrosis
- < 4weeks ⟶ Acute Peripancreatic Fluid Collection
- > 4weeks ⟶ Pseudocyst

Necrosis
- < 4weeks ⟶ Acute Necrotic Collection
- > 4weeks ⟶ Walled-Off Necrosis

Vascular Complications:
- Splenic Vein and Portal Vein Thrombosis
  - *Isolated gastric varices can be see secondary to splenic vein occlusion*
- Pseudo-aneurysm of the GDA and Splenic Arteries

Non-Vascular Complications:
- Abscess, Infection, etc... as discussed
- Gas, as a characteristic sign of an infected fluid collection, is detected in only 20% of cases of pancreatic abscesses.

Random Imaging Pearl:
- On Ultrasound, an inflamed pancreas will be *hypoechoic* (edematous) when compared to the liver (opposite of normal).

Pancreatic Divisum –

Anatomy Refresher: There are two ducts, a major (Wirsung), and a minor (Santorini). The way I remember this is that "Santorini is Superior", and "W" is in the back of the alphabet. "Santorini is also Small" , i.e. the minor duct.

Pancreatic Divisum is the most common anatomic variant of the human pancreas, and occurs when the main portion of the pancreas is drained by the minor or accessory papilla. The clinical relevance is an increased risk of Pancreatitis.

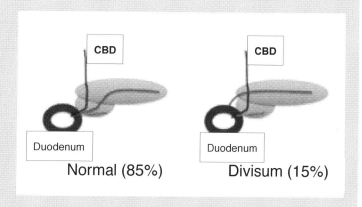

291

Chronic pancreatitis (CP) represents the end result of prolonged inflammatory change leading to irreversible fibrosis of the gland. Acute pancreatitis and chronic pancreatitis are thought of as different disease processes, and most cases of acute pancreatitis do not result in chronic disease. So, acute doesn't have to lead to chronic (and usually doesn't), but chronic can still have recurrent acute.

Etiology: Same as acute pancreatitis, the most common causes are chronic alcohol abuse and cholelithiasis which together result in about 90% of the cases.

Imaging Findings: Findings can be thought of as early or late:

Early:
- Loss of T1 signal *(pancreas is normally the brightest T1 structure in the body)*
- Delayed Enhancement
- Dilated Side Branches

Late:
- Commonly small, uniformly atrophic – but can have focal enlargement
- Pseudocyst formation (30%)
- **Dilation and beading of the pancreatic duct with calcifications ** *most characteristic finding of CP.*

This vs That: **Chronic Pancreatitis Duct Dilation vs Pancreatic Malignancy Duct Dilation**	
CP	**Cancer**
Dilation is Irregular	Dilation is uniform *(usually)*
Duct is < 50% of the AP gland diameter	Duct is > 50% of the AP gland diameter *(obstructive atrophy)*

Complications: Pancreatic cancer *(20 years of CP = 6% risk of Cancer)* is the most crucial complication in CP and is the biggest diagnostic challenge because focal enlargement of the gland induced by a fibrotic inflammatory pseudotumor may be indistinguishable from pancreatic carcinoma.

Uncommon Types and Causes of Pancreatitis				
Autoimmune Pancreatitis	Associated with elevated IgG4	Absence of Attack Symptoms	Responds to steroids	Sausage Shaped Pancreas, capsule like delayed rim enhancement around gland (like a scar)
Groove Pancreatitis	Duodenal and biliary obstruction, symptoms overlap with pancreatic cancer		Duodenal stenosis and /or strictures of the CBD in 50% of the cases	Soft tissue within the pancreaticoduodenal groove, with or without delayed enhancement
Tropic Pancreatitis	Young Age at onset, associated with malnutrition	Increased risk of adenocarcinoma		Multiple large calculi within a dilated pancreatic duct
Hereditary Pancreatitis	Young Age at Onset	Increased risk of adenocarcinoma	SPINK-1 gene	Similar to Tropic Pancreatitis
Ascaris Induced	Most commonly implicated parasite in pancreatitis			Worm may be seen within the bile ducts

When I Say - Auto Immune Pancreatitis	
I Say Auto Immune Pancreatitis	You Say IgG4
I Say IgG4	Autoimmune Pancreatitis Retroperitoneal Fibrosis Sclerosing Cholangitis Inflammatory Pseudotumor Riedel's Thyroiditis

This vs That: Auto Immune Pancreatitis vs Chronic Pancreatitis	
Auto Immune Pancreatitis	**Chronic Pancreatitis**
No ductal dilation	Ductal Dilation
No calcifications	Ductal Calcifications

Cystic Pancreatic Lesions

Pseudocyst: When you see a cystic lesion in the pancreas by far the *most common cause is going to be an inflammatory pseudocyst,* either from acute pancreatitis or chronic pancreatitis.

Simple Cysts: True epithelial lined cysts are rare, and tend to occur with syndromes such as VHL, Polycystic Kidney Disease, and Cystic Fibrosis.

Serous Cystadenoma *(Grandma):* The former term "microcystic adenoma" helps me think of a little old lady, which is appropriate for a lesion primarily found in elderly ladies. The lesion is benign, and classically described as heterogeneous mixed-density lesion made up of multiple small cysts, which resembles a sponge. They are more commonly (70%) located in the pancreatic head (*mucinous is almost always in the body or tail*). An additional key distinction is that it does NOT communicate with the pancreatic duct (*IPMNs do*). About 20% of the time they will have the classic central scar, with or without central calcifications (*mucinous calcifications are peripheral*).

Rarely, they can be unilocular. When you see a unilocular cyst with a lobulated contour located in the head of the pancreas, you should think about this more rare unilocular macrocystic serous cystadenoma subtype.

Trivia: Serous Cystadenoma is associated with von hippel lindau
Memory Aid: "GRANDMA Serous is the HEAD of the household"

Mucinous Cystic Neoplasm *(Mother):* This pre-malignant lesion is "always" found in women, usually in their 50s. All are considered pre-malignant and need to come out. They are found in the body and tail (*serous was more common in the head*). There is generally no communication with the pancreatic duct (*IPMNs will communicate*). Peripheral calcifications are seen in about 25% of cases (*serous was more central*). They are typically unilocular. When mutlilocular, individual cystic spaces tend to be larger than 2cm in diameter (*serous spaces are typically smaller than 2cm*).

Memory Aid: "MUCINOUS in the MOTHER"

IPMN – Intraductal Papillary Mucinous Neoplasm: These guys are mucin-producing tumors that arise from the duct epithelium. They can be either side branch, main branch, or both.

Side Branch:
- o Typically appear as a small cystic mass, often in the head or uncinate process
- o If large amounts of mucin are produced it may result in main duct enlargement
- o Lesions less than 3cm, as usually benign

Main Branch:
- o Produces diffuse dilation of the main duct
- o Atrophy of the gland and dystrophic calcifications may be seen – *mimicking Chronic Pancreatitis*
- o **Have a much higher % of malignancy compared to side branch**
- o All Main Ducts are considered malignant, and resection should be considered

Features Concerning For Malignancy:
- o Main duct >10mm (some sources say 1.5cm)
- o Diffuse or multifocal involvement
- o Enhancing nodules
- o Solid hypovascular mass

Solid Pseudopapillary Tumor of the Pancreas - *(Daughter)*: Very rare, low grade malignant tumor that occurs almost exclusively in young (30s) females (usually Asian or Black). It is typically large at presentation, has a predilection for the tail, and has a "thick capsule." Similar to a hemangioma it may demonstrate progressive fill in of the solid portions.

Cystic Pancreatic Lesion Summary:

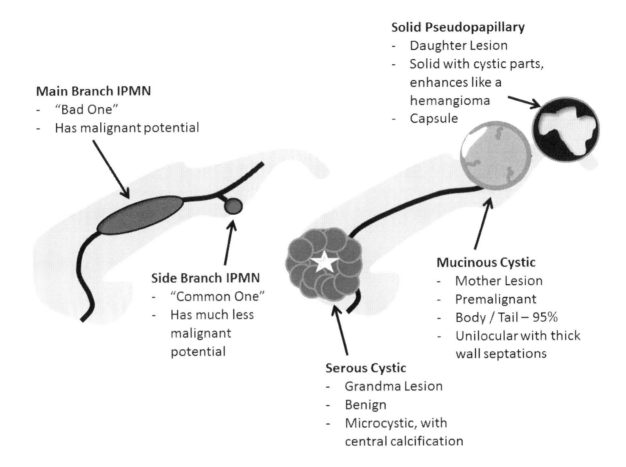

Solid Pseudopapillary
- Daughter Lesion
- Solid with cystic parts, enhances like a hemangioma
- Capsule

Main Branch IPMN
- "Bad One"
- Has malignant potential

Side Branch IPMN
- "Common One"
- Has much less malignant potential

Mucinous Cystic
- Mother Lesion
- Premalignant
- Body / Tail – 95%
- Unilocular with thick wall septations

Serous Cystic
- Grandma Lesion
- Benign
- Microcystic, with central calcification

Solid Pancreatic Lesions

Pancreatic Cancer basically comes in two flavors. (1) Ductal Adenocarcinoma – *which is hypovascular* and (2) Islet Cell / Neuroendocrine *which is hypervascular*.

Ductal Adenocarcinoma: In the setting of a multiple choice test, the finding of an enlarged gallbladder with painless jaundice is highly suspicious for pancreatic adenocarcinoma, especially when combined with migratory thrombophlebitis (*Trousseau's syndrome*). The peak incidence is in the 7th or 8th decade. The strongest risk factor is smoking.

Approximately, two thirds of these cancers arise from the pancreatic head. On ultrasound, obstruction of both the common bile duct, and the pancreatic duct is referred to as the "double duct sign". On CT, the findings are typically a hypovascular mass which is poorly demarcated and low attenuation compared to the more brightly enhancing background parenchyma.

The key to staging is assessment of the SMA and celiac axis, which if involved make the patient's cancer unresectable. Involvement of the GDA is ok, because it comes out with the whipple.

Additional Trivia Points about Pancreatic Adenocarcinoma:
* Tumor Marker = CA 19-9
* Hereditary Syndromes with Pancreatic CA:
    o HNPCC, BRCA Mutation, Ataxia-Telangiectasia, Peutz-Jeghers
* Small Bowel Follow Through: Reverse impression on the duodenum "Frostburg's Inverted 3 Sign" or a "Wide Duodenal Sweep." *They would have to actually find a case of the inverted 3 to show it, but could ask it in words. The "Wide Duodenal Sweep" Could actually be shown.*

Periampullary Tumor: Defined as originating within 2cm of the major papilla. It can be difficult to differentiate from a conventional pancreatic adenocarcinoma as both obstruct the bile duct, and present as a mass in the pancreatic head. Basically, all you need to know about them is they can try and treat them with a Whipple and they have a better prognosis than pancreatic adenocarcinoma.

Trivia: There is an increased incidence of ampullary carcinoma in Gardner's Syndrome

Islet Cell / Neuroendocrine:

Neuroendocrine tumors are uncommon tumors of the pancreas. Typically hypervascular, with brisk enhancement during arterial or pancreatic phase. They can be thought of as non-functional or functional, and then subsequently further divided based on the hormone they make. The can be associated with both MEN 1, and Von Hippel Lindau.

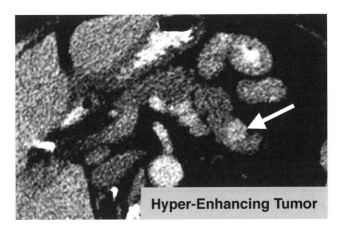

Hyper-Enhancing Tumor

Insulinoma: The most common type (about 75%). They are almost always benign (90%), solitary, and small (<2cm).

Gastrinoma: The second most common type overall, but <u>most common type associated with MEN</u>. They are malignant like 30-60%. They can cause increased gastric acid output and ulcer formation - Zolinger-Ellsion syndrome.

The buzzword is Jejunal Ulcer = Zolinger Ellison.

Non-Functional: The 3rd most common type, usually malignant (80%), and are usually large and metastatic at the time of diagnosis.

I say "non-functional," you say Large with Calcification

Intrapancreatic Accessory Spleen

It is possible to have a pancreatic mass that is actually just a piece of spleen. The typical scenario is that of post traumatic splenosis. Look for the question stem to say something like *"history of trauma."* Another hint may be the absence of a normal spleen.

Imaging Findings:
-Mass follows spleen on all image sequences (dark on T1, and bright on T2 - relative to the liver).
-It will restrict diffusion (just like the spleen).
-The classic give away, and most likely way it will be shown is as a <u>tiger stripped mass on arterial phase</u> (tiger striped like the spleen on arterial phase).

Trivia: Nuclear medicine tests - (1) Heat Treated RBC, and (2) Sulfur Colloid can be used to prove the mass is spleen (they both take up tracer — just like a spleen.

Surgical Correlates:

The Whipple Procedure:

The standard Whipple procedure involves resection of the pancreatic head, duodenum, gastric antrum, and almost always the gallbladder. A jejunal loop is brought up to the right upper quadrant for gastrojejunal, choledochojejunal or hepaticojejunal, and pancreatojejunal anastomosis.

An alternative method used by some surgeons is to perform a pancreatoduodenectomy to preserve the pylorus when possible. However, there is debate in the surgery literature with regard to which method should be the standard. In this pylorus-preserving pancreatoduodenectomy, the stomach is left intact and the proximal duodenum is used for a duodenojejunal anastomosis

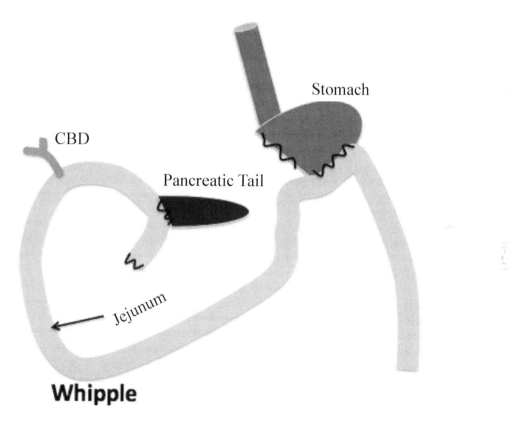

Whipple

Complications:

Delayed gastric emptying (*need for NG tube longer than 1- day*) and pancreatic fistula (*amylase through the surgical drain >50ml for longer than 7-10 days*), are both clinical diagnoses and are the most common complications after pancreatoduodenectomy. Wound infection is the third most common complication, occurring in 5%–20% of patients.

Transplant:

Pancreas transplant (usually with a renal transplant) is an established therapy for severe type 1 diabetes – which is often complicated by renal failure. The vascular anatomy regarding this transplant is quite complicated and beyond the scope of this text. Just know that the pancreas transplant receives arterial inflow from two sources: the donor SMA, (*which supplies the head via the inferior pancreaticoduodenal artery*) and the donor splenic artery, (*which supplies the body and tail*). The venous drainage is via both the donor portal vein and the recipient SMV. Exocrine drainage is via the bowel (*in older transplant via the bladder*).

The number one cause of graft failure is acute rejection. The number two cause of graft failure is splenic vein thrombosis. Splenic vein thrombosis usually occurs within the first 6 weeks of transplant. Venous thrombosis is much more common than arterial thrombosis in the pancreas, especially when compared to other transplants because the vessels are smaller and the clot frequently forms and propagates from the tied off stump vessels.
Both venous thrombosis and acute rejection can appear as reversed diastolic flow. Arterial thrombosis is also less of a problem because of the dual supply to the pancreas (via the Y graft). A point of trivia is that the resistive indices are not of value in the pancreas, because the organ lacks a capsule. The graft is also susceptible to pancreatitis, which is common < 4 weeks after transplant and usually mild. Increased rates of pancreatitis were seen with the older bladder drained subtype. "Shrinking Transplant" is a buzzword for chronic rejection, where the graft progressively gets smaller in size.

The Spleen

Normal Trivia

By the age of 15 the spleen reaches its normal adult size. The spleen contains both "red pulp" and "white pulp" which contribute to its tiger striped appearance during arterial phase imaging. The red pulp is filled with blood (a lot of blood), and can contain up to one liter of blood at any time. The spleen is usually about 20 HU more dense than the liver, and slightly more echogenic than the liver (equal to the left kidney). The splenic artery (which usually arises from the celiac trunk) is essentially an end vessel, with minimal collaterals. Occlusion of the splenic artery will therefore result in infarct of the spleen.

Pathology involving the spleen can be categorized as either congenital, acquired (as the sequella of trauma or portal hypertension), or related to a "mass." A general rule is that most things in the spleen are benign with exception of lymphoma or the rare primary angiosarcoma.

Normal Spleen on MRI:

The spleen is basically a <u>big watery lymph node.</u>

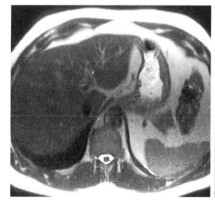 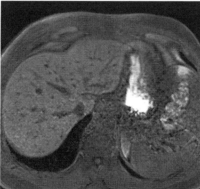 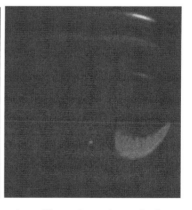

It's Bright on T2
-Relative to the liver

It's Dark on T1
-Relative to the liver

Just like a lymph node it
will restrict diffusion

Heterotaxia Syndromes

These lend themselves well to multiple choice test questions and are probably the highest yield topic to understand regarding the spleen. The major game played on written tests is "left side vs right side." So what the hell does that mean? I like to start in the lungs. The right side has two fissures (major and minor). The left side has just one fissure. So if I show you a CXR with two fissures on each side, (a left sided minor fissure), then the patient has two right sides. Thus the term "bilateral right sidedness." Well what else is a right sided structure? The liver. So, these patients won't have a spleen (the spleen is a left sided structure). The opposite is true, bilateral left sided patients have polysplenia.

Key trivia to know:

Right Sided	Left Sided
Two Fissures in Left Lung	One Fissure in Right Lung
Asplenia	Polysplenia
Cardiac Malformations	Biliary Atresia
Reversed Aorta / IVC	Azygous Continuation of IVC

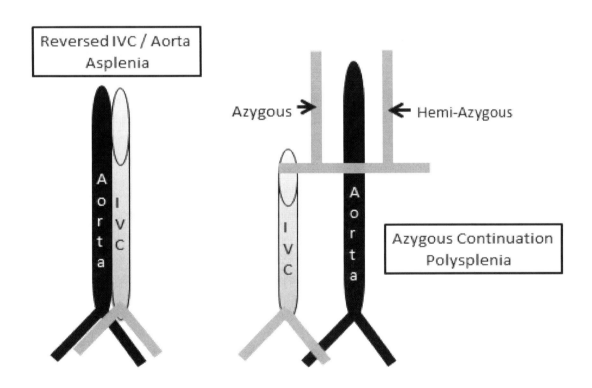

Accessory Spleens These are very common, we see them all the time. Some random trivia that might be testable includes the fact that sulfur colloid could be used to differentiate a splenule from an enlarged pathologic lymph node. Additionally, in the scenario where a patient is post splenectomy for something like ITP or autoimmune hemolytic anemia, an accessory spleen could hypertrophy and present as a mass. Hypertrophy of an accessory spleen can also result in a recurrence of the original hematologic disease process.

Wandering Spleen A normal spleen that "wanders" off and is in an unexpected location. Because of the laxity in the peritoneal ligaments holding the spleen, a wandering spleen is associated with abnormalities of intestinal rotation. The other key piece of trivia is that unusual locations set the spleen up for torsion and subsequent infarction. A chronic partial torsion can actually lead to splenomegaly or gastric varices.

Trauma The spleen is the most common solid organ injured in trauma. This combined with the fact that the spleen contains a unit or so of blood means splenic trauma can be life threatening. Remember the trauma scan is done in portal venous phase (70 second), otherwise you'd have to tell if that tiger stripped arterial phase spleen is lacked.

Splensosis: This occurs post trauma where a smashed spleen implants and then recruits blood supply. The implants are usually multiple and grow into spherical nodules typically in the peritoneal cavity of the upper abdomen (*but can be anywhere*). It's more common than you think and has been reported in 40-60% of trauma. Again, Tc Sulfur colloid (or heat treated RBC) can confirm that the implants are spleen and not ovarian mets or some other terrible thing.

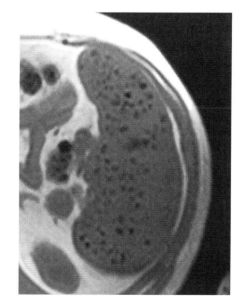

Gamma Gandy Bodies (Siderotic Nodule): These are small foci of hemorrhage in the splenic parenchyma that are usually associated with portal hypertension. They are T2 dark.

Gradient is the most sensitive sequence.

Sarcoidosis: Sarcoid is a disease of unknown etiology that results in noncaseating granulomas and forms in various tissues of the body (*complete discussion in the chest section of this text*). The spleen is involved in 50% - 80% of patients. Splenomegaly is usually the only sign. However, aggregates of granulomatous splenic tissue in some patients may appear on CT as numerous discrete 1-2cm hypodense nodules. Rarely, it can cause a massive splenomegaly and possibly rupture. Don't forget that the gastric antrum is the most common site in the GI tract.

Peliosis: This is a rare condition characterized by multiple blood filled cyst-like spaces in a solid organ (*usually the liver – peliosis hepatitis*). When you see it in the spleen it is usually also with the liver (isolated spleen is extremely rare). The etiology is not known, but for the purpose of multiple choice tests it occurs in women of OCPs, men on anabolic steroids, **people with AIDS, renal transplant patients** (up to 20%), and Hodgkin lymphoma. It's usually asymptomatic but can explode spontaneously.

Splenic Vascular Abnormalities

Splenic artery aneurysm is the most common visceral arterial aneurysm. Pseudoaneurysm can occur in the setting of trauma and pancreatitis. The incidence is higher in women of child bearing age who have had two or more pregnancies (*4x more likely to get them, 3x more likely to rupture*). It's usually sacular and in the mid to distal artery. They usually fix them when they get around 2-3cm. Major "F" up to avoid: Don't call them a hypervascular pancreatic islet cell mass and biopsy them.

Splenic vein thrombosis frequently occurs as the result of pancreatitis. Can also occur in the setting of diverticulitis or Crohns. Can lead to isolated gastric varices.

Infarction can occur from a number of conditions. On a multiple choice test the answer is sickle cell. The imaging features are classically a wedge-shaped, peripheral, low attenuation defect.

Splenic Infections

Most common radiologically detected splenic infection is histoplasmosis (with multiple round calcifications). Splenic TB can have a similar appearance (but much less common in the US). Another possible cause of calcified granuloma in the spleen in brucellosis, but these are usually solitary and 2cm or larger. They may have a low density center, encircled by calcification giving the lesion a "bull's eye" appearance.

In the immunocompetent patient, **splenic abscess** is usually due to an aerobic organism. **Salmonella is the classic bug** – which develops in the setting of underlying splenic damage (trauma, or sickle cell). In immunocompromised patient's, unusual organisms such as fungi, TB, MAI, and PCP can occur and usually present as multiple micro-abscesses. Occasionally, fungal infections may show a "bulls-eye" appearance on ultrasound.

Splenic Size - Too Big vs Too Small:

It's good to have a differential for a big spleen and a small spleen.

Small Spleen	Big Spleen
Sickle Cell	Passive Congestions (heart failure, portal HTN, splenic vein thrombosis)
Post Radiation	Lymphoma
Post Thorotrast	Leukemia
Malabsorption Syndromes (ulcerative colitis > crohns)	Gauchers

Felty's Syndrome – abnormality of granulocytes, with a triad of: (1) Splenomegaly, (2) Rheumatoid Arthritis, (3) Neutropenia

Benign Masses of the Spleen

Cysts:

Post traumatic cysts (pseudocysts) are the most common cystic lesion in the spleen. They can occur secondary to infarction, infection, hemorrhage or extension from a pancreatic pseudocyst. As a point of trivia they are "pseudo" cysts because they have no epithelial lining. They may have a thick wall or prominent calcifications peripherally.

Epidermoid cysts are the second most common cystic lesion in the spleen. They are congenital in origin. As a point of absolutely worthless trivia, they are "true" cysts and have an epithelial lining. They typically grow slowly and are usually around 10cm at the time of discovery. They can cause symptoms if they are large enough. They are solitary 80% of the time, and have peripheral calcifications 25% of the time.

Hydatid or Echinococcal cysts are the third most common cystic lesion in the spleen (most common worldwide). They are caused by the parasite Echinoccus Granulosus. Hydatid cysts consist of a spherical "mother cyst" that usually contains smaller "daughter cysts." Internal septations and debris are often referred to as "hydatid sand." Another sign described is the "water lily sign." The "water lily sign" is seen when there is detachment of the endocyst membrane resulting in floating membranes within the pericysts (looks like a water lily). This was classically described on CXR in pulmonary echinococcal disease.

Hemangioma is the most common benign neoplasm in the spleen. This dude is usually smooth and well marginated demonstrating contrast uptake and delayed washout. *The classic peripheral nodular discontinuous enhancement seen in hepatic lesions may not occur,* especially if the tumor is smaller than 2cm.

Lymphangiomas are rare entities in the spleen but can occur. Most occur in childhood. They may be solitary or multiple, although most occur in a subcapsular location. Diffuse lymphangiomas may occur (lymphangiomatosis).

Hamartomas are also rare in the spleen, but can occur. Typically this is an incidental finding. Most are hypodense or isodense and show moderate heterogeneous enhancement. They can be hyperdense if there is hemosiderin deposition.

Littoral Cell Angioma is a zebra that shows up occasionally in books and possibly on multiple choice tests. Clinical hypersplenism is almost always present. Usually presents as multiple small foci which are hypoattenuating on late portal phase. MR shows hemosiderin (low T1 and T2).

Malignant Masses of the Spleen

Most things that occur in the spleen are benign. Other than lymphoma (discussed below) it is highly unlikely that you will encounter a primary malignancy of the spleen (*but if you do it's likely to be vascular*). For the purposes of academic discussion (and possible multiple choice trivia) angiosarcoma is the most common.

Angiosarcoma: It is aggressive and has a poor prognosis. On CT it can manifest as a poorly defined area of heterogeneity or low density in an enlarged spleen. They can contain necrosis and get big enough to rupture *(spontaneous rupture occurs like 30% of the time)*. Contrast enhancement is usually poor. Yes, these can occur from prior thorotrast exposure.

Lymphoma is the most common malignant tumor of the spleen, and is usually seen as a manifestation of systemic disease. *Splenomegaly is the most common finding* (and maybe the only finding in low grade disease). Although both Hodgkins and Non-Hodgkins types can involve the spleen, Hodgkins type and high grade lymphomas can show discrete nodules of tumor. With regard to imaging, they are low density on CT, T1 dark, and are PET hot.

Metastatic disease to the spleen is rare. When it does occur, it occurs via common things (Breast, Lung, Melanoma).

Trivia: Melanoma is the most common primary neoplasm to met to the spleen

Blank for Scribbles / Notes

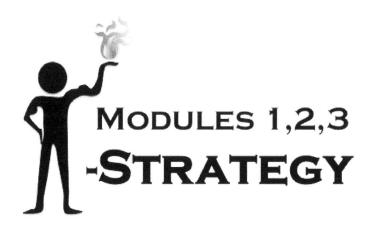 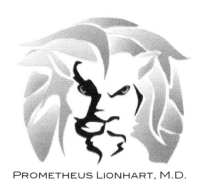

PROMETHEUS LIONHART, M.D.

MODULES 1,2,3 -STRATEGY

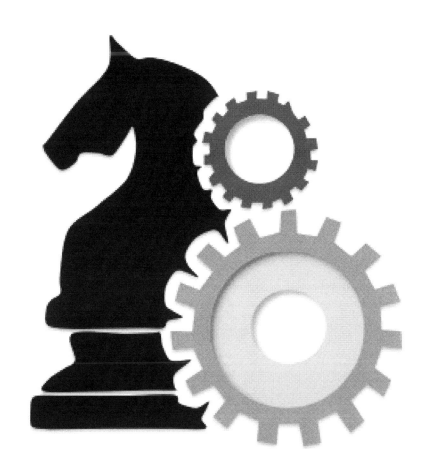

Section 1: Cardiac

When I Say This..... You Say That.....

- When I say "ALCAPA," you say Steal Syndrome
- When I say "Supra-valvular Aortic Stenosis" you say Williams Syndrome
- When I say "Bicuspid Aortic Valve and Coarctation" you say Turners Syndrome
- When I say "Isolated right upper lobe edema," you say Mitral Regurgitation
- When I say "Peripheral pulmonary stenosis," you say Alagille Syndrome
- When I say "Box shaped heart", you say Ebsteins
- When I say "Right Arch with Mirror Branching," you say congenital heart.
- When I say "hand/thumb defects + ASD," you say Holt Oram
- When I say "ostium primum ASD (or endocardial cushion defect)," you say Downs
- When I say "Right Sided PAPVR," you say Sinus Venosus ASD
- When I say "Calcification in the left atrium wall," you say Rheumatic Heart Disease
- When I say "difficult to suppress myocardium," you say Amyloid
- When I say "blood pool suppression on delayed enhancement," you say Amyloid
- When I say "septal bounce," you say constrictive pericarditis
- When I say "ventricular interdependence," you say constrictive pericarditis
- When I say "focal thickening of the septum - but not Hypertrophic Cardiomyopathy," you say Sarcoid.
- When I say "ballooning of the left ventricular apex," you say Tako-Tsubo
- When I say "fat in the wall of a dilated right ventricle," you say Arrhythmogenic Right Ventricular Cardiomyopathy (ARVC)
- When I say "kid with dilated heart and mid wall enhancement," you say Muscular Dystrophy
- When I say "Cardiac Rhabdomyoma," you say Tuberous Sclerosis
- When I say "Bilateral Atrial Thrombus," you say Eosinophilic Cardiomyopathy
- When I say "Diffuse LV Subendocardial enhancement not restricted to a vascular distribution," you say Cardiac Amyloid.
- When I say "Glenn Procedure," you say acquired pulmonary AVMs
- When I say "Pulmonary Vein Stenosis," you say Ablation for A-Fib
- When I say "Multiple Cardiac Myxomas," you say Carney's Complex
- Aliasing is common with Cardiac MRI. You can fix it by: (1) opening your FOV, (2) oversampling the frequency encoding direction, or (3) switching phase and frequency encoding directions.
- Giant Coronary Artery Aneurysms (>8mm) don't regress, and are associated with MIs.
- Wet Beriberi (thiamine def) can cause a dilated cardiomyopathy.

- Most common primary cardiac tumor in children = Rhabdomyoma.
- 2nd most common primary cardiac tumor in children = Fibroma
- Most common complication of MI is myocardial remodeling.
- Unroofed coronary sinus is associated with Persistent left SVC.
- Most common source of cardiac mets = Lung Cancer (lymphoma #2).
- A-Fib is most commonly associated with left atrial enlargement
- Most common cause of tricuspid insufficiency is RVH (usually from pulmonary HTN / cor pulmonale).

High Yield Trivia

- The right atrium is defined by the IVC.
- The right ventricle is defined by the moderator band.
- The tricuspid papillary muscles insert on the septum (mitral ones do not).
- Lipomatous Hypertrophy of the Intra-Atrial Septum - can be PET Avid (it's brown fat)
- LAD gives off diagonals
- RCA gives off acute marginals
- LCX gives off obtuse marginals
- RCA perfuses SA and AV nodes (most of the time)
- Dominance is decided by which vessel lives off the posterior descending - it's the right 85%
- LCA from the Right Coronary Cusp - always gets repaired
- RCA from the Left Coronary Cusp - repaired if symptoms
- Most common location of myocardial bridging is in the mid portion of the LAD.
- Coronary Artery Aneurysm - most common cause in adult = Atherosclerosis
- Coronary Artery Aneurysm - most common cause in child = Kawasaki
- Rheumatic heart disease is the most common cause of mitral stenosis
- Pulmonary Arterial Hypertension is the most common cause of tricuspid atresia.
- Double most common vascular ring is the double aortic arch
- Most common congenital heart disease is a VSD
- Most common ASD is the Secundum
- Infracardiac TAPVR classically shown with pulmonary edema in a newborn
- "L" Transposition type is congenitally corrected (they are "L"ucky).
- "D" Transposition type is doomed.
- Truncus is associated with CATCH-22 (DiGeorge)
- Rib Notching from coarctations spares the 1st and 2nd Ribs
- Infarct with 50% involvement is unlikely to recover function
- Microvascular Obstruction is NOT seen in chronic infarct
- Amyloid is the most common cause of restricted cardiomyopathy
- Primary amyloid can be seen in multiple myeloma
- Most common neoplasm to involve the cardiac valves = Fibroelastoma

- Most commonly the congenital absence of the pericardium is partial and involves the pericardium over the left atrium and adjacent pulmonary artery (*the left atrial appendage is the most at risk to become strangulated*).
- Glenn shunt - SVC to pulmonary artery (vein to artery)
- Blalock-Taussig Shunt - Subclavian Artery to Pulmonary Artery (artery - artery)
- Ross Procedure - Replaces aortic valve with pulmonic, and pulmonic with a graft (done for kids).

SECTION 2: VASCULAR

When I Say This..... You Say That.....

- When I say "vessel in the fissure of the ligamentum venosum," you say replaced left hepatic artery.
- When I say "vessel coursing of the pelvic brim," you say Corona Mortis
- When I say "ascending aorta calcifications," you say Syphilis and Takayasu
- When I say "tulip bulb aorta," you say Marfans
- When I say "really shitty Marfan's variant," you say Loeys-Dietz
- When I say "tortuous vessels," you say Loeys-Dietz
- When I say "renal artery stenosis with HTN in a child," you say NF-1
- When I say "nasty looking saccular aneurysm, without intimal calcifications" you say Mycotic.
- When I say "tree bark intimal calcification," you say Syphilitic (Luetic) aneurysm
- When I say "painful aneurysm in smoker, sparing the posterior wall," you say Inflammatory aneurysm.
- When I say "Turkish guy with pulmonary artery aneurysm," you say Behcets
- When I say "GI bleed with early opacification of a dilated draining vein," you say Colonic Angiodysplasia
- When I say "spider web appearance of hepatic veins on angiogram," you say Budd Chiari
- When I say "non-decompressible varicocele," you say look in the belly for badness
- When I say "right sided varicocele," you say look in the below for badness
- When I say "swollen left leg," you say May Thurner
- When I say "popliteal aneurysm," you say look for the AAA (and the other leg)
- When I say "most dreaded complication of popliteal aneurysm," you say distal emboli
- When I say "Great saphenous vein on the wrong side of the calf - lateral side," you say Marginal Vein of Servelle - which is supposedly pathognomonic for Klippel-Trenaunay Syndrome

- When I say "Asian," you say Takayasu
- When I say "Involves the aorta," you say Takayasu
- When I say "Kids with vertigo and aortitis," you say Cogan Syndrome
- When I say "Nasal perforation + Cavitary Lung Lesions," you say Wegners
- When I say "diffuse pulmonary hemorrhage," you say Microscopic Polyangitis
- When I say "Smoker + Hand Angiogram," you say Buergers
- When I say "Construction worker + Hand Angiogram," you say Hypothenar Hammer
- When I say "Unilateral tardus parvus in the carotid," you say stenosis of the innominate
- When I say "Bilateral tardus parvus in the carotids," you say aortic stenosis
- When I say "Bilateral reversal of flow in carotids," you say aortic regurg
- When I say "Lack of diastolic flow on carotid US," you say Brain Death

High Yield Trivia

- Artery of Adamkiewicz comes off on the left side (70%) between T8-L1 (90%)
- Arch of Riolan - middle colic branch of the SMA with the left colic of the IMA.
- Most common hepatic vascular variant = right hepatic artery replaced off the SMA
- The proper right hepatic artery is anterior the right portal vein, whereas the replaced right hepatic artery is posterior to the main portal vein.
- Accessory right inferior hepatic vein - most common hepatic venous variant.
- Anterior tibialis is the first branch off the popliteal
- Common Femoral Artery (CFA): Begins at the level of inguinal ligament
- Superficial Femoral Artery (SFA): Begins once the CFA gives off the profunda femurs
- Popliteal Artery: Begins as the SFA exits the adductor canal
- Popliteal Artery terminates as the anterior tibial artery and the tibioperoneal trunk
- Axillary Artery: Begins at the first rib
- Brachial Artery: Begins as it crosses the teres major
- Brachial Artery: Bifurcates to the ulnar and radial artery
- Intraosseous Branch: Typically arises from the ulnar
- Superficial Arch = From the Ulna, Deep Arch = From the Radius
- The "coronary vein," is the left gastric.
- Enlarged splenorenal shunts are associated with hepatic encephalopathy.
- Aortic Dissection, and intramural hematoma are caused by HTN (70%)
- Penetrating Ulcer is from atherosclerosis.

- Strongest predictor of progression of dissection in intramural hematoma = Maximum aortic diameter > 5cm.
- Leriche Syndrome Triad: Claudication, Absent/ Decreased femoral pulses, Impotence.
- Most common associated defect with aortic coarctation = bicuspid aorta (80%)
- Neurogenic compression is the most common subtype of thoracic outlet syndrome
- Splenic artery aneurysm - More common in pregnancy, more likely to rupture in pregnancy.
- Median Arcuate Compression - worse with expiration
- Colonic Angiodysplasia is associated with aortic stenosis
- Popliteal Aneurysm; 30-50% have AAA, 10% of patient with AAA have popliteal aneurysm, 50-70% of popliteal aneurysms are bilateral.
- Medial deviation of the popliteal artery by the medial head of the gastrocnemius = Popliteal Entrapment
- Type 3 Takayasu is the most common (arch + abdominal aorta).
- Most common vasculitis in a kid = HSP (Henoch-Schonlein Purpura)

SECTION 3: CHEST

When I Say This..... You Say That.....

- When I say "obliteration of Raider's Triangle," you say aberrant right subclavian
- When I say "flat waist sign," you say left lower lobe collapse
- When I say "terrorist + mediastinal widening," you say Anthrax
- When I say "bulging fissure," you say Klebsiella
- When I say "dental procedure gone bad, now with jaw osteo and pneumonia," you say Actinomycosis.
- When I say "culture negative pleural effusion, 3 months later with airspace opacity," you say TB
- When I say "hot-tub," you say Hypersensitivity Pneumonitis
- When I say "halo sign," you say Fungal Pneumonia - Invasive Aspergillus
- When I say "reverse halo or atoll sign," you say COP
- When I say "finger in glove," you say ABPA
- When I say "ABPA," you say Asthma
- When I say "septic emboli + jugular vein thrombus," you say Lemierre
- When I say "Lemierre," you say Fusobacterium Necrophorum
- When I say "Paraneoplatic syndromes with SIADH," you say Small Cell Lung CA

- When I say "Paraneoplatic syndromes with PTH," you say Squamous Cell CA
- When I say "Small Cell Lung CA + Proximal Weakness," you say Lambert Eaton
- When I say "Cavity fills with air, post pneumonectomy," you say Bronchopleural Fistula
- When I say "malignant bronchial tumor," you say carcinoid
- When I say "malignant tracheal tumor," you say Adenoid Cystic
- When I say "AIDS patient with lung nodules, pleural effusion, and lymphadenopathy," you say Lymphoma
- When I say "Gallium Negative," you say Kaposi
- When I say "Thallium Negative," you say PCP
- When I say "Macroscopic fat and popcorn calcifications," you say Hamartoma
- When I say "Bizarre shaped cysts," you say LCH
- When I say "Lung Cysts in a TS patient," you say LAM
- When I say "Panlobular Emphysema - NOT Alpha 1," you say Ritalin Lung
- When I say "Honeycombing," you say UIP
- When I say "The histology was heterogeneous," you say UIP
- When I say "Ground Glass with Sub pleural Sparing," you say NSIP
- When I say "UIP Lungs + Parietal Pleural Thickening," you say Asbetosis
- When I say "Cavitation in the setting of silicosis," you say TB
- When I say "Air trapping seen 6 months after lung transplant," you say Chronic Rejection / Bronchiolitis Obliterans Syndrome
- When I say "Crazy Paving," you say PAP
- When I say "History of constipation," you say Lipoid Pneumonia - inferring mineral oil use / aspiration.
- When I say "UIP + Air trapping," you say Chronic Hypersensitivity Pneumonitis
- When I say "Dilated Esophagus + ILD," = Scleroderma (with NSIP)
- When I say "Shortness of breath when sitting up," you say Hepatopulmonary syndrome
- When I say "Episodic hypoglycemia," you say solitary fibrous tumor of the pleura
- When I say "Pulmonary HTN with Normal Wedge Pressure," you say Pulmonary Veno-occlusive disease.
- When I say "Yellow Nails" you say Edema and Chylous Pleural Effusions (Yellow Nail Syndrome).
- When I say "persistent fluid collection after pleural drain/tube placement," you say Extrapleural Hematoma.
- When I say "Displaced extrapleural fat," you say Extrapleural Hematoma.
- When I say "Massive air leak, in the setting of trauma," you say bronchial or tracheal injury
- When I say "Hot of PET – around the periphery," you say pulmonary infarct
- When I say "Multi-lobar collapse," you say sarcoid
- When I say "Classic bronchial infection," you say TB
- When I say "Panbronchiolitis," you say tree in bud (not centrilobular or random nodules)
- When I say "Bronchorrhea," you say Mucinous BAC

High Yield Trivia

- The tricuspid valve is the most anterior
- The pulmonic valve is the most superior
- There are 10 lung segments on the right, and 8 lung segments on the left
- If it goes above the clavicles, it's in the posterior mediastinum (cervicothoracic sign)
- Azygos Lobe has 4 layers of pleura
- Most common pulmonary vein variant is a separate vein draining the right middle lobe
- Most common cause of pneumonia in AIDS patient is Strep Pneumonia
- Most common opportunistic infection in AIDS = PCP.
- Aspergilloma is seen in a normal immune patient
- Invasive Aspergillus is seen in an immune compromised patient
- Fleischner Society Recommendations do NOT apply to patient's with known cancers
- Eccentric calcifications in a solitary pulmonary nodule pattern is considered the most suspicious.
- A part solid nodule with a ground glass component is the most suspicious morphology you can have
- Most common lung CA to present as solitary nodule
- Stage 3B lung CA is unresectable (contralateral nodal involvement ; ipsilateral or contralateral scalene or supraclavicular nodal involvement, tumor in different lobes).
- The most common cause of unilateral lymphangetic carcinomatosis is bronchogenic carcinoma lung cancer invading the lymphatics
- There is a 20 year latency between initial exposure and development of lung cancer or pleural mesothelioma
- Pleural effusion is the earliest and most common finding with asbestosis exposure.
- Silicosis actually raises your risk of TB by about 3 fold.
- Nitrogen Dioxide exposure is "Silo Filler's Disease," gives you a pulmonary edema pattern.
- Reticular pattern in the posterior costophrenic angle is supposedly the first finding of UIP on CXR
- Sarcoidosis is the most common recurrent primary disease after lung transplant
- Pleural plaque of asbestosis typically spares the costophrenic angles.
- Pleural effusion is the most common manifestation of mets to the pleura.
- There is an association with mature teratomas and Klinefelter Syndrome.
- Injury close to the carina is going to cause a pneumomediastinum rather than a pneumothorax
- MRI is superior for assessing superior sulcus tumors because you need to look at the brachial plexus.
- Leiomyoma is the most common benign esophageal tumor (most common in the distal third).

- Esophageal Leiomyomatosis may be associated with Alport's Syndrome
- Bronchial / Tracheal injury must be evaluated with bronchoscopy
- If you say COP also say Eosinophilic Pneumonia
- If you say BAC also say lymphoma
- Bronchial Atresia is classically in the LUL
- Pericardial cysts MUST be simple, Bronchogenic cysts don't have to be simple
- PAP follows a rule of 1/3s post treatment; 1/3 gets better, 1/3 doesn't, 1/3 progresses to fibrosis
- Dysphagia Lusoria presents later in life as atherosclerosis develops
- Carcinoid is COLD on PET
- Wegener's is now called Granulomatosis with Polyangiitis – Wegener was a Nazi. Apparently he was not just a Nazi, he was a Nazi before it was "fashionable." Plus, I heard he was a real asshole, and a bad tipper (which is unforgivable).

SECTION 4: MSK

This vs That: Avulsion from where?

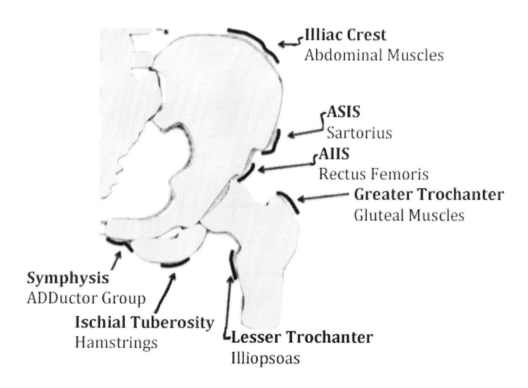

This vs That: Forearm Fractures:

Essex-Lopresti	Galeazzi Fracture (MUGR)	Monteggia Fracture (MUGR)
Fracture of the radial head + Anterior dislocation of the distal radial ulnar joint	Radial Shaft fracture, with anterior dislocation of the ulna at the DRUJ.	Fracture of the proximal ulna, with anterior dislocation of the radial head.

Shoulder - Bankart Spectrum

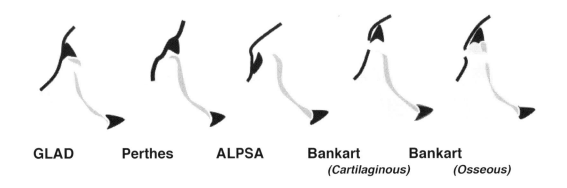

GLAD	Perthes	ALPSA	True Bankart
Superficial partial labral injury with cartilage defect	Avulsed anterior labrum (only minimally displaced). Inferior GH complex still attached to periosteum	Similar to perthes but with "bunched up" medially displaced inferior GH complex	Torn labrum
No instability	Intact Periosteum (lifted up)	Intact Periosteum	***Periosteum Disrupted***

When I Say This..... You Say That.....

- When I say, "Posterior elbow dislocation," you say Capitellum fracture
- When I say "Chondroblastoma in an adult", you say "Clear Cell Chondrosarcoma"
- When I say "Malignant epiphyseal lesion", you say "Clear Cell Chondrosarcoma"
- When I say "Permeative lesion in the diaphysis of a child" , you say "Ewings"
- When I say "T2 bright lesion in the sacrum" , you say "Chordoma"
- When I say "Lytic T2 DARK lesion" , you say "Fibrosarcoma"
- When I say "Sarcomatous transformation of an infarct", you say "MFH"
- When I say, "Epiphyseal Lesion that is NOT T2 Bright" , You say Chondroblastoma
- When I say, "short 4th metacarpal," You say pseudopseudohypoparathyroidism and Turner Syndrome
- When I say, "band like acro-osteolysis," You say Hajdu-Cheney
- When I say "fat containing tumor in the retroperitoneum," you say liposarcoma
- When I say "sarcoma in the foot" you say synovial sarcoma.
- When I say "avulsion of the lesser trochanter," you say pathologic fracture
- When I say "cross over sign," you say pincher type Femoroacetabular Impingement
- When I say "Segond Fracture," you say ACL tear
- When I say "Reverse Segond Fracture," you say PCL
- When I say "Arcuate Sign," you say fibular head avulsion or PCL tear
- When I say "Deep Intercondylar Notch," you say ACL tear
- When I say "Bilateral Patellar Tendon Ruptures," you say chronic steroids
- When I say "Wide ankle mortise," you say show me the proximal fibula (Maisonneuve).
- When I say "Bilateral calcaneus fractures," you say show me the spinal compression fracture ("lover's leap")
- When I say "Dancer with lateral foot pain," you say avulsion of 5th MT
- When I say "Old lady with sudden knee pain with standing," you say SONK
- When I say "Looser's Zones," you say osteomalacia or rickets (vitamin D)
- When I say "Unilateral RA with preserved joint spaces," you say RSD
- When I say "T2 bright tumor in finger," you say Glomus
- When I say "Blooming in tumor in finger," you say Giant Cell Tumor of Tendon Sheath (PVNS)
- When I say "Atrophy of teres minor," you say Quadrilateral Space syndrome
- When I say "Subluxation of the Biceps Tendon," you say Subscapularis tear
- When I say "Too many bow ties," you say Discoid Meniscus
- When I say "Celery Stalk ACL - T2" you say Mucoid Degeneration
- When I say "Drumstick ALC - T1" you say Mucoid Degeneration
- When I say "Acute Flat foot," you say Posterior Tibial Tendon Tear
- When I say "Boomerang shaped peroneus brevis," you say tear - or split tear

- When I say "Meniscoid mass in the lateral gutter of the ankle," you say Anteriolateral Impingement Syndrome
- When I say "Scar between 3rd and 4th metatarsals," you say Morton's neuroma
- When I say "Osteomyelitis in the spine," you say IV drug user
- When I say "Osteomyelitis in the spine with Kyphosis," you say TB (Gibbus Deformity)
- When I say "Unilateral SI joint lysis," you say IV Drug User
- When I say "Psoas muscle abscess," you say TB
- When I say "Rice bodies in joint," you say TB - sloughed synovium
- When I say "Calcification along the periphery," you say myositis ossificans
- When I say "Calcifications more dense in the center," you say Osteosarcoma - reverse zoning
- When I say "Permeative lesion in the diaphysis of a child," you say Ewings
- When I say "Long lesion in a long bone," you say Fibrous Dysplasia
- When I say "Large amount of edema for the size of the lesion," you say Osteoid Osteoma
- When I say "Cystic bone lesion, that is NOT T2 bright," you say Chondroblastoma
- When I say "Lesion in the finger of a kid," you say Periosteal chondroma
- When I say "looks like NOF in the anterior tibia with anterior bowing," you say Osteofibrous Dysplasia.
- When I say " RA + Pneumoconiosis," you say Caplan Syndrome
- When I say " RA + Big Spleen + Neutropenia," you say Felty Syndrome
- When I say "Reducible deformity of joints - in hand," you say Lupus.
- When I say "destructive mass in a bone of a leukemia patient," you say Chloroma

High Yield Trivia

- Arthritis at the radioscaphoid compartment is the first sign of a SNAC or SLAC wrist
- SLAC wrist has a DISI deformity
- The pull of the Abductor pollucis longus tendon is what causes the dorsolateral dislocation in the Bennett Fracture
- Carpal tunnel syndrome has an association with dialysis
- Degree of femoral head displacement predicts risk of AVN
- Proximal pole of the scaphoid is at risk for AVN with fracture
- Most common cause of sacral insufficiency fracture is osteoporosis in old lady
- Patella dislocation is nearly always lateral
- Tibial plateau fracture is way more common laterally
- SONK favors the medial knee (area of maximum weight bearing)
- Normal SI joints excludes Ank Spon
- Looser Zones are a type of insufficiency fracture
- T score of -2.5 marks osteoporosis
- First extensor compartment = de Quervains
- First and Second compartment = intersection syndrome
- Sixth extensor compartment = early RA
- Flexor pollicis longus goes through the carpal tunnel, flexor pollicis brevis does not
- The pisiform recess and radiocarpal joint normally communicate
- The periosteum is intact with both Perthes and ALPSA lesions. In a true bankart it is disrupted.
- Absent anterior/superior labrum, along with a thickened middle glenohumeral ligament is a Buford complex.
- Medial meniscus is thicker posterior.
- Anterior talofibular ligament is the most commonly torn ankle ligament
- TB in the spine - spares the disc space (so can brucellosis).
- Scoliosis curvature points away from the osteoid osteoma
- Osteochondroma is the only benign skeletal tumor associated with radiation.
- Mixed Connective Tissue Disease requires serology (Ribonucleoprotein) for Dx
- Medullary Bone Infarct will have fat in the middle
- Bucket Handle Meniscal tears are longitudinal tears

Section 5: GI

Problem Solving Through MRI

Different programs have variable volume with MRI. Some of you will be excellent at it. Some of you will suck at it. An important skill to have is to understand how to problem solve with different sequences. The best way to do this is to have a list of T1 bright things, T2 bright things, dark things, and things that restrict diffusion.

T1 Bright	T2 Bright	T1 and T2 DARK	Restricts Diffusion
Fat	Fat	Flow Void	Stroke
Melanin (Melanoma)	Water	Fibrosis / Scar	Hypercellular Tumor
Blood (Subacute)	Blood (Extracellular Methemoglobin)	Metal	Epidermoid
Protein Rick Fluid	Most Tumors	Air	Abscess (Bacterial)
Calcification (Hyalinized)			Acute Demyelination
Slow Moving Blood			CJD
Laminar Necrosis			T2 Shine Through

Be able to move through sequences and problem solve.

Think about a Lipoma for example. This will be T1 bright, T2 bright, and fat sat out. Another example might be something with layers in it. What can layer? Fat could layer, water could layer, blood could layer, pus could layer. Fat would be bright/ bright. Water would be dark on T1. Pus would be dark on T2. Blood could do different things depending on it's age. Fat would sat out. Pus may restrict diffusion (like a subdural empyema). You get the idea. Run through some scenarios in your mind. The key point is to know your differentials for this.

When I Say This..... You Say That.....

- When I say "narrowed B Ring," You say Schatzki *(Schat"B"ki Ring)*
- When I say "esophageal concentric rings," You say Eosinophilic Esophagitis
- When I say "shaggy" or "plaque like" esophagus, You say Candidiasis
- When I say "looks like candida, but an asymptomatic old lady," you say Glycogen Acanthosis
- When I say "reticular mucosal pattern," you say Barretts
- When I say "high stricture with an associated hiatal hernia," you say Barretts
- When I say "abrupt shoulders," you say cancer
- When I say "Killian Dehiscence," you say Zenker Diverticulum
- When I say "transient, fine transverse folds across the esophagus," you say Feline Esophagus.
- When I say "bird's beak," you say Achalasia
- When I say "solitary esophageal ulcer," you say CMV or AIDS
- When I say "ulcers at the level of the arch or distal esophagus," you say Medication induced
- When I say "Breast Cancer + Bowel Hamartomas," you say Cowdens
- When I say "Desmoid Tumors + Bowel Polyps," you say Gardners
- When I say "Brain Tumors + Bowel Polyps," you say Turcots
- When I say "enlarged left supraclavicular node," you say Virchow Node (GI Cancer)
- When I say "crosses the pylorus," you say Gastric Lymphoma
- When I say "isolated gastric varices," you say splenic vein thrombus
- When I say "multiple gastric ulcers," you say Chronic Aspirin Therapy.
- When I say "multiple duodenal (or jejunal) ulcers," you say Zollinger-Ellsion
- When I say "pancreatitis after Billroth 2," you say Afferent Loop Syndrome
- When I say "Weight gain years after Roux-en-Y," you say Gastro-Gastro Fistula
- When I say "Clover Leak Sign - Duodenum," you say healed peptic ulcer.
- When I say "Sand Like Nodules in the Jejunum," you say Whipples
- When I say "Sand Like Nodules in the Jejunum + CD4 <100," you say MAI
- When I say "Ribbon-like bowel," you say Graft vs Host
- When I say "Ribbon like Jejunum," you say Long Standing Celiac
- When I say "Moulage Pattern," you say Celiac
- When I say "Fold Reversal - of jejunum and ileum," you say Celiac
- When I say "Cavitary (low density) Lymph nodes," you say Celiac

- When I say "hide bound" or "Stack or coins," you say Scleroderma
- When I say "Megaduodenum," you say Scleroderma
- When I say "Duodenal obstruction, with recent weight loss," you say SMA Syndrome
- When I say "Coned shaped cecum," you say Amebiasis
- When I say "Lead Pipe," you say Ulcerative Colitis
- When I say "String Sign," you say Crohns
- When I say "Massive circumferential thickening, without obstruction," you say Lymphoma
- When I say "Multiple small bowel target signs," you say Melanoma
- When I say "Obstructing Old Lady Hernia," you say Femoral Hernia
- When I say "sac of bowel," you say Paraduodenal hernia.
- When I say "scalloped appearance of the liver," you say Pseudomyxoma Peritonei
- When I say "HCC without cirrhosis," you say Hepatitis B
- When I say "Capsular retraction," you say Cholangiocarcinoma
- When I say "Periportal hypoechoic infiltration + AIDS," you say Kaposi's
- When I say "sparing of the caudate lobe," you say Budd Chiari
- When I say "large T2 bright nodes + Budd Chiari," you say Hyperplastic nodules
- When I say "liver high signal in phase, low signal out phase," you say fatty liver
- When I say "liver low signal in phase, and high signal out phase," you say hemochromatosis
- When I say "multifocal intrahepatic and extrahepatic stricture," you say PSC
- When I say "multifocal intrahepatic and extrahepatic strictures + papillary stenosis," you say AIDS Cholangiopathy.
- When I say "bile ducts full of stones," you say Recurrent Pyogenic Cholangitis
- When I say "Gallbladder Comet Tail Artifact," you say Adenomyomatosis
- When I say "lipomatous pseudohypertrophy of the pancreas," you say CF
- When I say "sausage shaped pancreas," you say autoimmune pancreatitis
- When I say "autoimmune pancreatitis," you say IgG4
- When I say "IgG4" you say RP Fibrosis, Sclerosing Cholangitis, Fibrosing Medianstinitis, Inflammatory Pseudotumor
- When I say "Wide duodenal sweep," you say Pancreatic Cancer
- When I say "Grandmother Pancreatic Cyst" you say Serous Cystadenoma
- When I say "Mother Pancreatic Cyst" you say Mucinous
- When I say "Daughter Pancreatic Cyst," you say Solid Pseudopapillary

High Yield Trivia

- Most Common benign mucosal lesion of the esophagus = Papilloma
- Esophageal Webs have increased risk for cancer, and Plummer-Vinson Syndrome (anemia + web)
- Dysphagia Lusoria is from compression by a right subclavian artery (most patients with aberrant rights don't have symptoms).
- Achalasia has an increased risk of squamous cell cancer (20 years later).
- Most common mesenchymal tumor of the GI tract = GIST
- Most common location for GIST = Stomach
- Krukenberg Tumor = Stomach (GI) met to the ovary
- Menetrier's : involves fundus and spares the antrum
- The stomach is the most common location for sarcoid (in the GI tract)
- Gastric Remnants have an increased risk of cancer years after Billroth
- Most common internal hernia, Left sided paraduodenal
- Most common site of peritoneal carcinomatosis = retrovesical space
- An injury to the bare area of the liver can cause a retroperitoneal bleed
- Primary Sclerosing Cholangitis associated with Ulcerative Colitis
- Extrahepatic ducts are normal with Primary Biliary Cirrhosis
- Anti-mitochondrial Antibodies - positive with primary biliary cirrhosis
- Mirizzi Syndrome - the stone in the cystic duct obstructs the CBD.
- Mirizzi has a 5x increased risk of GB cancer.
- Dorsal pancreatic agenesis - associated with diabetes and polysplenia
- Hereditary and Tropical Pancreatitis - early age of onset, increased risk of cancer
- Felty's Syndrome - Big Spleen, RA, and Neutropenia
- Splenic Artery Aneurysm - more common in women, and more likely to rupture in pregnant women.
- Insulinoma is the most common islet cell tumor
- Gastrinoma is the most common islet cell tumor with MEN
- Ulcerative Colitis has an increased risk of colon cancer (if it involves colon past the splenic flexure). UC involving the rectum only does not increase risk of CA.

Notes / Scribbles

Notes / Scribbles

THE JOURNEY CONTINUES WITH CRACK THE FRCR VOL 2, WHICH INCLUDES MODULES 4, 5, 6

—-

What's Next For Prometheus Lionhart ? Check out TitanRadiology.com for updates

—Physics Review Course - Video Series - January 2016

—Expanded Stand Alone Physics Book - "The War Machine" - January 2016

—Flash Card Application - January 2016

—"TOP 100" - CORE Rapid Review Book - February 2016

—"Titan Radiology Video Lecture Series" - The Magnum Opus - April 2016

Printed in Germany
by Amazon Distribution
GmbH, Leipzig

16669547R00189